INSTANT LOSS

ON A BUDGET

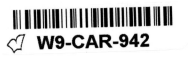

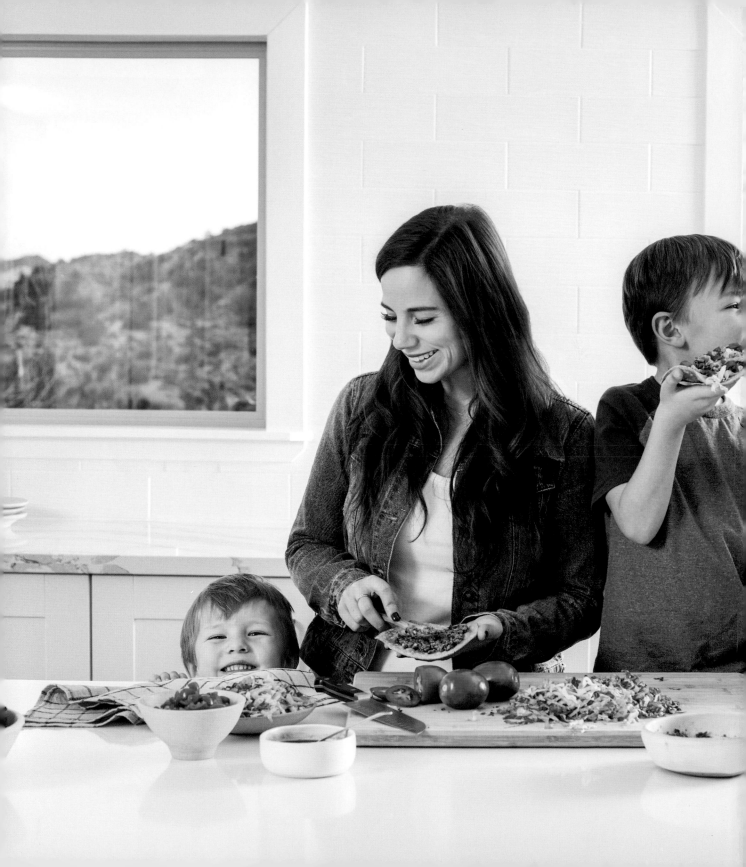

INSTANT LOSS
ON A BUDGET

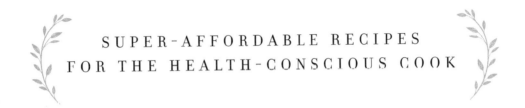

SUPER-AFFORDABLE RECIPES
FOR THE HEALTH-CONSCIOUS COOK

BRITTANY WILLIAMS

PHOTOGRAPHY BY
GHAZALLE BADIOZAMANI

HOUGHTON MIFFLIN HARCOURT
BOSTON   NEW YORK   2021

For information about permission to reproduce selections from this book, write to
trade.permissions@hmhco.com or to Permissions, Houghton Mifflin Harcourt Publishing Company,
3 Park Avenue, 19th Floor, New York, New York 10016.

hmhbooks.com

Library of Congress Cataloging-in-Publication Data is available.
ISBN 978-0-358-35392-8 (pbk)
ISBN 978-0-358-35391-1 (ebk)

Book design by Suet Chong

Printed in China
SCP 10 9 8 7 6 5 4 3 2 1

Unsung hero, you've been my biggest support from Day 1.

*Offering encouragement, jumping on board this crazy
roller-coaster adventure with positivity and never complaining.*

Putting your dreams on hold so that mine could be fully realized.

*Wearer of all the hats: dish-doer, laundry guru, kitchen builder,
best dad in the world. None of this would have been possible without you.*

*When asked how I've accomplished all that I have,
there are only two answers: God and Brady.*

Thank you for choosing me then and still.

How could I dedicate this book to anyone else?

For Brady.

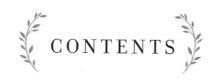

CONTENTS

FOREWORD

I first met Brittany at a breastfeeding support group, of all places. I was immediately drawn to her enthusiasm and zest for life—I realize this sounds cliché, but if you've met Brittany, or followed her on social media, you know what I'm talking about. She is funny, warm, and entertaining. After getting to know each other through several group meetings, we ventured out on our own for our first friend date—making homemade soap in a slow cooker at my house. While it would've been much easier to just buy organic, clean-ingredient soap, we wanted to do this the crunchy way and make it ourselves. This also shouldn't surprise you about Brittany (or me).

She showed up at my house early in the morning, little three-year-old Avey and toddler Ben in tow, and we set to work. We completely butchered our batch of soap, but we had the best time laughing, chatting, and watching our kids play together. It ended up being an all-day event, and when she left, I felt like I had made a new lifelong friend. I was right.

In January of 2017, when Brittany first announced her goal of cooking real food at home for an entire year, I was excited to follow her journey and cheer her on. She had been through the wringer and back over the past couple of years, and I could tell she was determined to leave the darkness behind and start looking ahead. And as we all know, she more than succeeded.

What has made her so successful, in my opinion, is not just her delicious recipes, drive, and enthusiasm for living a healthy lifestyle—but her passion for people. She sincerely cares about each and every person who has bought her books, tried her recipes, or reached out to her for encouragement. She wants everyone to succeed and she wants to be there to help every step of the way. I believe, deep down, that that's why she wrote her books. She can't physically be there for every single person out there like she was for herself, but her books can, and they have.

Now, with *Instant Loss on a Budget,* she continues to help people incorporate a simplistic, long-lasting, real-food lifestyle, but this time, she shows how to embrace these methods while keeping one eye on the checkbook. She has managed to create 135 amazing new recipes and delivers these delectable creations with her tried-and-true tips: Just Eat Real Food (JERF), exercise portion control, and listen to your body's cues. Each recipe has a dollar amount, so you know exactly how much each meal will cost and can plan your meals out for the week according to your budget. I find this incredibly helpful in combatting the "healthy food is too expensive" argument that often comes up when switching to a real-food lifestyle. When you set a budget and plan ahead, it is actually possible to eat real food on a budget. But in this case, Brittany has done all of the work for you! Now there really is no excuse to stop what you're doing and start your real food adventure now.

As a nutritional therapy practitioner, this book embodies so much of what I work on with my clients and what, I believe, is absolutely vital when it comes to finding your true happy weight. I can't wait to recommend yet another book of Brittany's to my friends, family, and clients to help them find success in their health journey.

—*Sloane Simon,*
Functional Nutritional Therapy Practitioner, Simon Says Real Food

THANK YOU

Instant Loss Fam

Book Three!!! Can you believe it? Thank you for encouraging me all those years ago to begin to share. As messy and unexperienced as I was, you've walked along beside me and helped me grow this into all it has become. I could never say thank you enough.

Avey, Ben, and Noah

You're the best part of every day. I'm so glad that I was chosen to be your mom. Spectacular little firecrackers that keep me on my toes and keep me striving to be the best person I can be, thank you for sharing me.

Mom and Dad

Your love, your support, your friendship, and loving my babies as your own. You're pretty much the best.

Aunt Kim

I'm glad you don't charge me for therapy. Thank you for always checking in, for planting the seeds, and for loving me since "caco." xx

Grandparents

Only a really blessed girl has so many wonderful grandparents. I love you so deeply, so much of me is made from what I learned from you.

Colin, Kyli, Kyle, Sarah, Bethany, Connor, Caleb, Tristan

I love our ever expanding 7 + 1's. Thank you for always being there and for being some of the best friends I'll ever have.

Katie and Roxanne

Who runs the world?? Ya'll do. Thanks for taking care of our community for the last four years. Day in and day out, you show up, you encourage, and you love the heck out of people. Your hearts are so big, and I am so blessed to know you both.

Sam

Thanks for taking me every way I come and always being there to step into exactly what I need at the moment. Who would have thought we'd be doing this twenty years ago? Life is funny, thanks for being my friend.

Lisa

Thank you for sprinkling your magic on this book, for testing every single recipe to ensure that my creations will actually work for other families, too. Your friendship keeps me sane during the development days and your wisdom makes everything so much better.

Heather, Jana, Rachel, Tracy, Shaylee, Candy, Sloane

My girls, thanks for making life fun.

Andy

Big sister, protector, friend, you are so much more to me than an agent. You see the vision in the crazy. Thanks for never letting me give up.

Photog Team: Ghazalle, Bridget, Stephanie, Carrie, Katherine, Aubrey, and Laura

Thank you for coming to my house! This was the first book photoshoot we have ever done on my home turf, and it makes everything so much more special. Thank you for living with us nine to five for a couple weeks, making all of the recipes shine in that special way that you do and lending your talents to my little heart project.

Thank you for bringing it all to life.

Cover Photography Team

Thank you for rushing in the 11th hour to shoot the cover of this book! I couldn't be happier and I am grateful for your willingness to be flexible and share your wonderful talents on this project.

HMH Team: Justin, Sarah, Marina, Tai, Shara, Jacqueline, the Sales Team, and more

Putting together something this big requires a whole heck of a lot of teamwork. I'm so blessed to have such a phenomenal team. The artwork, graphic design, publicity, all of the hours that go into marketing, managing the book within the accounts, dealing with printing errors, making itineraries, and dealing with crazy creatives, y'all are the real MVPs. Thank you for taking on this crazy creative once again. It's always such a pleasure to work with you.

Waterbury Publications
Thank you for being my second set of eyeballs and editing my recipes to make sure they all make sense. You make me look good.

Lord
You knew all that would be before it all began. Thank you for entrusting me with such an incredible task.

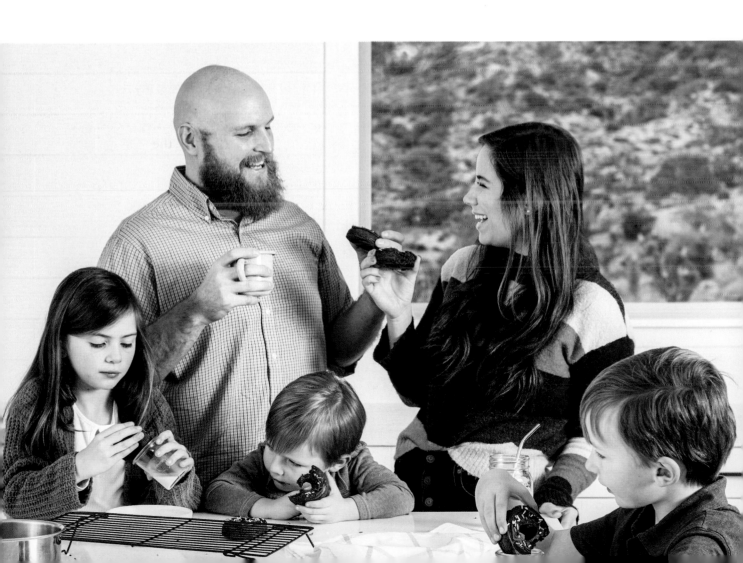

INTRODUCTION

"Eating healthy is too expensive." I can't tell you how many times I've heard that sentence over the last four years—and honestly, I used to agree. It was one of my favorite excuses to grab food off the dollar menu or the 69-cent box of mac and cheese at the grocery store.

I was right . . . to a certain extent. Eating well is more expensive in some regards. If you're comparing dollar-menu fast-food items to a salad on the menu, or if you're starting a new diet that requires a lot of expensive cuts of meat or strange ingredients that you don't have in your pantry, it can get quite pricey.

Instant Loss on a Budget isn't about eating the cheapest foods out there. It's about learning how to make an investment in your overall health and well-being that will yield a great return in the long run. Not only am I going to show you how eating well is actually cheaper than a processed-food diet, but I am going to show you how making an up-front investment can save you loads of money in the long term.

STARTING OUT

When I was single, I used to juggle two to three jobs while going to school full-time. After seeing my parents struggle with trying to pay off college debt, I decided I was going to try to pay for my college education as I went. This resulted in me working nearly all hours of the day, sleeping rarely, with no social life to speak of. Being so busy, I didn't have time to prep meals, so I usually ate whatever was cheap, available, or free. I ate a lot of pizza at church gatherings and a lot of dollar-menu items from McDonald's and Taco Bell, and utilized my free break-meal perks when I was waitressing. I was obese before I started college. After college, though, is when I became clinically, morbidly obese.

My body was a mess. I was tired all the time. I was always running on empty. Consuming copious amounts of caffeine and sugar still didn't pick me up. I even binged the occasional diet pills. This is when my doctor suggested that I try a program called Medifast. If you're unfamiliar, they're meal packets and shakes that only need water added. You eat three to six of them a day, and you lose weight.

So, even though I was broke, I invested $600 in this program. I stuck with it for about three days and then went on a massive fast-food binge. At the time, I was willing to spend any amount on a program if I ended up thinner as a result. I was in heavy pursuit of the next diet trend or magic pill. Surely it couldn't be as simple as just eating real food.

I was willing to invest money into a "sure thing" weight-loss cure, but paying $6 for a salad instead of $3 for my dollar-menu items? Out of the question. Asking them to lettuce-wrap my burger instead of putting it on a bun? Crazy talk! They still charged the same amount! What a rip-off! But a quick-and-easy way to lose weight? Here! Take my $600!

GETTING WISER

After Brady and I married, we were on a tight single-income budget. We didn't have a house, we were underneath Brady's student loan debt, and we had two car loans. It was not the way we wanted to start a family, but it's how we started anyway.

We had goals, though, and babies weren't going to derail those. "Live below your means" became our mantra. We seriously cut back on eating out, and we didn't have streaming apps or a DVR. We canceled our smartphone plans and downgraded to a $30/month family plan, talk and text only.

I don't think I bought new clothes or shoes for six years, I spent maybe $15 a year on makeup, and Brady stopped buying video games. We created our own plan and budgeted everything. Instead of putting the saved money back into our pocket, we aggressively paid off debt. We started with our lowest-balance loan, and when that was paid off, we snowballed that money into the next lowest.

When we had enough money for a down payment to purchase something of our own, instead of buying a starter home, we purchased a duplex. We lived in one side and rented the other side out to a tenant. This covered all but $300 of our mortgage payment. All the money we'd been spending previously on an apartment payment went into savings. We kept this up until we had a down payment for another house.

During this time, I realized how much cheaper eating at home was compared to eating out. We budgeted for pizza night once a week, usually about $10 for our little family, and the rest of the week we ate from home. Not always healthy meals, mind you. I made a lot of breads, lasagnas, and pastas, basically anything from the Pioneer Woman's website.

My weight yo-yoed a lot. It was also during these years that I began to learn about nutrition. I binged Netflix documentaries like *Fat, Sick & Nearly Dead*; *Forks Over Knives*; and *Food Matters*, and I began to understand the healing benefits of food. I mimicked a lot of these diets short-term, but none had lasting sustainability for me.

After our second baby became a toddler, I lost ninety pounds. I would drink a homemade smoothie for one meal a day, usually breakfast, and eat high-nutrient-dense meals the other two, with maybe one or two snacks. Not only did I begin to feel better, but our monthly food cost also went down. Inspired by the positive impact this change had on me, I decided to adapt a similar way of eating for my family. We first cut back on meat and dairy, then increased our vegetables, fruits, seeds, nuts, whole grains, and legumes. Not only did that not affect my weight loss but, again, it drastically reduced our family grocery budget.

When you're primarily plant-based and stay away from a lot of the boxed, prepackaged, and processed foods in the grocery store, your grocery budget will go down, just like ours did. Think about shopping the outside perimeter of the grocery store and avoid the inner aisles.

In recent years, it's become very popular to eat a more carnivore-style diet. This usually means lots of meat, and sometimes a lot of dairy. These are healthy foods, but good-quality meat and dairy are some of the most expensive things on your grocery list. Although currently a popular idea, you do not need to eat your body weight in meat protein to obtain wellness (see Let's Talk Protein below). Plants contain protein, too—usually not as much ounce-for-ounce as meat—but not eating a lot of meat doesn't mean you're protein-deficient.

With our current style of eating, our family typically spends $150 every two weeks on groceries—sometimes a

Thanks to the Instant Loss *books, our groceries last longer, all the food is used, and we rarely throw things away. It's been a real game-changer. We now have a better idea of what to spend monthly, and it's way cheaper than before. Even though we may be buying more expensive items, they are lasting longer, and we ultimately spend less. We used to spend $700 to $800 a month and now we spend $300!*

—JESSICA LUCIO

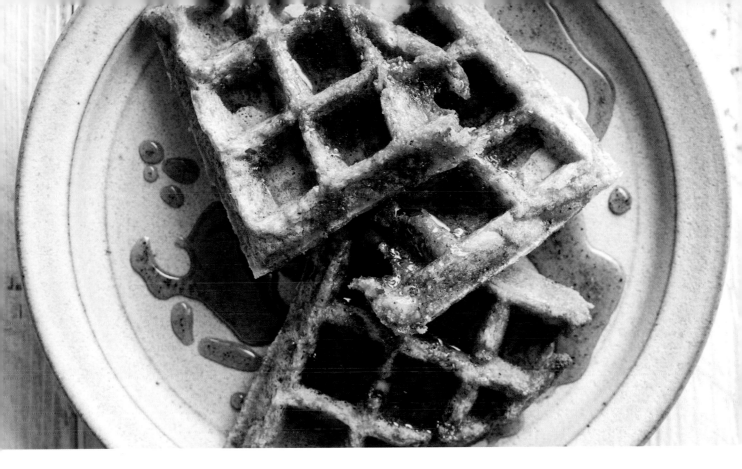

little closer to $200 if I'm buying things for a party, drinking a lot of sparkling water, or buying extra prepackaged snacks for the kids.

DIETING IS EXPENSIVE

When we say, "eating healthy is expensive," what we really mean is *dieting* is expensive. Let's get real: Most diets cut out some of the most cost-effective *healthy* foods in the grocery store! Foods like legumes and whole grains are filling and packed full of protein and other micronutrients that are great for the body—yet we cut them out because we're afraid of carbohydrates.

But I'm here to tell you that you don't have to be afraid of carbs! Simply put, a carb is a unit of energy. Consume too much, and your body will store the excess for future use. Consume the right amount, and your body will have just enough to get through the day without having to store any. Fat is used by the body in the same way.

I'm sure we've all experienced the drastic change in our shopping bill when we begin to adhere to a new way of eating. We have to buy new staple ingredients to restock the pantry, fridge, and freezer. Then there are the meals we buy in between because we're tired and don't want to cook. Half of the food spoils before we get to it, and it feels like throwing money in the garbage.

If you don't stick to this new way of eating for more than a week, it can seem like a waste of time and money. This is why I want to encourage you to stop dieting. Keep it simple! Eat real foods from the earth. Only buy stuff you're going to eat. I don't care what the meal plan says. You make the plans work for you, not the other way around.

Converting is expensive—*it just is*—especially if you're a novice cook and don't have an array of oils or spices to choose from. The first grocery trip can be quite a shock, but subsequent trips will rarely be as expensive as your first or second ones. Once you have a well-stocked pantry, fridge, and freezer, you'll find that you can eat well for very little week to week.

LET'S TALK PROTEIN

I'll say it again—you don't have to eat your body weight in meat protein in order to be healthy. We should, without doubt, invest in quality meat, but there's no need to eat hundreds of grams each day unless you're a bodybuilder. The average woman should consume about 46 grams; the average man about 56. On average, Americans typically consume 100 grams a day, twice the recommended value. You do not need protein shakes or supplements to be healthy, either. This whole protein movement is a marketing ploy. The fact of the matter is that protein can be found in many foods, not just meat!

MEATLESS MONDAY

When I first began participating in Meatless Monday, it was really to help cut down my family's food budget. Meat was absolutely the most expensive thing that we were purchasing in the grocery store because it was very important to me to purchase meats that were ethically and sustainably sourced, and these can be pricey.

At first, I started cutting down on our meat portions in different dishes. Instead of using a pound, I'd use half a pound or 3 ounces, and supplement the rest with finely chopped mushrooms. Doing this helped to stretch our meat a lot further.

Then I took it a step further and began participating in Meatless Mondays. That was revolutionary for me. As a single-income family of five, with a two-week grocery budget of $150, not only did it help me lower our grocery budget, but it also introduced me to a host of amazing new plant-based sources of nutrition and protein that I didn't even know existed. (Well, I knew they existed, I just didn't know they were great sources of protein!)

PLANT-BASED SOURCES OF PROTEIN

Adzuki beans (cooked)	1 cup	17.3 g	Lentils (cooked)	1 cup	17.9 g
Almond butter	2 tbsp	7 g	Mushrooms	1 cup	5 g
Almonds	¼ cup	7.6 g	Oatmeal (cooked)	1 cup	7 g
Asparagus	1 cup	4.3 g	Peas	½ cup	4.5 g
Avocado	1 medium	4 g	Pinto beans (cooked)	1 cup	15.4 g
Black beans (cooked)	1 cup	15.2 g	Potato	1 large	8 g
Black-eyed peas (cooked)	1 cup	27 g	Quinoa (cooked)	1 cup	8.1 g
Broccoli	1 cup	2.5 g	Sesame seeds	¼ cup	6.4 g
Cauliflower	1 cup	2 g	Spinach (cooked)	1 cup	5 g
Chia seeds	1 oz	4.7 g	Spirulina (dried)	1 tbsp	4 g
Chickpeas (cooked)	1 cup	14.5 g	Split peas (cooked)	1 cup	16.4 g
Corn	1 cup	4.6 g	Sunflower seeds	¼ cup	7.3 g
Edamame	1 cup	18.5 g	Sweet potato	1 cup	2.3 g
Flax seeds	1 tbsp	2 g	Walnuts	¼ cup	4.5 g
Hazelnuts	¼ cup	5 g	White beans (cooked)	1 cup	17.4 g
Hemp seeds	3 tbsp	9.5 g	Wild rice	1 cup	6.5 g
Kale	1 cup	3 g			

This is not an all-inclusive list. There are many more sources than listed here. I didn't even touch on fruit, which contains a lot of amino acids. Amino acids are, of course, the building blocks of protein.

Something to also consider—not only is this more sustainable for your budget, it's more sustainable for the environment, and it just might be easier on your gut, too!

MAKING HARD DECISIONS

First, I'd like to preface this section by saying: Please do not let these definitions overwhelm you. Just like I pick my battles with my kids and my spouse, I pick my battles with my grocery budget. Fine-tuning your diet, choosing which foods to buy, and trying to determine what is worth accommodating in your budget is such a process— *and it will always be.*

I don't feel like at any point I will have "arrived." I learn new things all the time. One of my favorite sayings is "Know better, do better." And sometimes, even when we know better, we are unable to do better because of financial predicaments, location difficulties, partner disagreements, or flat-out inconvenience.

I will be a work in progress for the rest of my life. Just as I am ever-evolving, so are my diet and dietary needs. Be flexible, be willing try new things, and be open to learn.

I don't know that you can discuss eating well and budgeting without at least touching on conventional vs. organic. You absolutely can eat conventionally raised and grown meat and produce and still be healthy and lose weight. However, it's important to know the differences between organically and conventionally raised and grown meat and produce. This can give you an understanding of why one might opt to purchase one over the other. It does not always boil down to cost, but can sometimes relate to ethics, overall health, and well-being.

So, without further ado . . .

What do these buzzwords mean?

GMO: Stands for "genetically modified organism." It's suspected that consuming GMOs in large quantities can lead to infertility, gluten disorders, allergies, and even cancer.

ORGANIC: When a food is labeled "100 percent organic," it means the food you are consuming hasn't been treated with synthetic pesticides or insecticides. It has been grown without the use of synthetic fertilizers, sewage sludge, or ionizing radiation and doesn't contain GMOs.

This is important because when you consume nonorganic produce, you could be taking in up to thirty different types of pesticides, which are then metabolized by your body and stored in your colon. People who consume more pesticides are more likely to develop cancer, Alzheimer's disease, ADHD, and have children with birth defects. These chemicals can harm the nervous system, the reproductive system, and the endocrine system.

THE DIRTY DOZEN AND THE CLEAN FIFTEEN: If you cannot afford to purchase all organic (I can't either), I'd encourage you to search these lists, found at www.ewg.org/foodnews, which change every year. They share the "dirtiest" chemically grown foods and the "cleanest" within the food industry. I loosely follow these guides and forgive myself the rest.

ETHICALLY RAISED: A process dedicated to promoting free range, cruelty free, and organic animal farming.

SUSTAINABLY SOURCED: Ingredients, whether agricultural produce or meat, that are sustainably farmed with more economic considerations. Organic agriculture can be a more efficient economic system for generating profit and reducing environmental impacts that end up costing consumers. Sustainable farmers consider the environmental and social impact of their faming activities.

CERTIFIED HUMANE: Meat, chicken, pork, eggs, pet food, and dairy products that come from farms where the standards for the humane treatment of farm animals are being met and implemented.

It is very important to me to purchase meats and seafood that are ethically and sustainably sourced, which can get pricey fast. It was difficult to adjust to paying higher prices for grass-fed, pasture-raised, wild-caught, and organic, so I didn't convert 100 percent originally. Even now, I am not 100 percent organic.

Sometimes we have to think about things in terms of better, not best. Take it one step at a time. It's difficult to overhaul your entire diet and way of thinking in an instant. So, don't. Absorb what resonates with you and leave the rest.

BEEF

GRASS-FED: This means that the cattle were allowed to forage on their own for fresh food. They are sometimes supplemented with very close substitutes like alfalfa during the winter. Unlike conventionally raised grain-fed animals, grass-fed cattle have a much more natural diet.

GRASS-FINISHED: This means the cows have received a grass or forage diet their entire lives. It differs from grass-fed because it means they never received supplemental grain feed.

HORMONE-FREE: Animals raised without being given additional hormones.

ANTIBIOTIC-FREE: Animals raised without antibiotics in their feed or water or via injections.

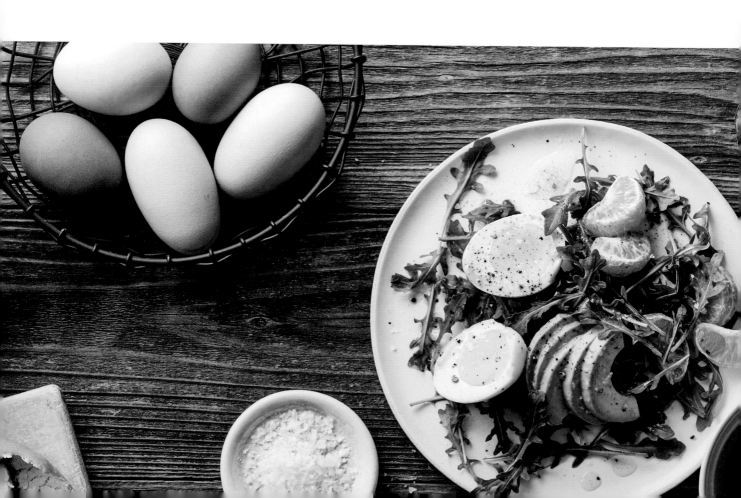

POULTRY

CAGE-FREE: Instead of cages, these chickens are packed by the thousands into multilevel aviaries, and they never get to see the outdoors. Due to poor indoor air quality, cannibalism, and high mortality rates, this is not much better than caging. Also, these operations cost 36 percent more to operate, which is a cost that is passed on to the consumer.

FREE-RANGE: This typically refers to poultry that is allowed to have freedom of movement while being kept in natural conditions. The opposite is the norm: 95 percent of eggs in the U.S. come from chickens raised in battery cages. As many as 100,000 birds can live in a single warehouse with less than 67 square inches for each to call its own. That's a little smaller than a laptop.

ORGANIC: According to the USDA, this means that the hens are "uncaged and free to roam in their houses and have access to the outdoors. The hens are fed an organic diet of feed produced without conventional pesticides or fertilizers."

PASTURE-RAISED: This is an unregulated term, but it means that chickens have plenty of time to forage and play outside. According to *Mother Earth News,* they have one-third less cholesterol than conventionally raised hens, one-fourth less saturated fat, two-thirds more vitamin A, twice as many omega-3 fatty acids, three times as much vitamin E, and seven times the amount of beta carotene.

FISH

FARM-RAISED: Fish that are raised in tanks, irrigation ditches, and ponds.

WILD-CAUGHT: Fish that come from seas, rivers, and other natural bodies of water.

SUSTAINABLY SOURCED: Seafood that is caught or farmed in ways that consider the long-term viability of harvested species and the well-being of the ocean, as well as the livelihoods of fishery-dependent communities.

INVESTING IN YOUR BODY IS A WORTHWHILE INVESTMENT

When you become a parent, you are charged with a tiny human's physical and mental well-being. You are also responsible for everything they eat, from the time they're born until the time they can go out and purchase food on their own.

I grew up on a processed-food diet. It consisted of things I could easily make myself: hot dogs, cereal, pizza pockets, and blue-box mac and cheese. I was allowed to choose my own school lunch, and I ate pizza, Hot Cheetos, and a package of cookies almost every day, usually with a Gatorade or soda. I was a child. I didn't realize the power that food had over a person's physical well-being. Food was food, wasn't it? As I got older, I realized that all food was not created equal. I realized that it has the power to heal or to harm.

As an adult, and as a new mother, I had to decide how I was going to navigate the land mine–laden field of health and nutrition. The minefield began with breastfeeding, first foods, and then what a day of food should like for a toddler after weaning. I began to read and research, I joined Facebook groups, and I spoke to other mothers I knew.

Everyone had an opinion. A different method or ideology that they followed. It was overwhelming. I felt like a failure before I'd even begun, so I decided to gather little truths and to listen, but to only absorb what sounded true for me and my family.

This is where I began to realize that our bodies are a worthwhile investment—or, at least, I believed my children's bodies were. I was willing to stay up late at night reading books about healthy foods. I was willing to pay a little extra so that they could have quality ingredients, and when we couldn't afford to pay extra, I spent the time to make baby food at home.

Don't get me wrong, I'm no Sanctimommy. My kids still got Cheerios, donuts at church on Sunday, and fast food occasionally. I didn't want to make those things diet staples for them, though. They were the exception, not the rule. This decision was born out of my own issues with the way that I was fed growing up.

Please do not misunderstand me here: My aim is never to shame or belittle other parents for their choices. We are all doing the best we can. The point in sharing this bit with you is that I did the best I could for my children, but was unwilling to extend that same love and care to my own body.

Just because we have the knowledge, doesn't mean that we always know how to implement it. I would spring for the healthy choice for my kiddos, but I'd buy cheap dollar-menu items for myself. It wasn't always about the money, though. Oftentimes it was simply because I was addicted. I didn't want the lean meat and vegetables, I wanted the greasy double cheeseburger with a large fries and a Mountain Dew.

But I had the knowledge. I knew what I was eating wasn't a great way to nourish myself, and one day things began to click. I had to begin to treat my body like it wasn't my own, because I didn't put any value on my own body. I had to treat it like it belonged to one of my children or a friend, people I knew how to love well. Our bodies are the only things that are with us from the time we're born until we pass away. They should be something we're willing to invest in—not only after we're sick, but before, preventatively.

It turned out we only had to extend our grocery budget for a couple of months. After our pantry was better equipped with whole-food ingredients, our grocery bill dropped significantly.

I was surprised to realize that our family of five was thriving on a whole-foods diet for $75 to $100 a week!

KEEPING COSTS DOWN

I love that eating well is becoming mainstream. No longer are we limited to pricey health food stores! Even Walmart has jumped on board, creating a gluten-free dairy and freezer section with alternative ingredients.

Where you shop is completely dependent on where you live and your ability to purchase things online. This will vary greatly from family to family so I decided to poll our 150,000-member community and ask where they shop to save money!

The two most recommended places, by a landslide, were ALDI and Costco. We do not have an ALDI close to us, but I have shopped at one before and their prices are remarkable. It's generally cheaper than Walmart and not a bulk seller like Costco. I really was impressed.

I try to avoid stores like Whole Foods unless I'm shopping for something that hasn't quite made it into the mainstream marketplace yet. There are many items that I can purchase at my local grocery store that are marked up as much as 100 percent at Whole Foods.

The online marketplace is also a great way to find cheaper prices on pantry items. My favorites are Thrive Market, Vitacost, and Amazon. Comparison shopping can take a little bit more time, but can yield great cost savings. Vitacost will frequently send out promo codes for 20 percent off your entire purchase, too, so make sure you're subscribed to their emails.

QUICK TIPS

* **LOOK FOR DISCOUNTS AND REBATES.** There are rebate and coupon apps now for many stores, as well as point systems for gas money, special sales, and coupons for frequent shoppers. Some stores will even price-match Amazon. Check the websites of your favorite stores—you could be missing out on some serious kickbacks!

* **SHOP ON A FULL STOMACH.** I spend so much more money when I go to the store hungry. I'm more prone to deviate from my list and grab whatever looks good. Not only is this bad for your budget, it can also be bad for your waistline.

* **SET ASIDE TIME FOR MEAL PLANNING.** Pick a few recipes out of this book to prepare for the week and then fill the rest of the week with easy throw-it-together meals like salads, soups, wraps, omelets, and smoothies!

* **BUY ONLY WHAT YOU NEED.** Have a clear plan of action for the week before you go shopping, and stick to it. Ordering online and opting for grocery pickup can help a lot if you struggle with this.

* **EAT MORE PLANTS!** Limit meat, dairy, and processed snacks. Do not cut out whole grains and legumes unless you have a health concern or allergy.

* **MEAL PREP TO REDUCE WASTE.** Often, we have the best of intentions at the beginning of the week. We buy all the good groceries, but by midweek we're tired, and it's easy to default back to poor food choices. Help eliminate these circumstances by prepping a few meals at the beginning of the week so there is something in the refrigerator ready to go on the nights you don't feel like cooking.

* **USE YOUR FREEZER.** If you wind up eating out a lot and can't get to your fresh produce before it goes bad, remember that almost anything can be frozen! Be proactive and freeze things before they spoil.

* **BUY FROZEN PRODUCE.** I purchase a lot of my fruit and vegetables frozen so I don't have to worry about them going bad. I find that buying them this way is usually cheaper, too!

* **STOP DIET HOPPING!** If you buy all the healthy food and then halfway through the week decide "Screw it!" and go back to the store to buy all of the junk, you're paying double! This isn't because healthy eating is expensive—it's because subscribing to two different types of eating at the same time is.

* **ONLY SHOP ONCE A WEEK.** I try to hit up the grocery store only once a week at the very most. It's usually more like once bi-weekly. Just by being in the store, I'm more prone to spend money. Even if I forget an ingredient or two, I try to work around it. Chances are, heading back to the store for that one $3 thing will yield a $50 oopsie-daisy, especially if I'm at a store like Target! Not only does staying away from the market save a lot of money, it forces me to get creative and advance my cooking skills when ingredients get tight.

* **PURCHASE IN BULK.** Things like spices, flours, nuts, seeds, grains, and so on are available in bulk. You'll especially save on spices. Buying tiny jars of spice blends at the grocery store adds up fast. Instead, buy the large containers at wholesale clubs or in one-pound bags online. If something you love goes on sale, stock up and freeze it!

* **GET CREATIVE!** I cannot stress this one enough. Part of becoming a great home cook is learning how to throw things together on the fly. Do not be afraid to use up the leftover bits and bobs in the refrigerator by making a salad or soup without a recipe!

* **GROW IT YOURSELF!** I grow fresh herbs all along the windowsills in my kitchen. The only thing I really buy in the store anymore is cilantro. I go through so much of it I have a difficult time growing as much as I use. Start a small garden with the things that grow best in your area, or if you don't have the space, start with an herb or two on the windowsill. You'll save a bundle on purchasing fresh in store all the time, and it will really brighten up your space!

My grocery bill is much less than when I bought processed boxed foods and junk. It's just me and my daughter, and honestly I spend $200 to $300 each month, and some months I spend nothing because I buy in bulk and once I freeze the recipes, we have plenty of food for several meals. I make my own chicken broth, stock, and vegetable broth. I freeze everything and waste nothing! I've saved over $175 to $200 a month in groceries since Instant Loss. I feel so much better after fixing, cooking, and preparing our meals. It's just a life change that I am going to stick with because my health is so important for my daughter with special needs. I have to be healthy to continue to care for her!

—BEV & BECKY HANNIBAL

✳ **REPLACE WHAT YOU CAN, WHEN YOU CAN.** When starting a new diet, it's customary to tear through your pantry and throw out all of the "bad food." I didn't do this. We used things up until they were gone and then we replaced them with healthier alternatives. This will cut down on your grocery budget tremendously to start.

CREATING A BUDGET

Creating a food budget for a family is a tricky thing. It will depend on your location, what stores you have available, how willing you are to shop sales and make comparisons, and if you are a one-stop shopper. It will depend on your family's size, your children's ages, and how many adults you have in the home. Allergies, food sensitivities, dietary restrictions, and medical issues will also influence your food budget.

Your budget is yours alone, and whatever number you decide is right for your family is no one else's business. My hope is that through sharing all of these tips, stories, and testimonies, eating healthy can be destigmatized. I hope you also realize that eating well can actually be quite affordable. It may not always be the cheapest option, but it is still an option.

SIMPLE, EASY, CHEAP

If you are making the lifestyle adjustment to eating well, it's best to keep things simple at first. This will also help keep your grocery budget in check. Roast a chicken breast, make a large salad, steam some sweet potatoes, and season them to taste.

I think we psych ourselves out a lot. We think eating well requires a lot of time, a lot of energy, and a lot of know-how—but it really doesn't. I don't make one of those spectacular recipes for every single meal. No one does.

Instead, I recommend that you pick one thing to make a day and find some simple, easy staples for the other two meals. Remember, you don't have to eat breakfast for breakfast! I can't even tell you how many times we've eaten scrambled eggs, toast, and bacon for dinner or leftovers for breakfast.

When in doubt, just eat real food. It's really that simple.

Turn the page for eight of my favorite things to throw together on the fly that don't require any cooking or prep time at all!

Chicken Salad

SERVES 2

8 ounces cooked chicken, cut into bite-size chunks
½ cup diced celery
½ cup quartered purple grapes
¼ cup chopped pecans, walnuts, or sunflower seeds
¼ cup mayonnaise
1 teaspoon dried dillweed
¼ teaspoon fine sea salt
⅛ teaspoon ground black pepper

Combine all of the ingredients in a medium-size bowl. Serve over rice cakes, salad, or in romaine lettuce leaves.

Egg Salad

SERVES 2

4 hard-boiled eggs, peeled and chopped
1 tablespoon mustard
1½ tablespoons mayonnaise
¼ cup diced dill pickles
¼ teaspoon apple cider vinegar
⅛ teaspoon ground paprika
⅛ teaspoon fine sea salt
⅛ teaspoon ground black pepper

Combine all of the ingredients in a medium-size bowl. Serve over rice cakes, salad, or in romaine lettuce leaves.

Tuna Salad

SERVES 2

1 (5-ounce) can wild-caught tuna, drained
¼ cup mayonnaise
¼ cup organic sweet relish
Fine sea salt, to taste
Ground black pepper, to taste

Combine all of the ingredients in a medium-size bowl. Serve over rice cakes, salad, or in romaine lettuce leaves.

Simple Salad

SERVES AS MANY AS NEEDED

Mixed greens and any vegetables or fruits you need to get rid of
Extra-virgin olive oil
Balsamic vinegar, apple cider vinegar, red wine vinegar, Dijon mustard, or horseradish
Fine sea salt, to taste
Ground black pepper, to taste

Combine all of the ingredients in a medium-size bowl. Serve immediately.

Eggs, Bacon, and Toast

('nuff said, no recipe needed!)

Vegetable Platter with Ranch

SERVES AS MANY AS NEEDED

Any vegetables you need to get rid of
Hard-boiled eggs
Cheese
Fruit
Whatever else your heart desires
Creamy Ranch Dressing (page 110)

Place the things on a large plate, put the ranch dressing a bowl in the center for dipping, and enjoy.

PB&J Rice Cake

SERVES 1

1 lightly salted brown rice cake
Nut or seed butter
Organic/low-sugar jelly
Veggies (carrots, cucumbers, celery, etc.), cut into sticks, for serving

Spread the butter and the jelly on the rice cake. Consume with a side of veggie sticks.

Popcorn and Smoothies

Home popped popcorn with sea salt and coconut oil
Your favorite smoothie

HOMEMADE FTW!

There are certain things that are cost-effective to make at home. When cooking with things like organic broths, condiments, and nondairy milks, it's best to keep your money in your pocket and simply make them from scratch!

You can find my favorite recipes for broths, sauces, and seasonings in the Basics chapter on page 321.

If you are dairy-free or purchasing a lot of raw or organic milk, costs can add up quickly! For this reason, my absolute favorite, cost-effective milk to use in my recipes is oat milk, which is very simple to throw together. The recipe for this and other nondairy milks is on page 288.

BUDGET-FRIENDLY SNACKS

Fruits

- Apples
- Applesauce
- Bananas
- Clementines (Cuties)
- Dried fruit
- Frozen berries
- Grapefruit
- Grapes
- Pineapple
- Watermelon

Vegetables

- Bell peppers
- Broccoli
- Carrots
- Celery
- Cherry tomatoes
- Cucumbers
- Edamame
- Small salad
- Sweet potato fries

Miscellaneous

- Apple chips
- Banana chips
- Corn tortilla chips
- Dill pickles
- Hard-boiled eggs
- Lunch meat (nitrate- and sugar-free)
- Muffins
- Plantain chips
- Popcorn
- Rice cakes
- Smoothie or juice
- Trail mix (create your own!)

Dips

- Avocado with lime, sea salt, and garlic powder
- Creamy Ranch Dressing (page 110)
- Hummus
- Nut/seed butters

ELECTRIC PRESSURE COOKER
COOK TIME CHEAT SHEET

MEAT AND FISH
Water is only needed when cooking under pressure, not when using the Sauté function.

o 6-quart pressure cooker: 1 cup water or broth
o 8-quart pressure cooker: 1½ cups water or broth

MEAT/FISH	WEIGHT	TIME	COOK	RELEASE
Beef, ground	1 lb	5 to 8 minutes	Sauté	Normal
Beef roast	3 to 4 lbs	90 minutes	High pressure	Natural release
Beef, stew meat (1-inch pieces)	1 to 2 lbs	35 minutes	High pressure	Natural release
Chicken breasts (whole or cubed)	1 lb	6 minutes	High pressure	Natural release
Chicken drumsticks	1 lb	10 minutes	High pressure	Natural release
Chicken, whole	3 lbs	25 minutes Note: Add 6 minutes per additional pound of chicken	High pressure	Natural release
Fish fillet	1 to 3 lbs	2 to 3 minutes	High pressure	Natural release
Mussels	1 to 3 lbs	1 to 2 minutes	High pressure	Natural release
Pork, loin, or rump roast	2 to 3 lbs	60 minutes	High pressure	Natural release
Ribs	1 to 3 lbs	25 minutes	High pressure	Natural release
Eggs, hard-boiled	1 dozen	5 minutes Note: 5 minutes ice bath after release	High pressure	Natural release (5 minutes)

BEANS

- Unsoaked: 1 cup beans to 3 cups water or broth
- Soaked: 1 cup beans to 2 cups water or broth

BEANS	SOAKED	UNSOAKED	COOK	RELEASE
Black beans	22 minutes	50 minutes	High pressure	Natural release
Black-eyed peas	10 minutes	38 minutes	High pressure	Natural release
Cannellini (white)	22 minutes	50 minutes	High pressure	Natural release
Chickpeas	25 minutes	50 minutes	High pressure	Natural release
Kidney beans	25 minutes	50 minutes	High pressure	Natural release
Lentils, brown	n/a	10 minutes	High pressure	Natural release
Lima beans	10 minutes	14 minutes	High pressure	Natural release
Navy beans	20 minutes	45 minutes	High pressure	Natural release
Pinto beans	25 minutes	50 minutes	High pressure	Natural release

RICE AND GRAINS

- 1 cup rice/grain to 1½ cups water or broth

RICE/GRAIN	TIME	COOK	RELEASE
Oats, old-fashioned	8 minutes	Manual high pressure	Quick release
Oats, steel-cut	10 minutes	Manual high pressure	Quick release
Pasta, brown rice/ quinoa/corn	6 minutes	Manual high pressure	Quick release
Quinoa	1 minute	High pressure	Natural release (10 minutes), then quick release
Rice, basmati	8 minutes	High pressure	Quick release
Rice, brown	28 minutes	High pressure	Quick release
Rice, jasmine	10 minutes	High pressure	Quick release
Rice, white	10 minutes	High pressure	Quick release
Rice, wild	28 minutes	High pressure	Quick release

VEGETABLES

o 6-quart pressure cooker: 1 cup water or broth

o 8-quart pressure cooker: 1½ cups water or broth

VEGETABLE	TIME	COOK	RELEASE
Asparagus	1 to 2 minutes	Low pressure	Quick release
Broccoli	1 minute	Low pressure	Quick release
Brussels sprouts	2 minutes	High pressure	Quick release
Butternut squash (2-inch pieces)	4 to 6 minutes	High pressure	Quick release
Cabbage (wedges)	2 minutes	High pressure	Quick release
Carrots (1-inch pieces)	3 minutes	High pressure	Quick release
Cauliflower (head)	2 minutes	High pressure	Quick release
Collard greens	10 minutes	High pressure	Quick release
Corn (on the cob)	2 minutes	High pressure	Quick release
Green beans	2 minutes	High pressure	Quick release
Potatoes (cubed)	8 minutes	High pressure	Natural release
Potatoes (whole, small)	15 minutes	High pressure	Natural release
Potatoes (whole, medium)	18 minutes	High pressure	Natural release
Potatoes (whole, large)	20 minutes	High pressure	Natural release

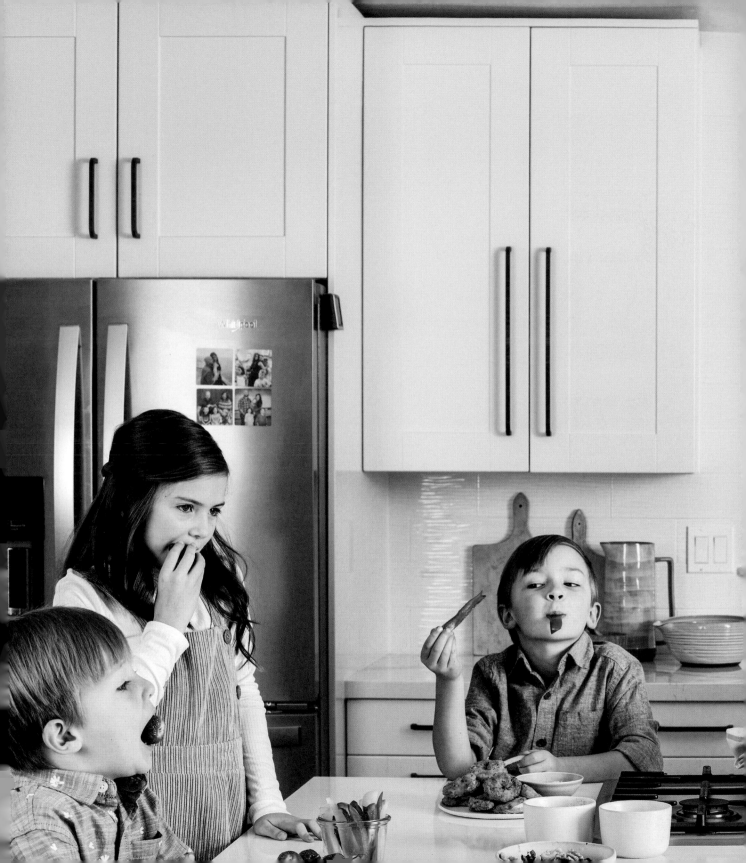

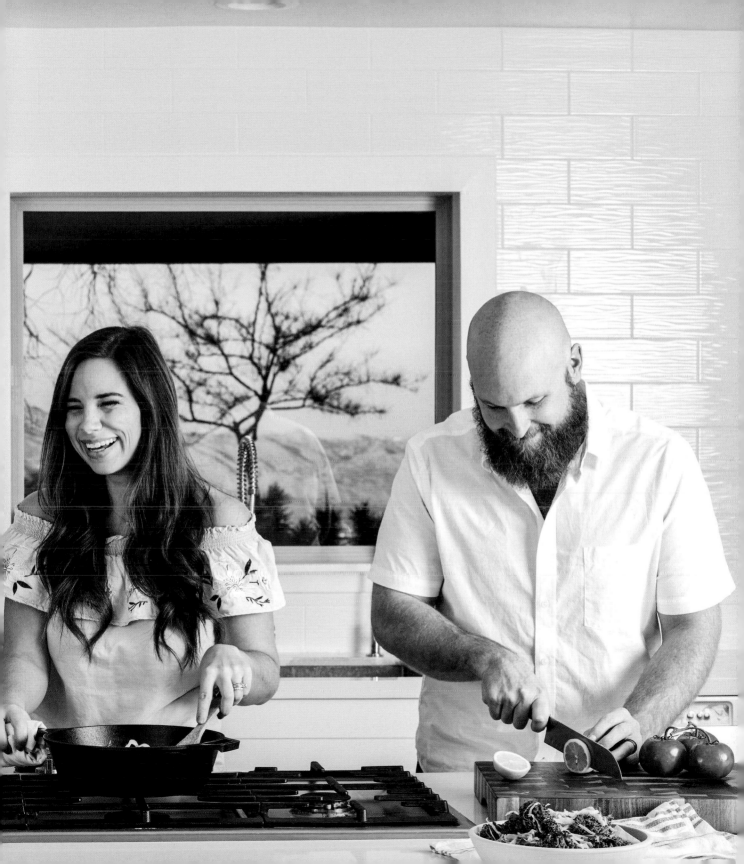

MEAL PLANS

PORTION SIZES

If you're not counting calories, how do you know how much to eat? I use my hand to guide correct food portions for each food group! (Per the Arizona State University School of Nutrition and Health.)

PROTEIN: It's customary to eat 3 to 4 ounces of a protein source at mealtime. A great way to judge how much you should eat is by using the palm of your hand as a portion guide, not including your fingers or thumb.

VEGETABLES: The perfect portion of a side of vegetables at mealtime is two hands cupped together.

FRUIT: A good portion guide for fruit is about one cupped hand.

STARCHES: Clench your hand to form a fist; that's as much starchy carbohydrates as you should eat for one portion. It's ½ to 1 cup.

FATS: I'm a fan of healthy fats. It's recommended that a healthy serving of fats such as peanut butter, mayo, or oil is equal to the size of your thumb. I'm a bit more indulgent than that, though, and often eat a little more.

PLANNING

I've found that organizing our meals into a meal plan allows me to be more efficient with my time and mindful of what we are going to eat that day. Even if we don't eat exactly what I have planned, at all times I have a week's worth of breakfast, lunch, and dinner ingredients on hand so that I am never left wondering what I should make.

The vast majority of the recipes in this book use the same ingredients, repurposed in different ways. This ensures that with just a few staple ingredients, you'll be able to make several different recipes and eliminate virtually all food waste.

Below you'll find a four-week meal plan that I hope helps you get organized! You don't have to follow these meal plans strictly. They're just a guide to show you what several weeks' worth of meals might look like for my family and how I'd prep accordingly.

These are only six-day meal plans because, inevitably, there will be days when you have leftovers, are on the go, or just don't flat feel like making what's on the meal plan. There will also be other things you'll need to purchase at the store, things for kids' lunches, and the random odd or end. These plans have been designed to get you as close as possible to under $100 a week total.

Note: Potatoes, onions, peppers, broth, etc. colors and varieties are all interchangeable for one another. As you work through these shopping lists and meal plans, feel free to swap one ingredient for another if you already have something on hand.

Note 2: All of these meals are interchangeable. Just be mindful not to consume several heavier meals in one day, i.e., pasta, rice, or bean dishes. Remember to make this plan work for you!

GROCERY LIST

These lists have all of the ingredients for your meals throughout the week. Pick a few items from the snack list on page 24 and add them to your shopping list. In addition, it's best to keep a tub of mixed greens on hand for small side salads, a quick breakfast or lunch, or throw-together meals when you don't feel like preparing one of these recipes.

MENU: WEEK 1

	DAY 1	DAY 2	DAY 3	DAY 4	DAY 5	DAY 6
BREAKFAST	Scrambled Eggs with Roasted Asparagus Toast (page 80) Cost: $5.20	Dinosaur Juice (page 292) Cost: $0.75 with a side of scrambled eggs (bacon/sausage optional)	Cinnamon Apple Granola Parfaits (page 85) Cost: $2.60	Simple breakfast salad (no recipe) or eggs/bacon/toast	Breakfast Hash (page 95) Cost: $6.20	Chocolate Brownie Donuts (page 58) Cost: $4.85
LUNCH	Simple mixed green salad with Hard-Boiled Eggs and Lemon Turmeric-Dressing (page 87) Cost: $1.75	The Best Vegetable Minestrone Soup (page 124) Cost: $7.80	Leftovers or mixed green salad with 3 ounces cooked salmon Cost: $3.00	Barbecue Chicken with Cilantro-Lime Coleslaw (page 249) Cost: $4.00	Panzanella (page 167) Cost: $2.00	Chicken Waldorf Salad (page 151) Cost: $5.20
DINNER	Thai Red Curry with Potatoes and Lentils (page 241) Cost: $7.50	Barbacoa Lettuce Wrap Tacos (page 274) Cost: $8.50	Poblano Pepper–Potato Stew (page 232) Cost: $5.80	Zucchini Spaghetti with Meatballs (page 191) Cost: $8.85	Easy Weeknight Chicken and Potatoes (page 262) with simple side salad or steamed broccoli Cost: $6.40	The Ultimate Veggie Thin-Crust Pizza (page 234) Cost: $5.80

TOTAL COST FOR THE WEEK: $86.20

SHOPPING LIST: WEEK 1

Fruit

- 4½ apples
- ½ banana
- 1 Medjool date
- 1 cup purple seedless grapes
- 1 lemon
- 4 limes

Vegetables

- 1 bunch of asparagus
- 1 small head green cabbage
- 1½ cups shredded purple cabbage
- 2 large carrots
- 6 stalks celery
- ½ medium cucumber
- 1 medium jalapeño
- 1 bunch kale
- 1 large head butterleaf lettuce
- 2 large heads romaine lettuce
- 6 cremini mushrooms
- 5 green onions
- 1 red onion
- 3 medium yellow onions
- 1 medium orange bell pepper
- 1 red bell pepper (¼ cup)
- 2 fresh poblano peppers
- 1½ pounds baby creamer potatoes
- 10 ounces gold potatoes
- ¾ cup red baby potatoes
- 1 pound sweet potatoes
- 9 cups baby spinach
- 3 large zucchini
- 12 cherry tomatoes
- 2 medium Roma tomatoes

Herbs

- ¼ cup fresh basil
- ½ cup fresh cilantro leaves
- 11 cloves garlic
- 1 small knob of fresh ginger

Frozen

- 2 cups frozen corn
- ½ cup frozen strawberries

- 2 cups frozen mixed vegetables (peas, carrots, corn)

Meat, Eggs, and Dairy

- 4 strips nitrate-free bacon
- 1 pound beef stew meat
- 1 pound lean ground beef
- 3 pounds boneless, skinless chicken breasts
- 1 pound pork sausage or ground turkey
- 8 large eggs
- Oat Milk (page 288) or other milk (3¼ cups)
- Oat Milk Yogurt (page 84) or other yogurt (3 cups)
- 1 cup Homemade Mayo (page 330) or store-bought

Dry Goods

- ¾ cup dry black beans
- 1½ cups cubed Olive Oil and Herb Focaccia (page 67) or gluten-free French style bread
- 4 slices whole-grain bread or Oat Bread (page 65)
- 1 cup Super-Simple Granola (page 323) or store-bought
- 1 cup red lentils
- 1 cup gluten-free fusilli pasta
- 1 cup quinoa
- ½ cup shelled sunflower seeds

Canned/Jarred Goods

- 1 (15-ounce) can cannellini beans
- 1 (15-ounce) can red kidney beans
- 1 (14-ounce) can full-fat coconut milk
- 1 jar Thai red curry paste
- 2 (15-ounce) cans crushed tomatoes
- 3 (15-ounce) can diced tomatoes
- 3½ tablespoons tomato paste
- 1 (15-ounce) can tomato sauce

Flours, Powders, and Sugars

- Garbanzo bean flour (1⅓ cups)
- Arrowroot powder (1 tablespoon)
- Aluminum-free baking powder
- Cacao powder (½ cup)
- Coconut sugar (½ cup)
- Baking soda
- Unfortified nutritional yeast (Sari Foods brand) (3 tablespoons)

Miscellaneous

- ½ cup low-sodium beef broth or Bone B
- Raw honey (¾ cup)
- 1 teaspoon liquid smoke
- 100 percent pure maple syrup (1 tablespoon plus 1 teaspoon)
- 3⅔ cup low-sodium vegetable or chicken stock (store-bought or homemade)
- ¼ cup sun dried tomatoes
- Pure vanilla extract (1 teaspoon)
- 1½ teaspoons reduced-sodium Worcestershire sauce

With the help of Instant Loss, I am able to feed my active family of four on a $75 budget each week! The lunch and dinner meals are easy and quick to put together. For example, for under $10, I made lunches for five days, as well as a dinner for my family. I could barely get two kids fast food meals for that before. The meal prep took me about twenty-five minutes. Cooking healthy for the family does not need to be complicated, time-consuming, or pricey. I watch the ads each week and plan my Instant Loss recipes around what is on sale. I'm a full-time working mom and wife, running after my two elementary-aged kiddos. I've lost 17 pounds in three months and my husband has lost 25 pounds.

—REBECCA EDLER

Oils and Vinegars

- Cooking oil spray
- Avocado oil (¼ cup)
- Extra-virgin coconut oil (¼ cup)
- Extra-virgin olive oil
- Apple cider vinegar (1 tablespoon plus 4 teaspoons)
- Red wine vinegar (3 tablespoons)

Spices

- o Chili powder
- o Chipotle chili powder
- o Coriander
- o Cumin
- o Dried basil
- o Dried minced onion
- o Dried oregano
- o Dried parsley
- o Dried rosemary
- o Dried thyme
- o Fine sea salt
- o Garlic powder
- o Ground black pepper
- o Ground cinnamon
- o Ground nutmeg
- o Ground turmeric
- o Onion powder
- o Paprika
- o Red pepper flakes

Optional Ingredients

- o Eggs and bacon, breakfast Day 2 and Day 4
- o Eggs for hard-boiled eggs, Day 1 salad (1 or 2 per person)
- o 1 large container mixed greens, side and breakfast salads throughout the week
- o 3 ounces salmon, Day 3

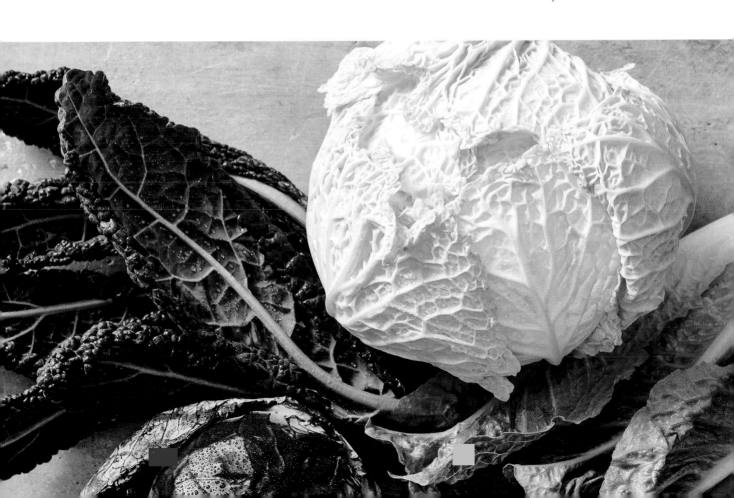

MENU: WEEK 3

	DAY 1	DAY 2	DAY 3	DAY 4	DAY 5	DAY 6
BREAKFAST	Soft-Boiled Eggs with Citrus-Arugula Salad and Lemon-Turmeric Dressing (page 87) Cost: $7.40	Caprese Frittata (page 89) Cost: $3.10	Blueberry-Banana Cream of Oat (page 99) Cost: $0.30	Mini Everything Bagels (page 62) with a small side salad and a soft- or hard-boiled egg Cost: $1.50	Dinosaur Juice (page 292) with leftover Mini Everything Bagel (page 62) Cost: $0.75	Eggs and bacon (no recipe)
LUNCH	Two-Bean and Lentil Chili (page 237) Cost: $5.50	Greek Lemon-Chicken Soup (page 133) Cost: $5.85	Salsa Verde Chicken Nachos [prepared with Mexican Lasagna] (page 258) Cost: $5.90	Tuna Salad (page 22) on a rice cake Cost: $2.45	Kale and Cabbage Chicken-Bacon Salad (page 149) Cost: $7.30	Cilantro-Lime Quinoa Salad (page 164) Cost: $4.50
DINNER	Lemon Pasta Pesto Primavera (page 201) Cost: $6.75	Cajun Popcorn Shrimp (page 113) with mixed green side salad Cost: $8.75	Sesame-Chili Turkey Meatballs (page 252) Cost: $6.00 Optional: Serve with rice and steamed broccoli	Mexican Lasagna (page 258) Cost: $0 (prepared yesterday)	Sausage Pizza Pasta (page 194) Cost: $8.10	Brittany's California Burgers (page 208) Cost: $8.00

TOTAL COST FOR THE WEEK: $82.15

SHOPPING LIST: WEEK 2

Fruit

o 1 large avocado

o 2 bananas

o ½ cup blueberries (optional)

o 1 Medjool date

o 3 lemons

o 1 lime

o 2 mandarin oranges

Vegetables

- o 5 ounces arugula
- o 1 red bell pepper
- o 2 large carrots
- o 4 stalks celery
- o 2 cups shredded green cabbage
- o 4 cups mixed greens
- o 2 medium jalapeños
- o 4½ cups kale
- o 1 large head butterhead lettuce
- o 2 cups shredded romaine lettuce
- o 1 green onion
- o ½ small red onion
- o 5 medium/large yellow onions
- o 1 medium red potato
- o 3 cups baby spinach
- o ¾ cup cherry tomatoes
- o 5 Roma tomatoes

Herbs

- o 2 cups fresh basil
- o 1 bunch fresh cilantro
- o 9 cloves garlic

Frozen

- o 1½ cups frozen yellow corn
- o 3 cups frozen peas
- o ½ cup frozen strawberries

Meat, Eggs, and Dairy

- o 4 strips nitrate-free bacon
- o 1 pound lean ground beef
- o 3 pounds boneless, skinless chicken breasts
- o 1 pound ground sausage
- o 1 pound small shrimp (36/40 count), peeled and deveined
- o 1 pound ground turkey
- o 16 large eggs
- o Oat Milk Yogurt (page 84) or other yogurt (2½ cups)
- o ¾ cup Homemade Mayo (page 330) or store-bought

Dry Goods

- o ¾ cup dried kidney beans
- o ¾ cup dried pinto beans
- o ¾ cup raw cashews
- o 1½ tablespoons chia seeds
- o 3 ounces corn tortilla chips
- o ½ cup green or brown lentils
- o 4 ounces gluten-free fusilli pasta
- o 20 ounces gluten-free penne pasta
- o 1 cup quinoa
- o 1 package lightly salted brown rice cakes
- o 10 corn tortillas
- o 2 tablespoons chopped raw walnuts (optional)

Canned/Jarred Goods

- o 1 (15-ounce) can black beans
- o 2 tablespoons sugar-free mild hot sauce
- o Naturally sweetened ketchup
- o Organic dill or sweet pickles
- o ¼ cup plus 2 tablespoons organic sweet relish
- o 1 cup sugar-free salsa verde or jalapeño salsa

- Sriracha
- 1 (5-ounce) can wild-caught tuna
- 2 (15-ounce) cans diced tomatoes
- 2 tablespoons tomato paste
- 2 (15-ounce) cans tomato sauce

Flours, Powders, and Sugars

- Cassava flour (from Amazon) (¾ cup)
- 3¼ cup oat flour, or gluten-free old-fashioned rolled oats if you blend your own
- Aluminum-free baking powder
- Unfortified nutritional yeast (2½ tablespoons)

Miscellaneous

- 1½ tablespoons coconut aminos
- 1 teaspoon Red Boat fish sauce
- 1 tablespoon raw honey
- ½ teaspoon liquid smoke
- 1 tablespoon 100 percent pure maple syrup
- 1 tablespoon Dijon mustard
- 2¾ cups low-sodium vegetable or chicken stock (store-bought or homemade)

Oils and Vinegars

- Cooking oil spray
- Avocado oil (⅔ cup)
- Extra-virgin olive oil

- Sesame oil (½ teaspoon)
- Apple cider vinegar (2½ tablespoons)
- Balsamic vinegar (2 tablespoons)
- 1½ tablespoons rice vinegar (or any vinegar you have on hand)

Spices

- Cajun Seasoning (page 328) or store-bought
- Chili powder
- Chipotle chili powder
- Dried basil
- Dried minced onion
- Dried oregano
- Dried parsley
- Everything Bagel seasoning
- Fine sea salt
- Garlic powder
- Ground cinnamon
- Ground cumin
- Ground black pepper
- Ground turmeric
- Onion powder
- Sesame seeds
- Taco Seasoning (page 325) or store-bought

Optional Ingredients

- 1 pound frozen broccoli
- Extra eggs for hard-boiling
- Eggs and bacon, breakfast Day 6
- 1 cup brown rice or cauliflower rice

MENU: WEEK 3

	DAY 1	DAY 2	DAY 3	DAY 4	DAY 5	DAY 6
BREAKFAST	Peanut Butter Meal-Replacement Smoothie (page 294) Cost: $0.70	Migas (page 207) Cost: $6.45	Savory Garlic-Herb Chicken Waffles with Maple-Chili Syrup (page 205) Cost: $3.00	Smoothie Bowl Parfaits (page 76) Cost: $2.40	Banana Coffee Cake (page 69) Cost: $2.85	Plantain Pancakes with Caramel Sauce (page 92) Cost: $2.15
LUNCH	Asian Chicken Salad (page 152) Cost: $7.00	Carrot-Ginger Soup (page 131) Cost: $2.60	Dry-Rubbed Chili Chicken Wings (page 117) Cost: $4.35 Optional: side salad	Creamy Kale and Tomato Pasta (page 192) Cost: $4.20	No-Potato Potato Soup (page 142) Cost: $3.25	Cabbage Steaks (page 244) with simple salad Cost: $2.50
DINNER	Lasagna Soup with Cashew Ricotta Cheese (page 136) Cost: $7.50	Black Bean Tostadas (page 220) Cost: $3.20	Low-Country Shrimp Boil (page 210) Cost: $9.00	Easy Steak Bites with Peppers (page 276) Cost: $9.50	Kung Pao Chickpeas with Veggie Lo Mein (page 215) Cost: $5.00	Salisbury Steak with Mushroom Gravy (page 281) Cost: $4.15

TOTAL COST FOR THE WEEK: $79.80

SHOPPING LIST: WEEK 3

Fruits

- o 1 large avocado
- o 4 bananas
- o 1 Medjool date
- o 3 lemons
- o 1 lime
- o 1 large orange, for juicing
- o 1 mandarin orange
- o 2 large ripe plantains
- o 2 cups grape tomatoes
- o 3 medium to large Roma tomatoes

Vegetables

- o 1 medium to large head green cabbage
- o 2 cups shredded green cabbage

- 2 cups finely shredded red cabbage
- 4½ large carrots
- 4 stalks celery
- 3 ears corn
- 1 bunch kale
- 2 large heads romaine lettuce
- 1 cup mushrooms
- 7 green onions
- ½ medium red onion
- 4½ medium to large yellow onions
- ½ medium orange bell pepper
- 3 medium red bell peppers
- 2 medium jalapeños
- 1½ pounds small red potatoes
- 1 cup baby spinach
- 3 medium to large zucchini

Herbs

- ½ cup fresh basil
- Fresh chives
- 1 bunch fresh cilantro
- 15 cloves garlic
- 1 medium knob fresh ginger

Frozen

- ½ cup frozen blueberries
- 1 cup frozen riced cauliflower
- ½ cup frozen peaches
- 6 frozen strawberries

Meat, Eggs, and Dairy

- 2 pounds lean ground beef
- 1 cup shredded, unseasoned, cooked chicken breast
- 1 pound boneless, skinless chicken breasts

- 1 pound chicken wings
- ½ pound smoked andouille sausage
- 1 pound medium shrimp, deveined, shells left on
- 1 pound sirloin steak strips
- 18 large eggs
- 1 cup Almond Milk (page 288) or other milk
- 2 cups Oat Milk (page 288) or water

Dry Goods

- 2 tablespoons slivered almonds
- 1 cup dried black beans
- 1 cup raw cashews or unsalted sunflower seeds
- 1 cup dried chickpeas
- 12 corn tortillas
- ½ cup shelled hemp seeds or hearts
- 1 cup red lentils
- 4 ounces brown rice macaroni noodles
- 2½ cups gluten-free old-fashioned rolled oats
- 10 ounces gluten-free penne pasta

Canned/Jarred Goods

- ½ cup canned full-fat coconut milk
- Yellow mustard (1 tablespoon)
- Organic peanut butter (or other nut/ seed butter) (3 tablespoons)
- 1 cup Creamy Ranch Dressing (page 110) or store-bought
- Tahini
- 1 (15-ounce) can diced tomatoes
- 1 tablespoon tomato paste
- 1 cup sugar-free salsa

Flours, Powders, and Sugars

- o Superfine almond flour (¾ cup)
- o Arrowroot flour or corn starch (1 tablespoon)
- o Aluminum-free baking powder
- o Baking soda
- o Coconut flour (½ cup)
- o Unfortified nutritional yeast (1 tablespoon)

Miscellaneous

- o ¾ cup low-sodium beef broth
- o Coconut aminos (⅓ cup plus 3 tablespoons)
- o 2 teaspoons unsweetened coconut flakes
- o ½ cup coconut water
- o 1 cup Super-Simple Granola (page 323) or store-bought
- o Raw honey (2 tablespoons)
- o 100 percent pure maple syrup (⅔ cup)
- o Pure vanilla extract (1 tablespoon)
- o 8¾ cups low-sodium vegetable or chicken stock (store-bought or homemade)

Oils and Vinegars

- o Cooking oil spray
- o Avocado oil (5 tablespoons)
- o Extra-virgin coconut oil (½ cup)
- o Extra-virgin olive oil (1¼ cups)
- o Sesame oil (5 teaspoons)
- o Apple cider vinegar (2 teaspoons)
- o Balsamic vinegar (2 tablespoons)
- o Rice vinegar (1 tablespoon)

Spices

- o Bay leaves
- o Cajun Seasoning (page 328), or store-bought
- o Cayenne pepper
- o Chili powder
- o Dried basil
- o Dried minced onion
- o Dried parsley
- o Dried rosemary
- o Fine sea salt
- o Garlic powder
- o Ground black pepper
- o Ground cumin
- o Ground ginger
- o Old Bay seasoning
- o Onion powder
- o Paprika
- o Red pepper flakes
- o Sesame seeds
- o Taco Seasoning (page 325), or store-bought
- o Turmeric

Optional Ingredients

- o Cocktail sauce
- o 1 tablespoon collagen peptides
- o 1 tablespoon ghee
- o Hot sauce
- o Fresh parsley
- o Salad greens
- o Tartar Sauce (page 212)
- o ¾ cup chopped raw walnuts

MENU: WEEK 4

	DAY 1	DAY 2	DAY 3	DAY 4	DAY 5	DAY 6
BREAKFAST	Veggie-Lover's Quiche (page 77) Cost: $4.00	Baked Grapefruit with Honeyed Yogurt and Granola Sprinkle (page 82) Cost: $2.40	French Toast Rice Porridge (page 100) Cost: $3.90	Eggs and bacon (no recipe)	Peanut Butter Meal-Replacement Smoothie (page 294) Cost: $0.70	Blueberry Muffins (page 57) Cost: $2.70
LUNCH	Cauliflower Cheese Bisque (page 134) Cost: $6.40	Salmon Burgers with Broccoli Slaw (page 269) Cost: $6.50	Curried Chickpea Salad Cups (page 154) Cost: $2.10	Summer Pineapple Chicken over Cauliflower Rice (page 257) Cost: $7.60	Italian Pasta Salad (page 157) Cost: $6.20	Spicy Buffalo Cauliflower with Creamy Ranch Dressing (page 108) served with a side salad Cost: $2.85
DINNER	Spicy Mexi-Rice Bowls (page 239) with side salad Cost: $3.90	Balsamic-Dijon Chicken over Zucchini Noodles (page 197) Cost: $8.50	Lemon-Garlic Drumsticks (page 251) with Bacon and Broccoli (page 179) Cost: $9.25	Beijing Beef with Steamed Broccoli (page 217) served over rice or cauliflower rice Cost: $8.50	Cilantro-Lime Chicken with Casamiento (page 267) Cost: $5.90	Shredded Beef Taquitos with No-Queso Queso (page 114) Cost: $5.60

TOTAL COST FOR THE WEEK: $87.00

SHOPPING LIST WEEK 4

Fruits

o ½ Gala apple
o 1 medium avocado
o ½ ripe banana
o 1 Medjool date

o 2 large grapefruits
o 4 lemons
o 3 limes
o 1 pineapple

Vegetables

- o 3½ pounds broccoli florets
- o 2 cups broccoli slaw (I buy Trader Joe's bagged salad mixes)
- o 1 small head purple cabbage
- o 2 large carrots
- o 2 large heads cauliflower
- o 6 stalks celery
- o ½ medium cucumber
- o 8 cups mixed greens
- o 2 medium to large heads romaine lettuce
- o 1 medium red onion
- o 1½ medium yellow onions
- o ½ medium red bell pepper
- o 1 medium yellow bell pepper
- o 1 green onion
- o ⅓ small jalapeño
- o 2½ cups baby spinach
- o 2 large zucchini
- o 2 cups cherry tomatoes
- o 3½ Roma tomatoes

Herbs

- o 1 bunch fresh cilantro
- o Fresh chives
- o 10 cloves garlic
- o 1 small knob ginger

Frozen

- o ¼ cup frozen blueberries
- o 1 cup frozen carrots
- o 4 cups frozen riced cauliflower
- o 1 cup frozen corn
- o ½ cup frozen peaches
- o 2 cups frozen peas

Meat, Eggs, and Dairy

- o 2 pounds boneless, skinless chicken breasts
- o 1 to 1¼ pounds chicken drumsticks
- o 1 pound boneless, skinless chicken tenders
- o 14 ounces salmon fillets
- o 1 pound skirt or flank steak
- o 8 ounces beef stew meat
- o 8 large eggs
- o Oat Milk (page 288) or other milk (1½ cups)
- o 2 cups Oat Milk Yogurt (page 84) or other yogurt
- o 1 cup Homemade Mayo (page 330) or store-bought

Dry Goods

- o 2½ cups brown rice
- o 1½ cups raw cashews or shelled unsalted sunflower seeds
- o 8 to 10 corn tortillas
- o 1 cup Super-Simple Granola (page 323) or store-bought
- o 1 tablespoon hemp hearts
- o 1 cup dried kidney beans
- o 12 ounces gluten-free fusilli pasta

Canned/Jarred Goods

- o 1 (8-ounce) can black olives
- o 1½ cups canned full-fat coconut milk

- 2 (15-ounce) cans chickpeas
- Creamy Ranch Dressing (page 110) or store-bought
- Italian Dressing (page 158) or store-bought
- Organic peanut butter or other nut/seed butter (1 tablespoon)
- 2 cups mild hot sauce or sugar-free salsa
- Sriracha (½ cup)
- Homemade Tahini (page 329) or store-bought

Flours, Powders, and Sugars

- Superfine almond flour (1½ cups)
- Arrowroot powder (½ cup plus 2 teaspoons)
- Cassava flour (¼ cup)
- Coconut flour (¼ cup)
- Aluminum-free baking powder
- Coconut sugar (2 tablespoons)
- Baking soda
- Unfortified nutritional yeast (½ cup)

Miscellaneous

- ¼ cup low-sodium beef broth or Bone Broth (page 331)
- ⅔ cup coconut aminos
- Cooking oil spray
- Raw honey (9 tablespoons)
- 100 percent pure maple syrup (¼ cup)
- Dijon mustard (3 tablespoons)
- 2½ cups low-sodium vegetable or chicken stock (store-bought or homemade)

Oils and Vinegars

- Extra-virgin coconut oil (¼ cup)
- Extra-virgin olive oil (1¾ cups)
- Sesame oil
- Apple cider vinegar
- Balsamic vinegar
- Red wine vinegar
- Rice vinegar

Spices

- Cayenne pepper
- Chipotle chili powder
- Curry powder
- Dried basil
- Dried dill (optional)
- Dried minced onion
- Dried oregano
- Dried parsley
- Dried thyme
- Fine sea salt
- Garlic powder
- Ground black pepper
- Ground cinnamon
- Ground ginger
- Lemon pepper
- Mustard powder
- Onion powder
- Paprika
- Taco Seasoning (page 325)

Optional Ingredients

- Collagen peptides
- Eggs and bacon, breakfast Day 4
- Red pepper flakes
- Rice or cauliflower rice, dinner Day 4

INGREDIENTS

There may be many ingredients in this book that you are unfamiliar with. As my family began to make over our mindset concerning food, our pantry also had a makeover. Use this as a guide to better understand why I use the ingredients I use and what substitutions you can make if you have an allergy or don't have a particular ingredient on hand!

Please note that all the recipes in this book were tested with the ingredients listed in the recipe. If you make a substitution that isn't suggested, you may end up with a different result than intended.

Eggs

All of the recipes in this book call for large eggs, I prefer to buy free-range or pasture-raised organic eggs that are certified humane and antibiotic free. I like Costco's Kirkland organic brand. Costco has partnered with small farms throughout the country to ensure that their hens are treated well and that they provide quality eggs.

With egg allergies becoming more prevalent, I made sure to test the baked goods in this book with egg substitutes. There are two egg substitutes I've found that work best.

> **FLAX EGG:** Stir together 1 tablespoon ground flaxseed and 3 tablespoons water. Let sit for 5 to 10 minutes, or until gelatinous. This makes enough to substitute for one egg.

> **AQUAFABA:** This is the thick cooking liquid left over from legumes. Chickpeas are highly recommended and the only source of aquafaba substitute tested in

these recipes. It has a slight yellow tinge to it and has an egg-white/jellylike texture. You can use the liquid from canned or home-cooked chickpeas. Use 3 tablespoons of aquafaba to substitute for 1 large egg.

Fats

Fats have gotten a bad rap throughout the years. Much like carbohydrates, they are an energy source that the body relies on to function properly. Our cell structure needs healthy fats to thrive! The fats listed below are full of heart-healthy micronutrients that help keep our cell membranes strong. Healthy fats help boost your nutrient absorption and are an essential for healthy living!

I prefer to use organic, minimally processed fats in my cooking like extra-virgin olive oil, avocado oil, and extra-virgin coconut oil. These oils can usually be used interchangeably. When a recipe calls for a specific oil, it's because that is the oil that tastes the best in that recipe.

Flours

I am a big fan of alternative flours. Most of the traditional wheat in the U.S. is fortified and enriched with folic acid. Folic acid is the oxidized form of folate. Unfortunately, my family has a difficult time processing it because of a common gene mutation we all share. To learn more, visit instantloss.com/lets-talk-mthfr. For this reason, we use alternative flours in most of our cooking, and all of the recipes in this book are gluten-free.

If you do not have a gluten sensitivity, wheat flour is absolutely healthy to consume in modest portions! Just be mindful, as wheat can be inflammatory, and wheat flour is not an adequate 1:1 substitution for the alternative flours in any of the recipes in this book.

Since I started using Instant Loss recipes for our family of five in January, I am spending $100 to $125 weekly on groceries. That being said, almost all of it is now natural or organic also, whereas before it rarely was. We don't feel like we have to eat out anymore, which has saved us a few hundred dollars a week, as before we ate out multiple times a week. The initial startup was a bit more, and at first it seemed overwhelming to buy all of the flours, nutritional yeast, chia seeds, etc. (I wish I would have realized how much cheaper Costco was than the grocery store, so make sure you stock up there!) Not only have we been saving a bunch of money, but we have also been feeling better, enjoying the food more, and getting healthier along the way. My preschooler is back to eating veggies again and choosing to do so. As for exactly how much we spent on groceries before making the change—I'm not sure. But it would be $200+ a week and then eating out multiple days costing $50+ per meal. It's a lot of savings and a lot of health!

—KELLY ZAKRAJSEK

These alternative flours can be tricky to substitute so I highly recommend using the flour suggested in each recipe.

ALMOND FLOUR: Using a blanched, superfine grind of almond flour will yield the best results for baked goods. This flour is best stored in the freezer because it can go rancid quickly. If you have a nut allergy, you can substitute ½ cup cassava flour for every 1 cup almond flour. Almond flour can be pricey, so I highly recommend purchasing it at your local big box store like Costco or shopping online sales.

GARBANZO BEAN FLOUR: This flour is packed full of protein and relatively low in carbohydrates. It's also inexpensive! If you cannot consume legumes, you can substitute 1¼ cups superfine, blanched almond flour for every 1 cup garbanzo bean flour.

ARROWROOT POWDER: Arrowroot powder, also known as arrowroot flour or arrowroot starch, helps give baked goods elasticity. It's also a marvelous thickener that can be used in place of cornstarch. If you do not have any on hand, you can substitute tapioca starch or cornstarch 1:1 for arrowroot powder.

COCONUT FLOUR: Super-absorbent, a little bit of coconut flour goes a long, long way. Because it's unique, substituting it in large quantities is not recommended, unless you're looking for a science experiment! If you have a coconut allergy, you can substitute ¼ cup arrowroot powder for every 1 tablespoon coconut flour.

OAT FLOUR: All oats are gluten-free, but not all of them are processed in a gluten-free facility. If you have celiac disease, be mindful and make sure you purchase oats with a gluten-free label to ensure there is no cross contamination. I make my oat flour at home. Use a high-powered blender like a Vitamix to grind your oats fresh for an extra boost of nutrient content! 1 cup oats equals 1 cup oat flour.

CASSAVA FLOUR: Rich in minerals like calcium, potassium, magnesium, and iron, cassava flour is made from the whole root of the yucca plant and is nonallergenic. This grain-free flour can be a little hard to find, though, so I order mine through Amazon. If you're not gluten-free, cassava flour can be substituted 1:1 with whole-wheat flour.

UNFORTIFIED NUTRITIONAL YEAST: Highly nutritious and full of protein, vitamins, minerals, and antioxidants, nutritional yeast is an excellent source of B_6 and contains 8 grams of protein per serving. It's a cheesy-tasting powder that's dairy-free. I use it in recipes to give a big cheesy boost. You can also sprinkle it on home-popped popcorn with sea salt and coconut oil for a delicious snack, or top soups and salads with it. It's a fabulous ingredient. Note that this ingredient *cannot* be substituted with active dry yeast; it's a deactivated strain of yeast that looks like yellow flakes or powder. I purchase the Sari Foods brand from Amazon. One bag will last you forever!

Sweeteners

MAPLE SYRUP: One hundred percent pure maple syrup is not the same thing as pancake syrup. Pure maple syrup is made from the sap of maple trees, which is boiled to reduce the water content and concentrate the sweetness. Pancake syrup is usually made from high-fructose corn syrup or corn syrup and uses artificial flavorings to make it taste more like maple syrup. The real thing is pricey, and it's sometimes tempting to substitute a cheap alternative— but in this case, you really do get what you pay for! Look for pure maple syrup that does not have any added ingredients. Buying pure maple syrup in bulk at Costco saves me a bundle. If you still can't bite the bullet, you can substitute 1:1 with raw honey or, as a last resort, agave nectar.

COCONUT SUGAR: Also known as palm sugar, this sweetener is made from the sap of flower buds from the coconut palm tree. It's dark, coarse, and a fabulous brown sugar substitute. Can be subbed 1:1 with raw organic cane sugar.

RAW HONEY: Most of the honey that you encounter in the grocery store is made with artificial sugars like corn syrup and contains little, if any honey. It's always best to find a local source of raw honey. Local honey is a great way to battle seasonal allergies, but if you can't source it locally, any raw, organic honey will do!

Milks

OAT MILK is by far the most cost-effective milk to make at home, coming in at just a few cents per quart. Store-bought oat milk, however, is one of the most expensive alternative milks you can purchase. See page 288 for a guide on how to make your own milks at home. Any time milk is called for in a recipe, it can be subbed 1:1 with your milk of choice.

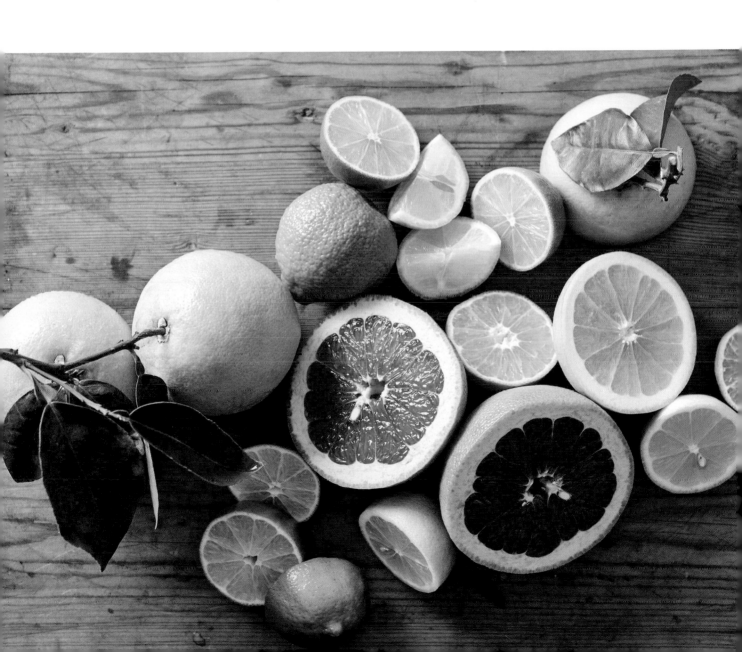

KITCHEN TOOLS

My kitchen didn't come together overnight. I've acquired all of these kitchen gadgets and tools over the last ten years as my family's budget permitted. The top two things I'd advise that you invest in first are an **electric pressure cooker** and a **high-powered blender,** preferably a Vitamix. If you cannot afford to invest in a quality blender, that's okay. I tested all of the recipes in this book with a $30 Magic Bullet, and that will suffice.

Investing in your kitchen by having the proper equipment will help you to work faster and more efficiently. It will enable you to make many more things from scratch—and quickly, too. This will end up saving you more in the long run and drastically reducing the time (and money) you spend inside the kitchen.

ELECTRIC PRESSURE COOKER: All of the recipes in this book were tested with the 6-quart Instant Pot 7-in-1 Duo. I have several different electric pressure cookers, and this is by far the brand and model that I love best. If you are using an 8-quart electric pressure cooker, you will need to adjust the recipes according to the manufacturer's specifications, specifically the liquids. This might require you to double some of the recipes.

AIR FRYER: All of the air-fryer recipes in this book were tested with the PowerXL 5.3-quart Air Fryer. Results with other air-fryer brands may vary.

BLENDER: Some of the recipes in this book call for a blender. Brady grew up with a Vitamix, so we pinched pennies and used birthday money to invest in one ten years ago. It was one of the best kitchen investments we've ever made. It makes it easy to make our own flours and nut/seed milks at home, and we even grind our own spices! However, I realize that the Vitamix is not very budget-friendly and therefore I tested the recipes in this book with a Magic Bullet. You can get one for as little as $30 at Costco or Walmart. These little power houses are small, compact, and get the job done.

IMMERSION BLENDER: This is a super-budget-friendly kitchen gadget. Typically for $20 to $30, you can get a machine that will make pureeing soups, dressings, and things like mayo an absolute breeze.

FOOD PROCESSOR: You don't need a big ole to-do. I bought a 10-cup $40 food processor on Amazon. I use the Hamilton Beach (70760) model. This machine makes chopping veggies, grating cheese, and blending things that are hard to dig out of a blender, like doughs and hummus, a breeze! If you can't afford one right now, that's okay. Having a food processor is not a requirement for this book; it's just something nice to have.

KNIVES: I love cheap knives! Twelve dollars for a pack of Cuisinart at Costco? That's my jam! Last year I invested in a couple really good knives and was sad to realize that they dulled just as quickly as my cheapies. Now we make it a habit to buy new cheap knives every few years when ours become really beat up. Just don't try to chop with dull ones—an exercise in frustration.

DONUT PAN: I highly recommend using a silicone donut pan for the donut recipes in this book.

BAKING SHEETS: I used stainless steel baking sheets for the recipes in this book. If you have dark-bottom pans, your results may vary.

INSTANT POT MINI BUNDT PAN: Sam's Club and Amazon both carry an Instant Pot–safe mini Bundt pan.

SPIRALIZER: These are fairly inexpensive on Amazon. You can usually snag one for under $20 and it'll save you a bundle, rather than paying a premium for spiralized veggies at the store.

POTS AND PANS: I stick with stainless steel or cast-iron pans for all of my cooking. Some of these pieces are an investment.

Your ideal kitchen will not come together overnight. It's been ten years and I'm still building mine. Use what you have, and upgrade when you can.

BEFORE YOU GET STARTED

WHY I DON'T LIST NUTRITION INFORMATION

There are several reasons that I do not list nutrition information with the recipes, the first being the negative effects that viewing food as numbers can have on an individual. I spent years tracking calories, carbs, points, and macros. It never led to sustainable long-term success because tracking, for me, was not sustainable.

It also tended to put me in "diet mode." Initially my focus was to try to fit as much crummy food into my number goals as possible. My focus was not on actual nourishment or nutrition but getting the numbers correct while continuing to consume food that was of poor quality.

I knew that I needed to find a different way to regulate portions. It seemed reasonable enough to me to look back to a time before the obesity epidemic. They didn't have calorie counters and trackers and society, as a whole, was in a healthy weight range.

They ate real food, in smaller portion sizes, and their bodies took care of the rest. I had to retrain my brain. I had to stop thinking about food as numbers and begin to think about it as fuel.

The second, probably more important, reason I don't include nutrition information is because, depending on the brand, nutritionals can vary greatly. If you need to

Our grocery budget has gone down about $400 a month since we started following Instant Loss. Before we bought a lot of processed alternatives for our son's food allergies. We made a few Instant Loss recipes and really liked how they tasted better and were much cheaper than the alternative options at the grocery stores!

—BRITTANY NEUJAHR

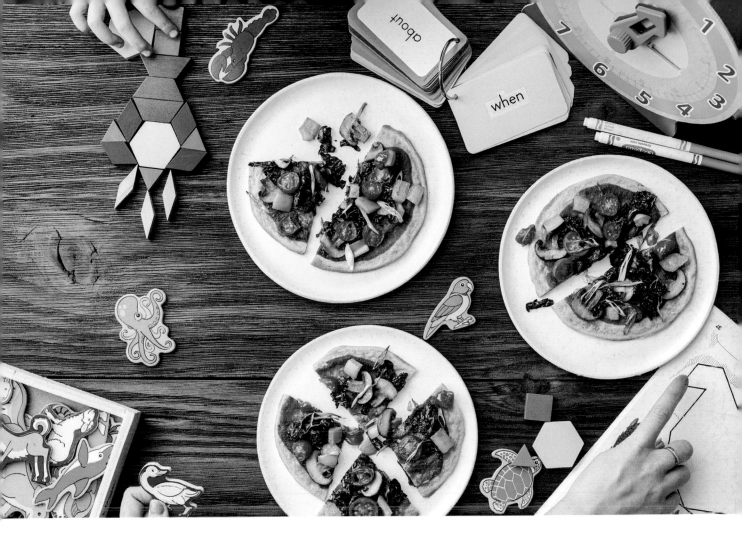

track nutritionals because you have a medical condition, it's best to calculate nutritional information yourself with your own ingredients.

Cost Breakdown

Each recipe shows the total cost I've calculated at the top of page. But keep in mind that prices will vary depending on location and availability of ingredients. In general, the lower numbers reflect buying a majority of conventional ingredients; the higher numbers reflect pricing with organic ingredients. All costs include meat that was humanely sourced and eggs that are pasture raised. All costs are in U.S. dollars.

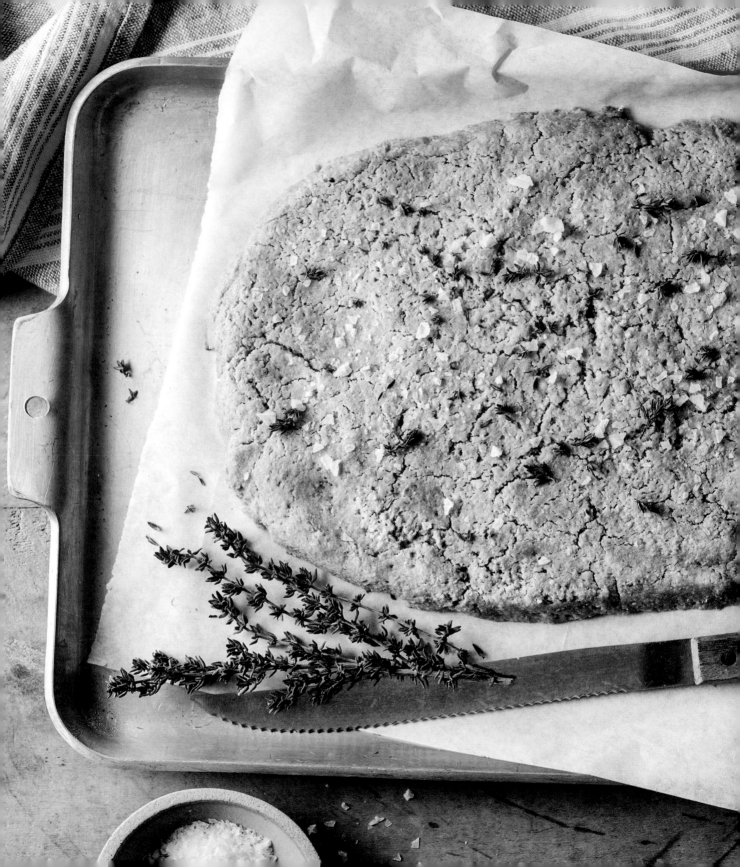

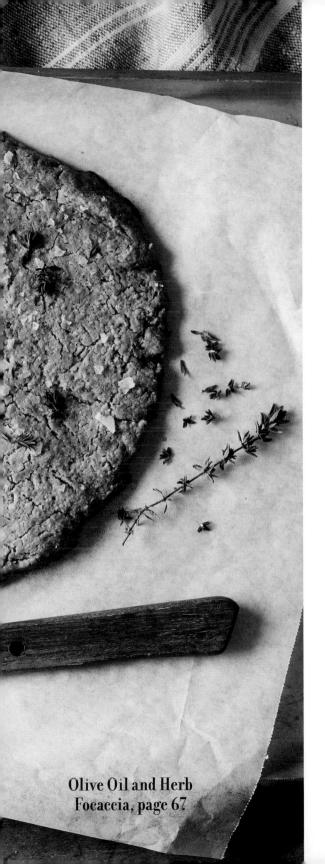

Olive Oil and Herb Focaccia, page 67

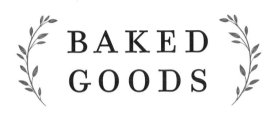

BAKED GOODS

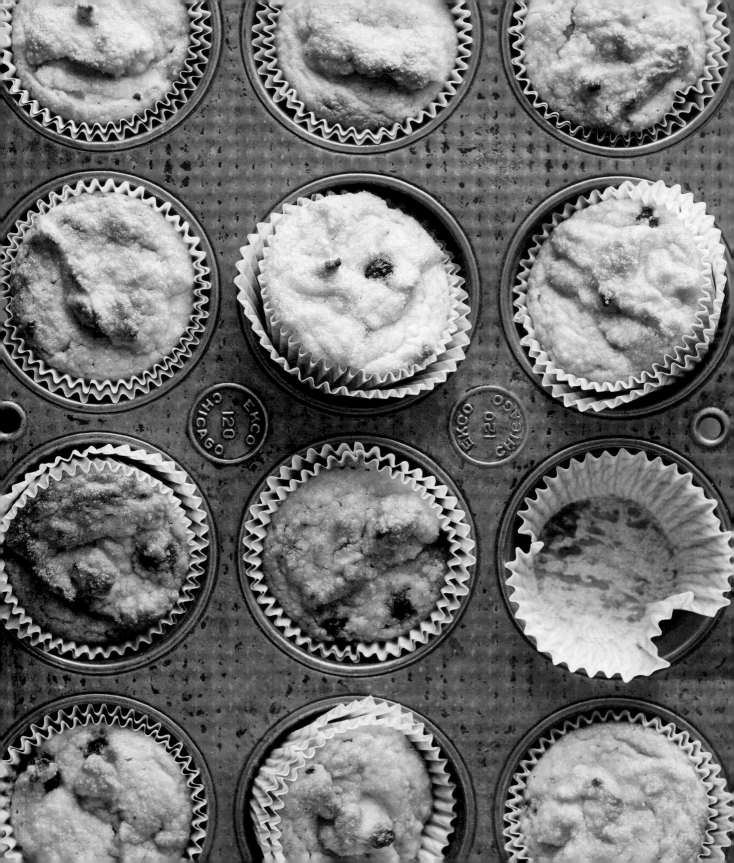

BLUEBERRY MUFFINS

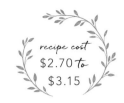
recipe cost
$2.70 *to*
$3.15

The perfect breakfast on the go! These grain-free muffins are a delightful accompaniment to a morning smoothie or juice. They are light and fluffy and absolutely scrumptious buttered. Serve them fresh out of the oven or freeze them for up to four months. Set them out on the counter the night before you want to enjoy one for breakfast!

MAKES 12 MUFFINS

Cooking oil spray (optional)

1 cup tightly packed superfine almond flour

½ cup water

¼ cup coconut flour

2 large eggs

3 tablespoons raw honey

2 tablespoons extra-virgin olive oil

¼ teaspoon fine sea salt

⅛ teaspoon baking soda

¼ cup fresh or frozen blueberries

1. Preheat the oven to 350°F. Lightly grease a 12-cup muffin pan with cooking oil spray or line with paper liners.

2. In a large bowl, whisk together the almond flour, water, coconut flour, eggs, honey, olive oil, salt, and baking soda until a thick batter forms. Stir in the blueberries.

3. Transfer the batter to the prepared muffin pan, filling each muffin cup three-fourths full. Bake for 30 minutes, or until a toothpick inserted into the centers of the muffins comes out clean.

4. Let cool for 5 minutes in the pan before transferring to a wire rack to cool completely.

5. Once cool, store in an airtight container at room temperature up to 3 days or in the freezer for up to 4 months.

CHOCOLATE BROWNIE DONUTS

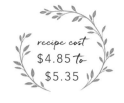

recipe cost
$4.85 to
$5.35

Enjoy dessert for breakfast with these chocolate brownie donuts! Decadent, delicious, and 100 percent kid-loved and approved. I use the large silicone donut pan by Unicorn Glitter from Amazon. It's not pricey and it's still like new three years in! Don't let the garbanzo bean flour throw you. It is flour made out of chickpeas and it's great for baking! You can buy it on Amazon or at your local health food store. Vitacost.com usually carries it at a discount, too.

MAKES 9 DONUTS

Cooking oil spray
1⅓ cups garbanzo bean flour
½ cup cacao powder
½ cup coconut sugar
¼ cup raw honey
⅓ cup extra-virgin olive oil
3 large eggs
1 teaspoon pure vanilla extract
1 teaspoon baking powder
½ teaspoon baking soda
½ teaspoon fine sea salt

1. Preheat the oven to 375°F. Spray a standard donut pan with cooking oil spray.

2. In a food processor, combine the flour, cacao powder, coconut sugar, honey, olive oil, eggs, vanilla, baking powder, baking soda, and salt. Process on high until well combined, about 30 seconds.

3. Transfer the batter to a piping bag fitted with a large tip. (If you don't have a piping bag, transfer the batter to a quart-size plastic bag and cut one corner off.) Pipe the mixture into the prepared pan.

4. Bake for 13 to 16 minutes, or until a toothpick inserted into the donuts comes out clean.

5. Set on top of a wire rack and let cool in pan completely, about 35 minutes, before serving.

TIDBIT: If you're in the mood for a more extravagant donut, frost with Chocolate Frosting (page 322) and sprinkle with natural sprinkles!

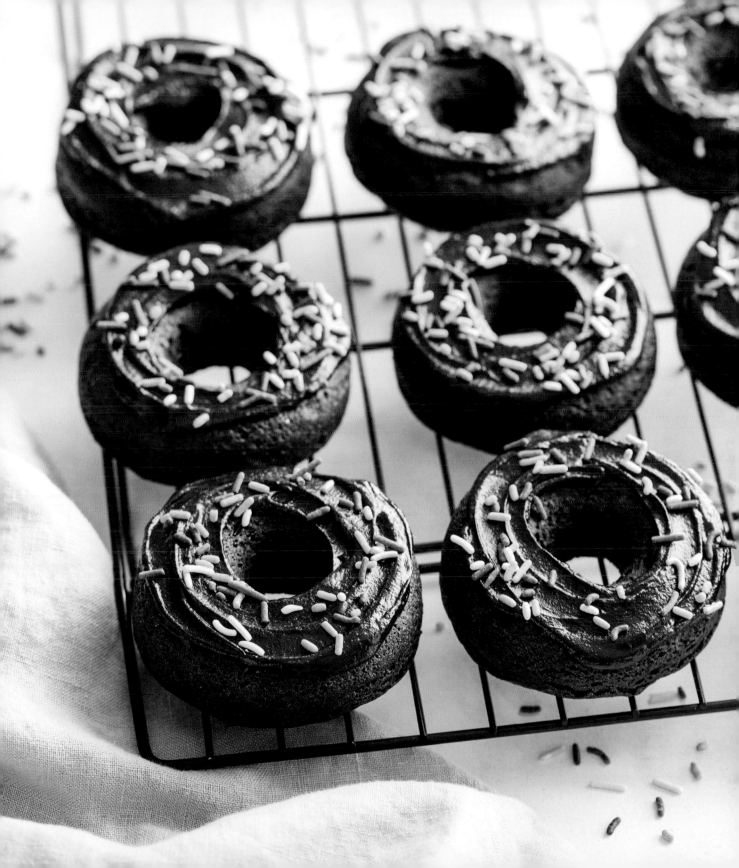

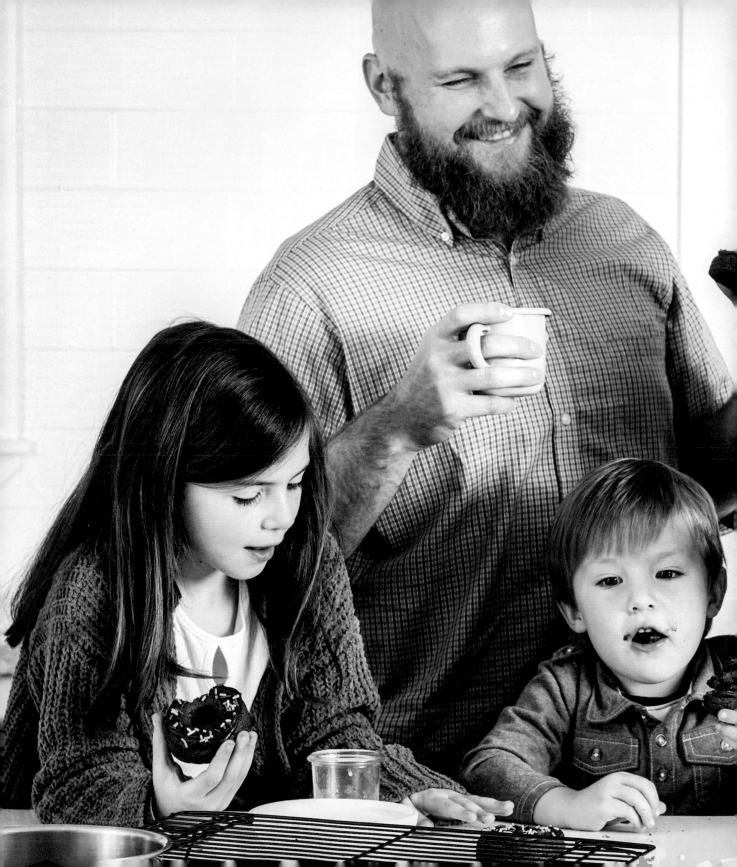

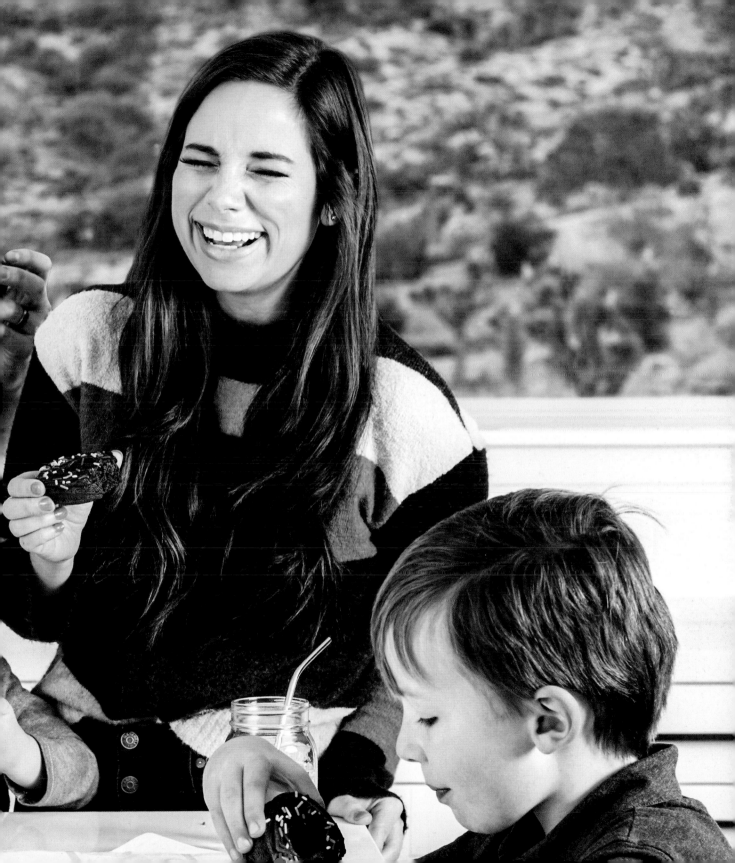

MINI EVERYTHING BAGELS

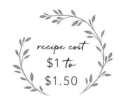

recipe cost
$1 to
$1.50

Stop what you're doing right now and make these bagels. I make them in large batches and freeze them for quick grab-and-go breakfasts. They keep well in the freezer for up to six months.

MAKES 9 BAGELS

Cooking oil spray

2¼ cups gluten-free oat flour

1½ cups Oat Milk Yogurt (page 84) or favorite plain yogurt

1½ tablespoons chia seeds

1½ tablespoons aluminum-free baking powder

1¼ teaspoons fine sea salt

1 to 2 tablespoons Everything Bagel Seasoning

1. Preheat the oven to 350°F. Spray a standard donut pan with cooking oil spray.

2. In a large bowl, combine the flour, yogurt, chia seeds, baking powder, and salt. Transfer the batter to a piping bag with a large tip. (If you don't have a piping bag, transfer the batter to a quart-size plastic bag and cut one corner off.) Pipe the mixture into the prepared pan. Sprinkle the tops with the bagel seasoning.

3. Bake for 35 minutes, or until a toothpick inserted into the centers of the bagels comes out clean.

4. Let cool for about 5 minutes in the pan, then turn over onto a wire rack. Let cool completely before serving.

5. Once cool, store in an airtight container at room temperature for up to 3 days or in the freezer for up to 4 months.

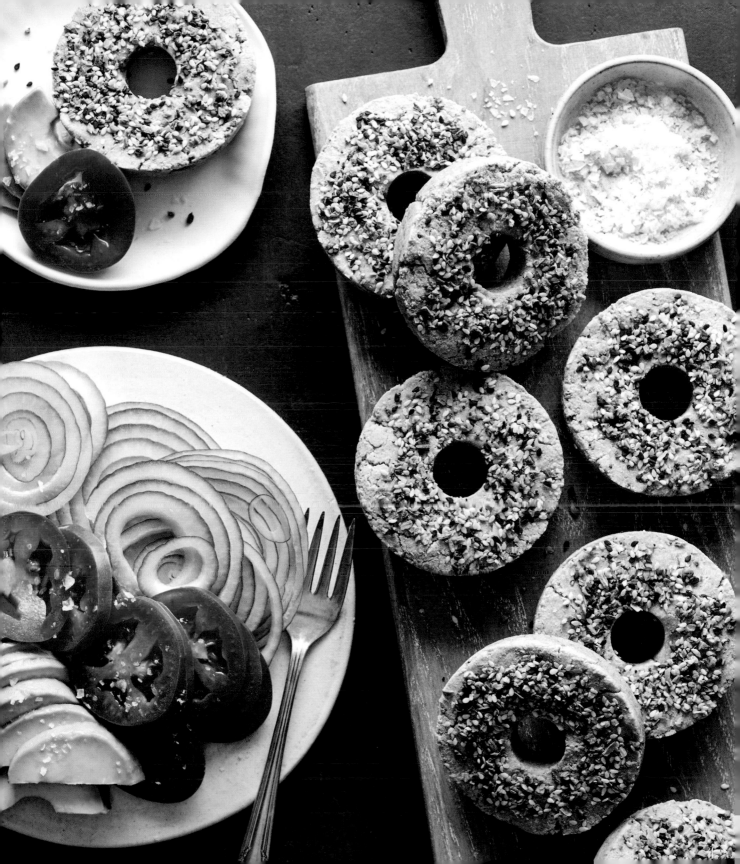

SAVORY DINNER MUFFINS

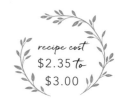

recipe cost
$2.35 to
$3.00

This is not your traditional dinner muffin; it has veggies interspersed throughout. Kid-approved, these muffins are the perfect addition to any of the soups starting on page 123. These are budget-friendly and cook up in no time!

MAKES 12 MUFFINS

Cooking oil spray

1½ cups gluten-free old-fashioned rolled oats

½ cup water

¼ cup Oat Milk Yogurt (page 84) or favorite plain yogurt

¼ cup extra-virgin olive oil

2 large eggs

1 tablespoon aluminum-free baking powder

1 teaspoon dried parsley flakes

½ teaspoon garlic powder

½ teaspoon fine sea salt

¼ teaspoon dried oregano

¾ cup frozen mixed vegetables (peas, carrots, corn)

1. Preheat the oven to 350°F. Lightly grease a 12-cup muffin pan with cooking oil spray or line with paper liners.

2. In a blender, combine the oats, water, yogurt, olive oil, eggs, baking powder, parsley, garlic powder, salt, and oregano. Blend on high until the mixture becomes a thick batter, about 60 seconds. Stir in the mixed vegetables.

3. Transfer the batter to the prepared muffin pan, filling each muffin cup three-fourths full. Bake for 30 minutes, or until a toothpick inserted into the centers of the muffins comes out clean.

4. Let cool in the pan for 5 minutes before transferring to a wire rack to cool completely.

5. Once cool, store in an airtight container at room temperature for up to 3 days or in the freezer for up to 4 months.

OAT BREAD

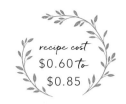

recipe cost
$0.60 to
$0.85

Store-bought gluten-free breads can be $6 a loaf and online recipes often have a laundry list of ingredients. This bread requires only seven ingredients that you probably already have on hand. It makes one small loaf, or the recipe can be doubled if you're serving a crowd.

1. Spray a standard loaf pan with cooking oil spray.

2. In a blender, combine the egg, water, olive oil, honey, oats, yeast, and salt.

3. Blend on high until the mixture forms a wet dough, about 60 seconds. Transfer the dough to the prepared loaf pan. Let rise, uncovered, in a warm dry place for 45 minutes, or until doubled in size.

4. Preheat the oven to 375°F.

5. Bake until the top is lightly browned around the edges, about 30 minutes. Remove from the oven. Cool in the pan on a wire rack for 10 minutes. Remove from the pan and let cool completely on the rack before slicing.

6. Once cool, store in an airtight container at room temperature for up to 3 days or in the freezer for up to 4 months.

MAKES 1 LOAF

Cooking oil spray

1 large egg

1 cup warm water

1½ teaspoons extra-virgin olive oil

2 tablespoons raw honey

1½ cups gluten-free steel-cut oats or gluten-free old-fashioned rolled oats

1 teaspoon active dry yeast

¾ teaspoon fine sea salt

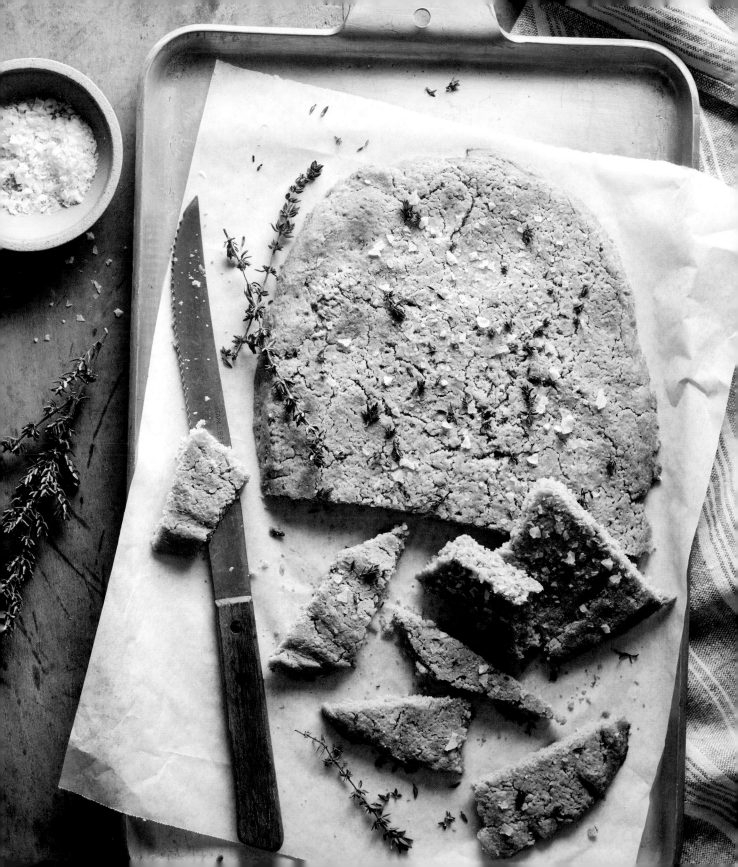

OLIVE OIL *and* HERB FOCACCIA

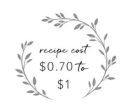

recipe cost
$0.70 *to*
$1

Who doesn't love bread? When I discovered that I was gluten-intolerant I felt like it was a death sentence—no more bread, no more pasta, no more fun. But I was wrong—there are so many amazing alternatives on the market today. They are just not all budget-friendly. This bread is budget-friendly and comes together quickly. I anticipate it'll quickly become a staple in your home!

MAKES 1 LOAF

2½ cups gluten-free old-fashioned rolled oats

1 cup warm water

2 tablespoons raw honey

1 teaspoon active dry yeast

1 large egg

1½ teaspoons extra-virgin olive oil, plus more for brushing

1¼ teaspoons fine sea salt, plus more for sprinkling

Cooking oil spray

1 tablespoon fresh thyme leaves

1. In a high-powered blender, combine the oats, water, honey, yeast, egg, olive oil, and salt. Blend on high until the mixture forms a wet dough, about 60 seconds.

2. Transfer the dough to a large bowl. Let rise in a warm dry place for about 1 hour, or until doubled in size.

3. Preheat the oven to 375°F. Lightly grease a baking sheet with cooking oil spray.

4. On the prepared pan, shape the dough into a flat, ¾-inch-thick oval. Brush the top with some olive oil. Sprinkle with the thyme and a little bit of salt.

5. Bake the bread for 30 minutes, or until the top is lightly browned around the edges. Remove from the oven and brush the top with more olive oil. Transfer to a wire rack and cool completely before slicing.

6. Once cool, store in an airtight container at room temperature for up to 3 days or in the freezer for up to 4 months.

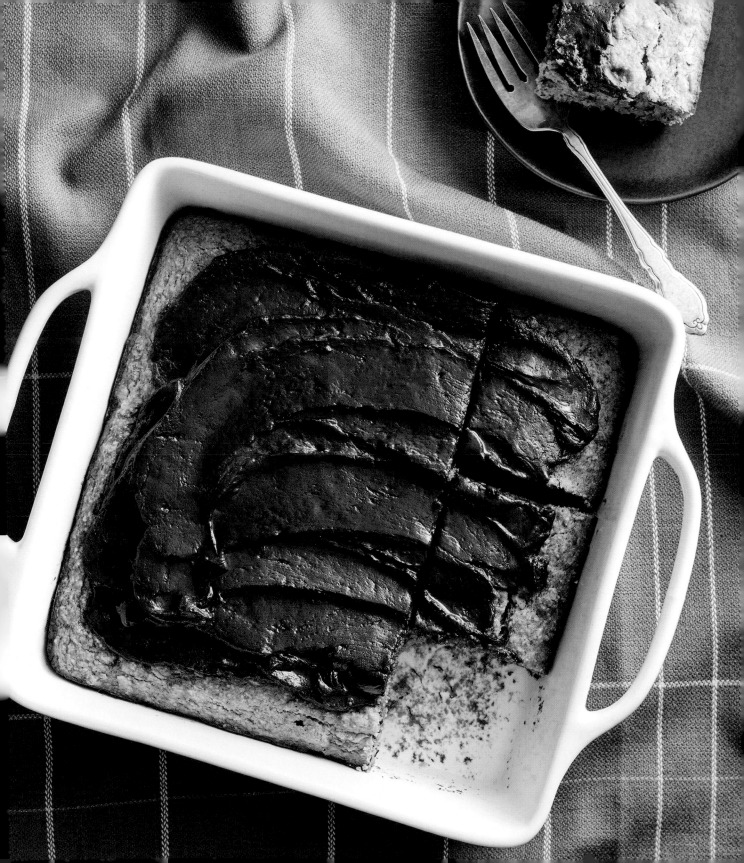

BANANA COFFEE CAKE

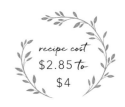

recipe cost $2.85 *to* $4

Banana bread lovers, look no further! My Aunt Kim always made the tastiest banana bread but, since going gluten- and dairy-free, it's been difficult to find the perfect combination of ingredients to make something just as good. Instead of a traditional bread, I decided to develop a cake. Eat it plain or frost it with the Chocolate Frosting on page 322—either way it's absolutely delicious!

SERVES 12

Cooking oil spray

1½ cups gluten-free rolled oats

3 medium very ripe bananas, peeled and mashed

¼ cup extra-virgin coconut oil

¼ cup 100 percent pure maple syrup

1 large egg

1 teaspoon pure vanilla extract

¾ cup superfine almond flour

1 teaspoon baking powder

½ teaspoon baking soda

¼ teaspoon fine sea salt

¾ cup chopped raw walnuts (optional)

1. Preheat the oven to 350°F. Spray an 8×8-inch baking pan with cooking oil spray.

2. Blend the oats in a high-powered blender on high until they become flour, about 30 seconds.

3. In a large bowl or stand mixer, combine the bananas, coconut oil, maple syrup, egg, and vanilla.

4. Using a hand mixer or stand mixer, mix on medium-low until well combined.

5. Add the oat flour, almond flour, baking powder, baking soda, and salt. Mix on medium-low until the ingredients are well-incorporated and a batter forms. If desired, gently stir in the walnuts.

6. Pour the batter into the prepared dish. Bake for 35 to 40 minutes, or until a toothpick inserted into the center of the cake comes out clean.

7. Remove the cake from the oven and let cool for 15 minutes before serving.

CINNAMON BUN CAKE *with* CINNAMON SWIRL

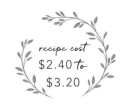

recipe cost $2.40 *to* $3.20

This tasty cake is perfect for breakfast or dessert. It's little, but packs big flavor and tastes just little a cinnamon roll! Top with a little bit of dairy-free whipped cream (see Note page 316) if you're feeling extra fancy! A lovely addition to a brunch spread when entertaining, your guests would never know it's refined sugar-free and healthy!

1. **MAKE THE CAKE:** Spray a 7-inch round pan with cooking oil spray.

2. In a large bowl, combine the oat flour, almond flour, oat milk, cassava flour, applesauce, maple syrup, flax meal, vanilla, baking powder, vinegar, baking soda, and salt. Using a hand mixer, mix on medium-low until well combined. Pour the batter into the prepared pan.

3. **MAKE THE CINNAMON SWIRL:** In a small bowl, combine the maple syrup, oat milk, tahini, cinnamon, and salt. Stir well with a spoon.

4. Pour the mixture into the cake batter. Use a spoon to swirl it through the batter. Place the pan in a 5.3-quart air-fryer basket and bake at 310°F for 30 minutes, or until a toothpick inserted into the center of the cake comes out clean. Carefully remove the pan from the basket and let cool for 10 minutes before serving.

NOTE: If you do not have an air fryer, you can bake the cake in a conventional 350°F oven for 35 minutes.

SERVES 6

FOR THE CINNAMON BUN CAKE
Cooking oil spray
½ cup oat flour
½ cup superfine almond flour
½ cup Oat Milk (page 288) or other milk
¼ cup cassava flour
¼ cup sugar-free applesauce
¼ cup 100 percent pure maple syrup
1 tablespoon flax meal
1½ teaspoons pure vanilla extract
1 teaspoon baking powder
½ teaspoon apple cider vinegar
¼ teaspoon baking soda
¼ teaspoon fine sea salt

FOR THE CINNAMON SWIRL
2 tablespoons 100 percent pure maple syrup
1 tablespoon Oat Milk (page 288) or other milk
1 teaspoon Homemade Tahini (page 329) or store-bought
1 teaspoon ground cinnamon
⅛ teaspoon fine sea salt

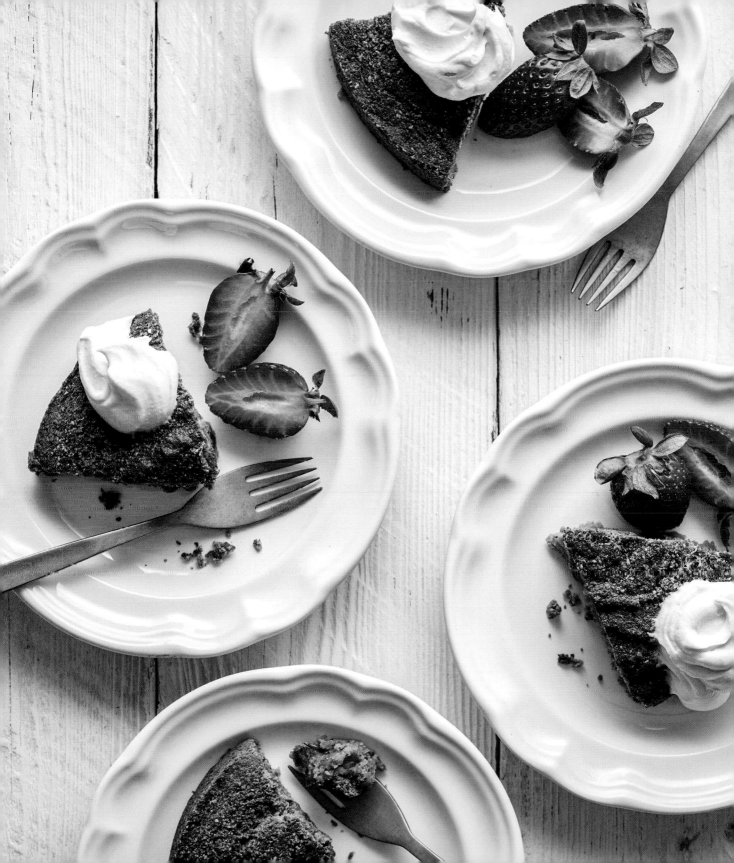

CHOCOLATE PECAN COOKIES

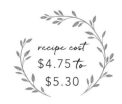

recipe cost
$4.75 to
$5.30

I love finding new ways to make delicious treats in a more healthful way! These cookies are dairy, grain, and refined-sugar free. The best part is you'd never know they were made without cane sugar! Make sure to pack your almond flour tightly into the cup, like you would brown sugar.

MAKES 16 COOKIES

½ cup extra-virgin olive oil

⅓ cup raw honey

1 large egg

1 teaspoon pure vanilla extract

1 cup tightly packed almond flour

¼ cup cassava flour

¼ cup coconut flour

¼ cup coconut sugar

2 teaspoons ground cinnamon

¾ teaspoon baking powder

½ teaspoon baking soda

½ teaspoon fine sea salt

½ cup dairy-free chocolate chips

¼ cup chopped raw pecans

¼ cup unsweetened coconut flakes

1. Preheat the oven to 350°F. Line a large baking sheet with parchment paper (see Note).

2. In a food processor, combine the olive oil, honey, egg, and vanilla. Process until well combined, 10 to 15 seconds. Add the almond flour, cassava flour, coconut flour, coconut sugar, cinnamon, baking powder, baking soda, and salt. Process for another 10 to 15 seconds. Stir in the chocolate chips, pecans, and coconut flakes.

3. Using a 1½-tablespoon cookie scoop, portion the dough onto the prepared baking sheet, arranging the cookies about ½ inch apart. Bake for 10 to 12 minutes, or until the cookies are very lightly browned.

4. Let cool for 10 minutes on the baking sheet before transferring to a wire rack to cool completely.

NOTE: Dark baking sheets will give you a dark color on the bottom of the cookies. I recommend using a light-colored or stainless steel baking sheet.

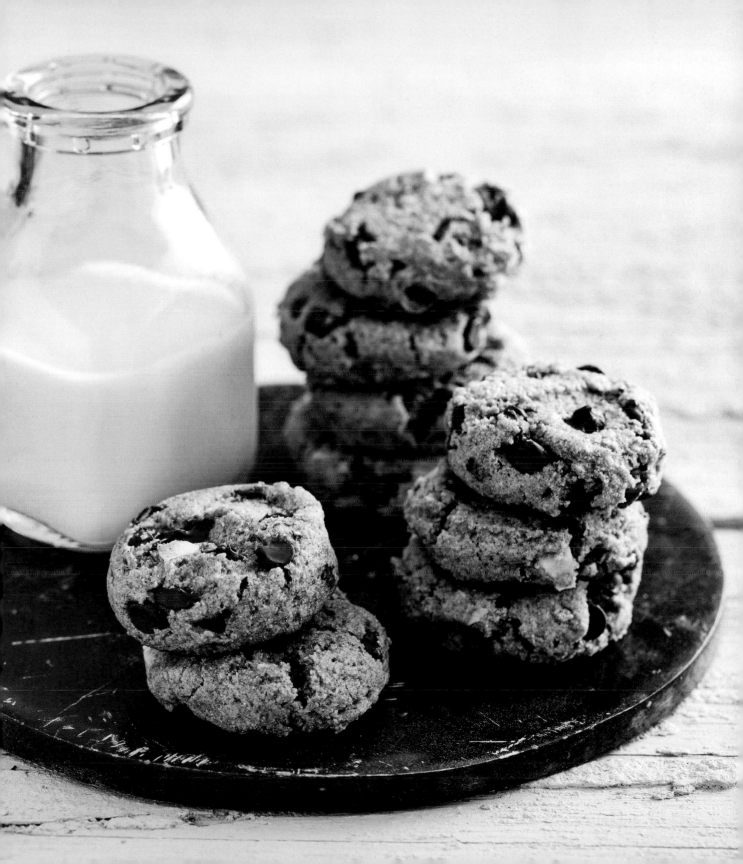

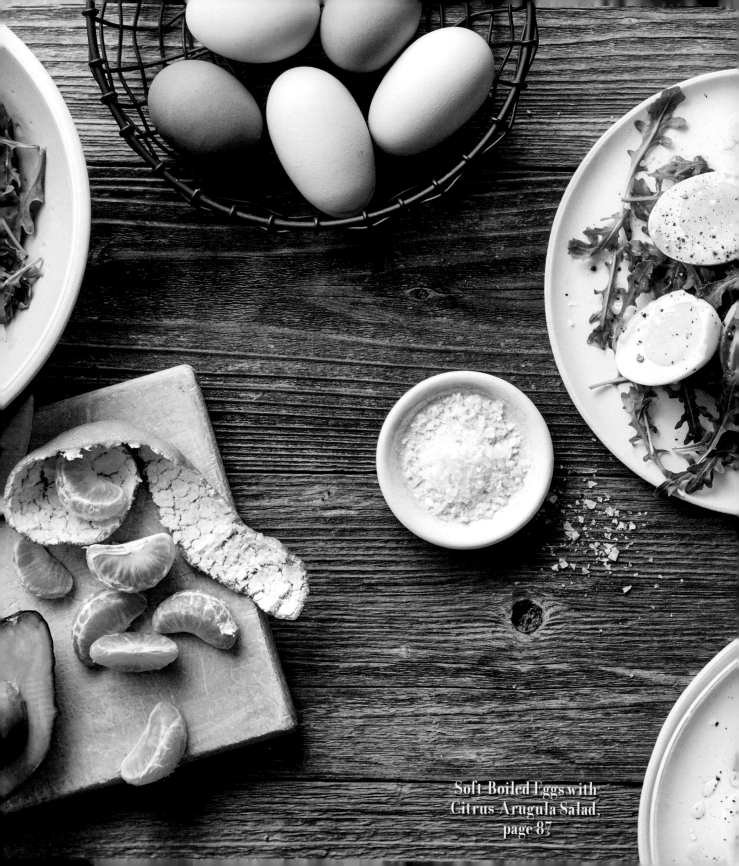

Soft-Boiled Eggs with
Citrus-Arugula Salad,
page 87

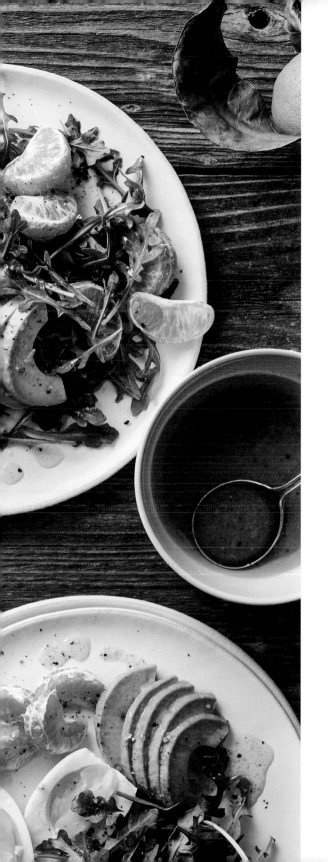

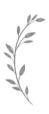 # BREAKFAST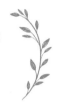

SMOOTHIE BOWL PARFAITS

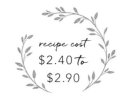

recipe cost
$2.40 *to*
$2.90

These light little parfaits are a nontraditional take on a healthy breakfast staple. Instead of using a dairy yogurt base, I created a plant-based smoothie substitute that tastes just like the real thing! I prefer not to make these ahead of time and find they taste best when served right away.

SERVES 2

1 cup frozen riced cauliflower
½ cup frozen blueberries
½ cup coconut water
6 small frozen strawberries
½ ripe banana, peeled
3 tablespoons hemp hearts
1 cup Super-Simple Granola (page 323)
2 teaspoons coconut flakes

1. In a high-powered blender, combine the cauliflower, blueberries, coconut water, strawberries, banana, and hemp hearts. Blend on high until smooth, about 30 seconds.

2. In each of two medium bowls, place ¼ cup Super-Simple Granola and ½ teaspoon coconut flakes. Divide the berry mixture between the bowls. Sprinkle the tops with the remaining ½ cup Super-Simple Granola and 1 teaspoon coconut flakes. Serve immediately.

VEGGIE-LOVER'S QUICHE

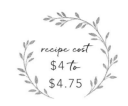

recipe cost
$4 to
$4.75

This is one of those great base recipes where the sky is the limit. Don't have broccoli? Use asparagus! No spinach? Use kale! Don't like tomatoes? Leave them out! I tell people all the time that you don't work for this lifestyle, you make it work for you. That's part of making this sustainable. Make this recipe at the beginning of the week and you will have breakfast all week long. If you have beautiful fresh herbs on hand that need using, like basil, thyme, oregano, chives, cilantro, or parsley, feel free to add what you have or sprinkle them on top at the end!

SERVES 4 TO 6

Cooking oil spray

5 large eggs

2 tablespoons extra-virgin olive oil

½ cup arrowroot powder

½ cup almond flour

½ teaspoon fine sea salt

¼ cup water

¼ teaspoon baking powder

¼ teaspoon onion powder

¼ teaspoon dried thyme

⅛ teaspoon chipotle chili powder

⅛ teaspoon ground black pepper

1½ cups baby spinach

1 cup roughly chopped broccoli

½ small Roma tomato, cored and diced

1. Spray a 6-cup baking dish that fits inside an electric pressure cooker or a 7-inch round oven-safe dish with cooking oil spray.

2. Separate the yolk from the white of one of the eggs.

3. In a food processor, combine the egg white, olive oil, arrowroot powder, almond flour, and ¼ teaspoon of the salt. Process on high until the mixture turns into a crumbly dough, about 15 seconds.

4. Press the dough firmly into the bottom and up the sides of the prepared dish.

5. In a large bowl, vigorously whisk the remaining egg yolk, 4 eggs, water, baking powder, onion powder, thyme, chipotle powder, remaining ¼ teaspoon salt, and black pepper until light and frothy. Stir in the spinach, broccoli, and tomato. Pour the egg mixture into the pie crust. Cover with foil and set on a trivet.

6. Pour 1 cup water into the cooker and carefully lower the trivet and dish into it.

(recipe continues)

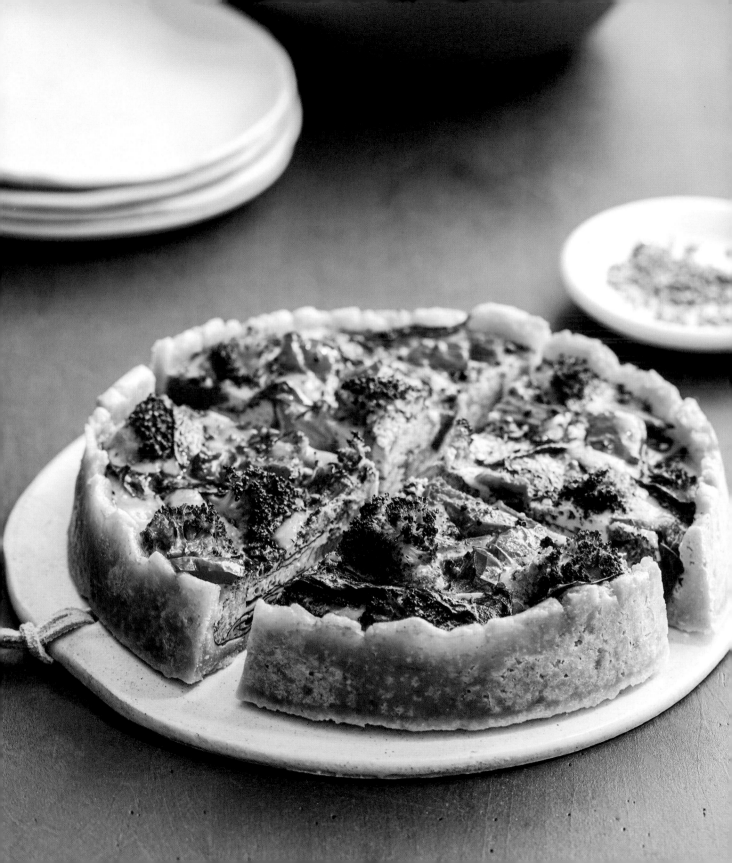

7. Place the lid on the cooker and make sure the vent valve is in the SEALING position. Using the display panel, select the MANUAL/PRESSURE COOK function and HIGH PRESSURE. Use the +/− buttons until the display reads 30 minutes.

8. When the cooker beeps, let it naturally release the pressure until the display reads LO:10. Switch the vent valve from the SEALING to the VENTING position. Use caution while the steam escapes.

9. Remove the quiche from the cooker and discard the foil. Let stand for 5 minutes before serving.

SCRAMBLED EGGS *with* ROASTED ASPARAGUS TOAST

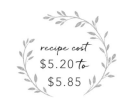

recipe cost $5.20 *to* $5.85

This is an excellent way to start your morning! The perfect mixture of energizing carbohydrates and protein—this is a toast to remember! If your asparagus is skinny like a pencil, it will only take 5 to 6 minutes to cook. If it's very thick, it'll require closer to 10 minutes.

SERVES 4

- 1 bunch asparagus, trimmed and cut into thirds
- 1 tablespoon extra-virgin olive oil
- ¾ teaspoon fine sea salt
- ½ teaspoon ground black pepper
- ¼ teaspoon garlic powder
- 4 large eggs
- 2 tablespoons Oat Milk (page 288) or other milk
- 4 slices whole-grain bread or Oat Bread (page 65), toasted
- 1 tablespoon sliced green onion

1. Place the asparagus in a large bowl and drizzle with 1½ teaspoons of the olive oil. Sprinkle with ½ teaspoon of the salt, ¼ teaspoon of the black pepper, and garlic powder and toss to coat.

2. Place the asparagus in a 5.3-quart air-fryer basket and bake at 370°F for 10 minutes.

3. While the asparagus cooks, heat a nonstick pan over medium heat.

4. In a large bowl, whisk together the eggs, oat milk, remaining ¼ teaspoon salt, and remaining ¼ teaspoon black pepper.

5. Add the remaining 1½ teaspoons olive oil to the preheated pan. Pour in the egg mixture and cook, stirring continuously, until the eggs are scrambled and fluffy, 2 to 3 minutes.

6. Place a piece of toasted bread on each of four plates. Top with eggs, asparagus, and green onion.

NOTE: If you do not have an air fryer, you can roast the asparagus in a conventional oven at 400°F for 15 to 20 minutes.

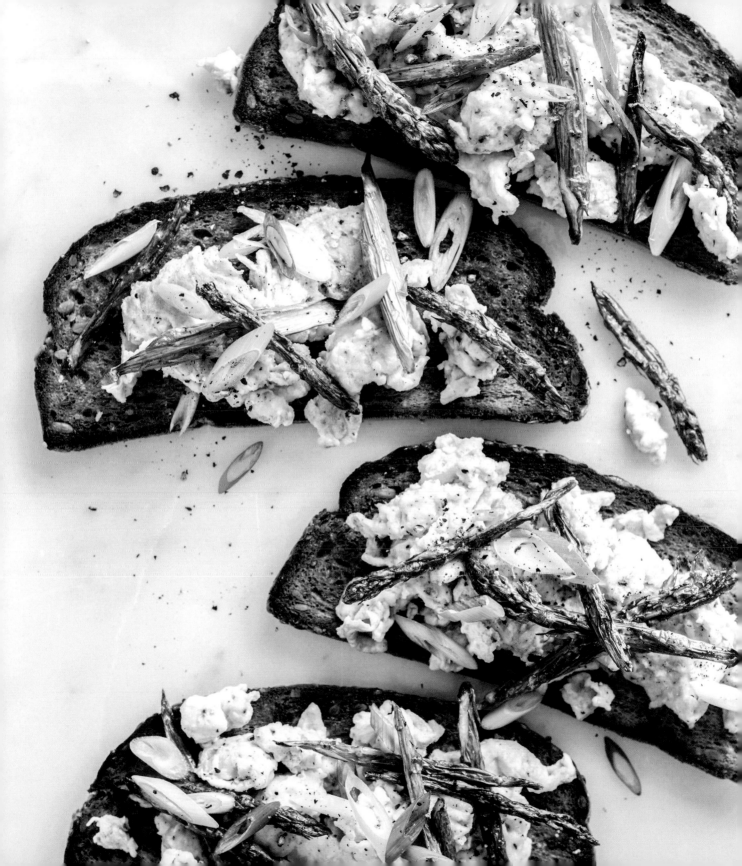

BAKED GRAPEFRUIT *with* HONEYED YOGURT *and* GRANOLA SPRINKLE

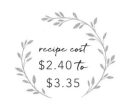

recipe cost
$2.40 *to*
$3.35

Grapefruit is an amazing food to eat for breakfast for its hydrating, filling, and immunity-boosting antioxidants! It also has a beneficial effect on blood sugar and insulin levels. This recipe takes the super-healthy grapefruit and makes it a true indulgence. It's a fresh and delicious way to start the day.

SERVES 4

2 large grapefruits

2 tablespoons coconut sugar

⅛ teaspoon ground ginger

⅛ teaspoon ground cinnamon, plus more for sprinkling

⅛ teaspoon fine sea salt

2 cups Oat Milk Yogurt (page 84) or favorite plain yogurt

2 tablespoons raw honey

1 cup Super-Simple Granola (page 323)

1. Slice ¼ inch off of the top and bottom of each grapefruit (this will help them to sit flat and not roll around), then cut them in half. Carefully run a small sharp knife between the flesh and the peel of the grapefruits, then cut between the natural segment breaks. Place the grapefruits in a 5.3-quart air-fryer basket.

2. In a small bowl, combine the coconut sugar, ginger, cinnamon, and salt. Sprinkle the grapefruit with the sugar mixture and bake at 400°F for 7 minutes.

3. In a large bowl, combine the yogurt and honey.

4. Using tongs, carefully remove each grapefruit half. Place one half on each of four plates. Top each grapefruit with ½ cup yogurt and sprinkle with ¼ cup granola.

NOTE: If you do not have an air fryer, the grapefruits can be broiled in a conventional oven for 7 to 10 minutes.

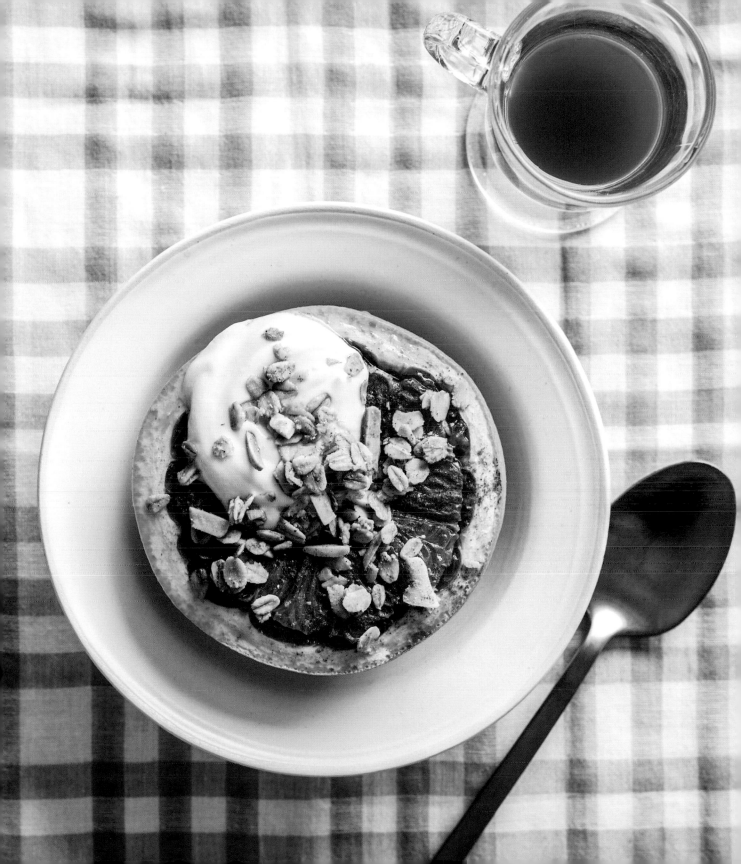

OAT MILK YOGURT

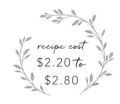

recipe cost
$2.20 *to*
$2.80

I love making plant-based yogurts, not just for eating but for using in other recipes. I made coconut milk yogurt for a long time, but the cost adds up! This Oat Milk Yogurt is a thick, Greek-style yogurt. I highly recommend using your sweetener of choice in it or blending it up with some berries before serving, as it isn't naturally sweet. It's absolutely fantastic for using in recipes (the Mini Everything Bagels on page 62, particularly!) I use Zint brand gelatin, one of the more cost-effective brands, and Renew Life Ultimate Flora Probiotic capsules.

MAKES 6 CUPS

- 1 cup gluten-free old-fashioned rolled oats
- 2 probiotic capsules, powder reserved, capsule discarded
- ¼ cup gelatin powder
- 4 pitted Medjool dates or 2 tablespoons raw honey
- 4 cups water

1. In a blender, combine the oats, probiotic powder, gelatin, dates, and water. Blend on high until the mixture is completely smooth, about 60 seconds. Pour the mixture into an electric pressure cooker. (You can strain the mixture through a nut milk bag or a fine-mesh strainer to get rid of any remaining sediment, if you like, but it's not necessary.)

2. Place the lid on the cooker and make sure the vent valve is in the VENTING position. Using the display panel, select the YOGURT function. Use the +/− buttons until the display reads 12 hours.

3. When the cooker beeps, remove the lid and pour the contents back into the blender. (The mixture will have thickened a little but will still be very runny.) Blend on high for 15 seconds to eliminate any separation. Transfer the yogurt to a large container with a lid.

4. Chill for 8 hours before serving to allow the yogurt to thicken.

5. Store in the refrigerator for up to 1 week.

CINNAMON APPLE GRANOLA PARFAITS

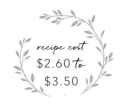

recipe cost
$2.60 *to*
$3.50

I love parfaits for breakfast—it's just an extra-special (and fancy!) way to begin the day. I also enjoy them as an afternoon snack or an after-dinner dessert. This one has a special bit of extra flair and is reminiscent of an apple crumble.

SERVES 4

4 apples, cored and sliced

1 tablespoon 100 percent pure maple syrup

1½ teaspoons ground cinnamon

1 cup water

2 cups Oat Milk Yogurt (page 84) or favorite plain yogurt

1½ tablespoons raw honey

⅛ teaspoon ground nutmeg

1 cup Super-Simple Granola (page 323)

1. In a 7-inch round heatproof dish that fits inside an electric pressure cooker, combine the apples, maple syrup, and cinnamon. Cover with foil and set on a trivet.

2. Pour the water into the cooker and carefully lower the trivet and dish into the cooker.

3. Place the lid on the pressure cooker and make sure the vent valve is in the SEALING position. Using the display panel, select the MANUAL/PRESSURE COOK function and LOW PRESSURE. Use the +/− buttons until the display reads 2 minutes.

4. When the cooker beeps, switch the vent valve from the SEALING to the VENTING position. Use caution while the steam escapes.

5. In a small bowl, combine the yogurt, honey, and nutmeg. Divide half of the yogurt mixture among 4 cups. Divide half of the apples among the cups, followed by half of the granola. Repeat with remaining apples, yogurt mixture, and granola. Serve immediately.

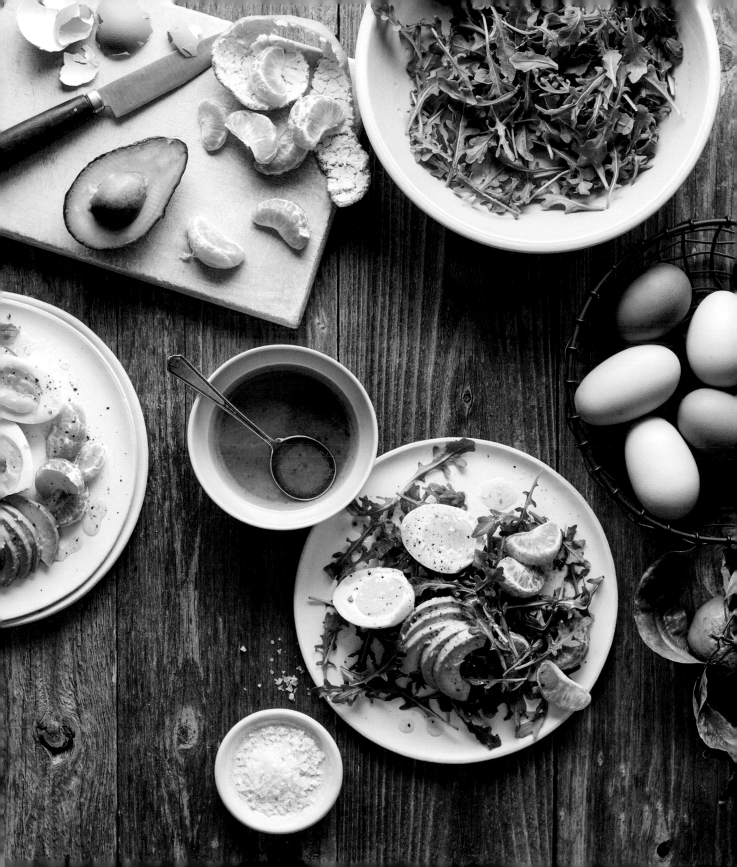

SOFT-BOILED EGGS *with* CITRUS-ARUGULA SALAD *and* LEMON-TURMERIC DRESSING

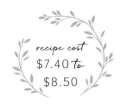

During my photography trip for *Instant Loss: Eat Real, Lose Weight*, the entire team would eat breakfast together every morning. I really hadn't enjoyed soft-boiled eggs until that point, but with the addition of some arugula, citrus, and a store-bought turmeric dressing, I was pleased to find myself having them for breakfast almost every morning for two weeks! Try this delicious homemade version and you can enjoy them yourself.

SERVES 4

FOR THE SOFT-BOILED EGGS

1 cup water

8 large eggs (see Note)

FOR THE CITRUS-ARUGULA SALAD

5 ounces arugula

2 mandarin oranges, peeled and sectioned

1 large avocado, pitted, peeled, and sliced

FOR THE LEMON-TURMERIC DRESSING

¼ cup avocado oil

¼ cup water

1 tablespoon fresh lemon juice

½ teaspoon garlic powder

Fine sea salt

¼ teaspoon onion powder

¼ teaspoon ground turmeric

Ground black pepper

1. **MAKE THE EGGS:** Pour the water into an electric pressure cooker and place a trivet inside. Carefully set the eggs on the trivet.

2. Place the lid on the cooker and make sure the vent valve is in the SEALING position. Using the display panel, select the MANUAL/PRESSURE COOK function and LOW PRESSURE. Use the +/− buttons until the display reads 3 minutes.

3. While the eggs cook, prepare an ice bath to place them in when they're finished cooking.

4. **MAKE THE SALAD:** Evenly divide the arugula among four plates. Top with mandarin oranges and avocado slices.

5. **MAKE THE DRESSING:** In a wide-mouth jar, combine the avocado oil, water, lemon juice, garlic powder, ½ teaspoon salt, onion powder, turmeric, and ⅛ teaspoon black pepper. Screw the lid on tightly and shake vigorously.

6. When the cooker beeps, switch the vent valve from the SEALING to the VENTING position, administering a quick release. Use caution while the steam escapes.

(recipe continues)

7. Using tongs, carefully remove the eggs from the cooker and plunge them into the ice bath. Let chill for 5 minutes.

8. Peel the eggs and carefully cut each in half. Place four egg halves on each plate. Sprinkle with salt and black pepper to taste. Drizzle with dressing and serve.

NOTE: If your eggs are extra-large, they'll require 1 more minute in the pressure cooker.

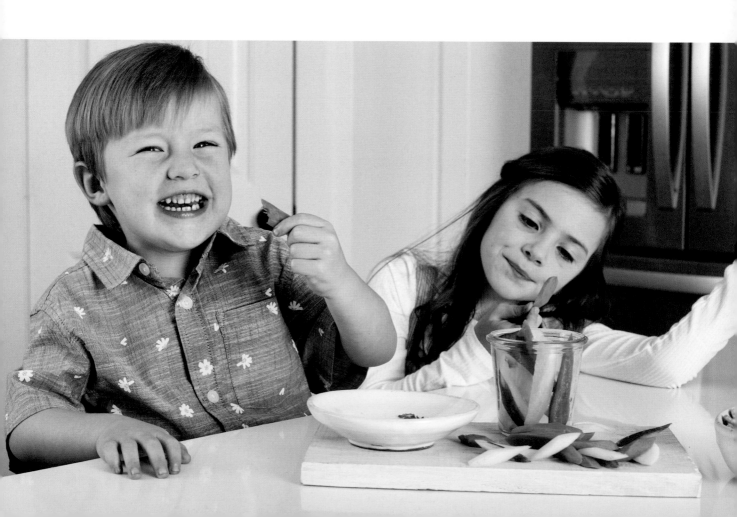

CAPRESE FRITTATA

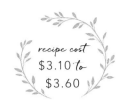

recipe cost
$3.10 *to*
$3.60

A frittata is an easy breakfast or brunch meal that jazzes up the ordinary. It keeps well in an airtight container in the refrigerator and reheats nicely. I like to spritz mine with a bit of water and cover with a paper towel before reheating to preserve the moisture.

SERVES 4 TO 6

1 tablespoon extra-virgin olive oil

1 medium red potato, cut into ¼-inch pieces

½ medium yellow onion, diced

7 large eggs

¼ cup water

¾ teaspoon onion powder

¾ teaspoon garlic powder

¾ teaspoon dried basil

¾ teaspoon dried oregano

½ teaspoon fine sea salt

½ teaspoon ground black pepper

Cooking oil spray

¾ cup halved cherry tomatoes

2 tablespoons balsamic vinegar

2 tablespoons chopped fresh basil (optional)

1. Preheat an electric pressure cooker using the SAUTÉ function and adjust the heat to MORE (see Note page 95). When the display reads HOT, add the olive oil, potato, and onion. Cook, stirring occasionally, until the onion softens and becomes translucent and the potato is tender, about 5 minutes.

2. In a high-powered blender, combine the eggs, water, onion powder, garlic powder, dried basil, oregano, salt, and black pepper. Blend on high until frothy, about 30 seconds. (If you do not have a blender, you can whisk the mixture in a large bowl.)

3. Spray a 7-inch round baking dish with cooking oil spray.

4. Layer the potato mixture and ½ cup of the cherry tomatoes on the bottom of the dish. Pour the egg mixture on top. Cover the pan with foil and set on a trivet.

5. Pour 1 cup water into the cooker and carefully lower the trivet and dish into the cooker.

6. Place the lid on the cooker and make sure the vent valve is in the SEALING position. Using the display panel, select the MANUAL/PRESSURE COOK function and HIGH PRESSURE. Use the +/− buttons until the display reads 30 minutes.

(recipe continues)

7. In a small bowl, toss the remaining ¼ cup cherry tomatoes with the vinegar.

8. When the cooker beeps, switch the vent valve from the SEALING to the VENTING position, administering a quick release. Use caution while the steam escapes.

9. Remove the frittata from the cooker and top with the cherry tomato mixture. Sprinkle with fresh basil, if desired, and serve.

COOKER TIP: You do not have to clean your cooker liner in between sautéing and baking the frittata. The water will steam the inner liner while the frittata bakes so all you have to do is rinse it out at the end!

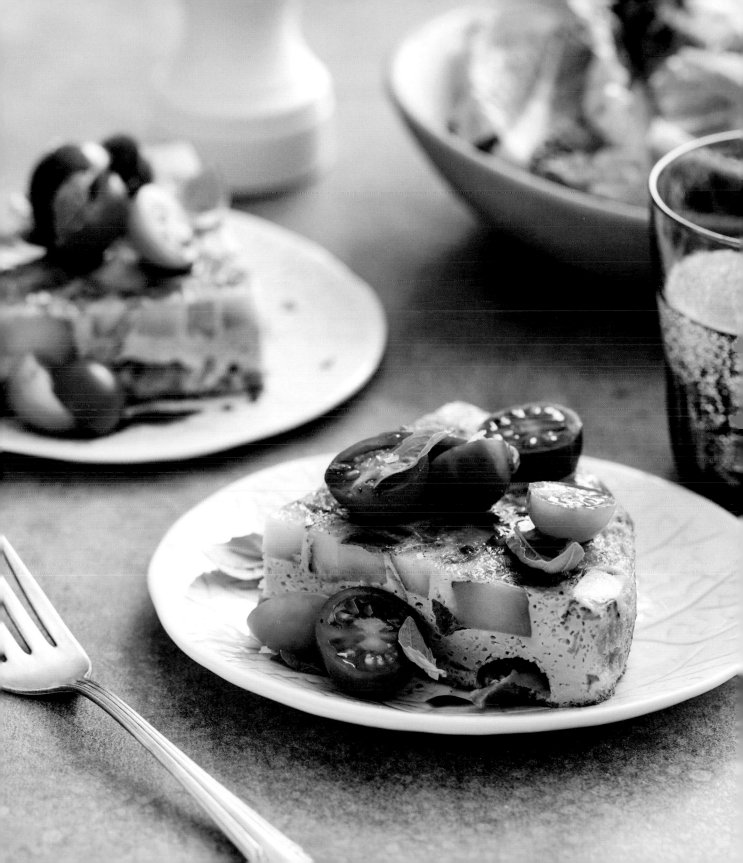

PLANTAIN PANCAKES *with* CARAMEL SAUCE

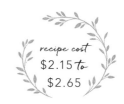

recipe cost
$2.15 *to* $2.65

I have several pancake recipes, but this one is my favorites. These are magic pancakes! Make them and I promise you're going to be amazed. Plantains are like a sister to a banana, oftentimes referred to as a "cooking banana." They are larger and a little more starchy, which makes them an optimal base with the perfect hint of sweetness.

SERVES 4

2 large ripe plantains, peeled
4 large eggs
2 teaspoons pure vanilla extract
½ teaspoon baking soda
¼ teaspoon fine sea salt
Cooking oil spray
Caramel Sauce (page 306)

1. Preheat an electric griddle to 350°F or heat a large skillet over medium heat.

2. In a high-powered blender, combine the plantains, eggs, vanilla, baking soda, and salt. Blend on high until a smooth batter forms, about 30 seconds.

3. Once the griddle is hot, spray with cooking oil spray. Using a ¼-cup measuring cup, spoon batter for each pancake onto the griddle. (Cook in batches if necessary. You will get about 14 small pancakes.)

4. Cook until the bottoms are lightly golden, 1 to 2 minutes. Flip and cook the other side for 1 minute. Transfer the pancakes to a plate and keep warm in a 200°F oven until all pancakes are cooked.

5. Serve with Caramel Sauce.

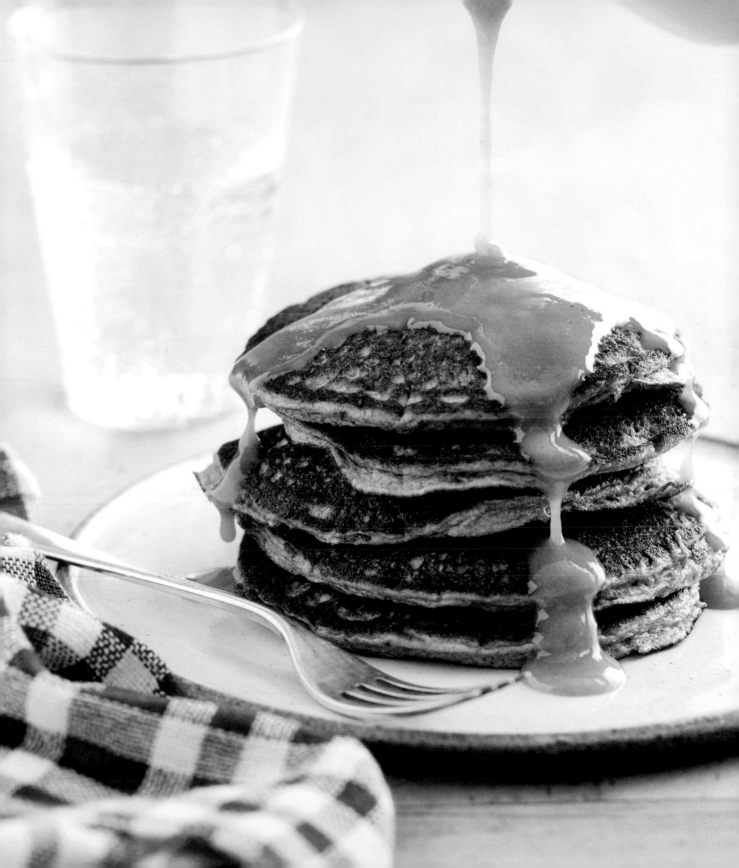

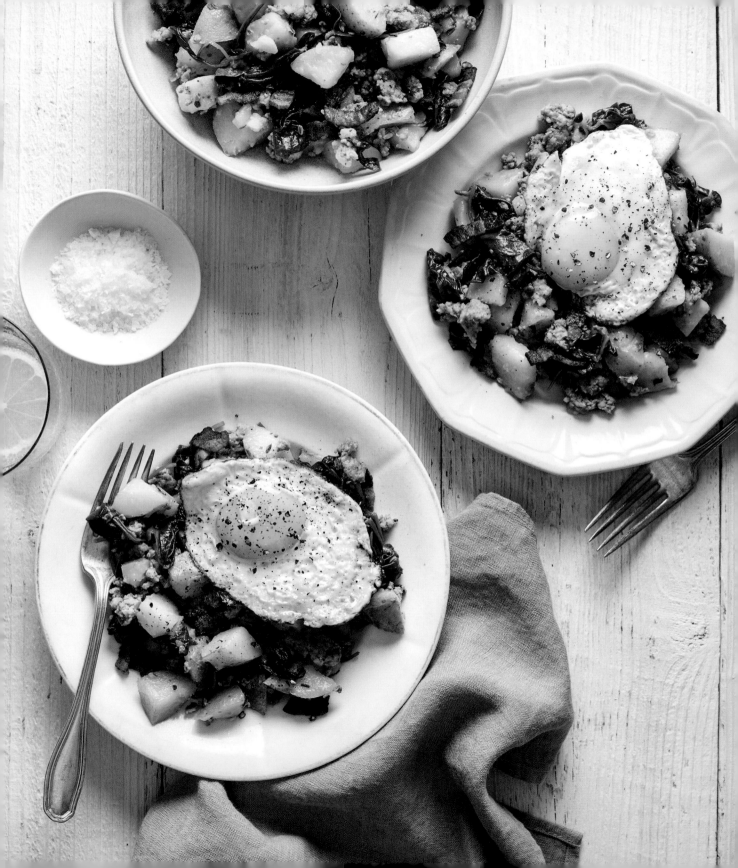

BREAKFAST HASH

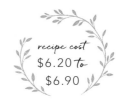

This is such a hearty breakfast. I enjoy it by itself, but my husband loves it with an egg on top or as the filling for his breakfast burrito.

SERVES 4

1 pound pork sausage or ground turkey

4 strips nitrate-free bacon, thinly sliced

1 tablespoon extra-virgin olive oil (optional)

4 cups packed baby spinach

1 teaspoon fine sea salt

½ teaspoon ground black pepper

½ teaspoon garlic powder

½ teaspoon dried parsley flakes

½ teaspoon dried basil

¼ teaspoon dried oregano

¼ teaspoon red pepper flakes (optional)

⅓ cup Vegetable Broth (page 332) or store-bought

10 ounces gold potatoes, cut into 1-inch cubes

1. Preheat an electric pressure cooker using the SAUTÉ function and adjust the heat to MORE (see Note). When the display reads HOT, add the sausage and bacon. (If using turkey in place of sausage, add the olive oil.) Cook, stirring occasionally, for about 5 minutes. Add the spinach, salt, black pepper, garlic powder, parsley, basil, oregano, and red pepper flakes (if using). Stir well and continue cooking until the sausage is browned, about 5 minutes.

2. Carefully remove the sausage mixture from the cooker and transfer to a large bowl.

3. Pour the broth into the cooker and scrape up any browned bits. Add the potatoes. Place the lid on the cooker and make sure the vent valve is in the SEALING position. Using the display panel, press the CANCEL button to turn off the SAUTÉ function, then select the MANUAL/PRESSURE COOK function and LOW PRESSURE. Use the +/− buttons until the display reads 6 minutes.

4. When the cooker beeps, switch the vent valve from the SEALING to the VENTING position, administering a quick release. Use caution while the steam escapes.

5. Add the potatoes to the sausage mixture, toss, and serve.

NOTE: Your cooker might not have an ADJUST button; if that is the case, just press the SAUTÉ button until MORE is highlighted.

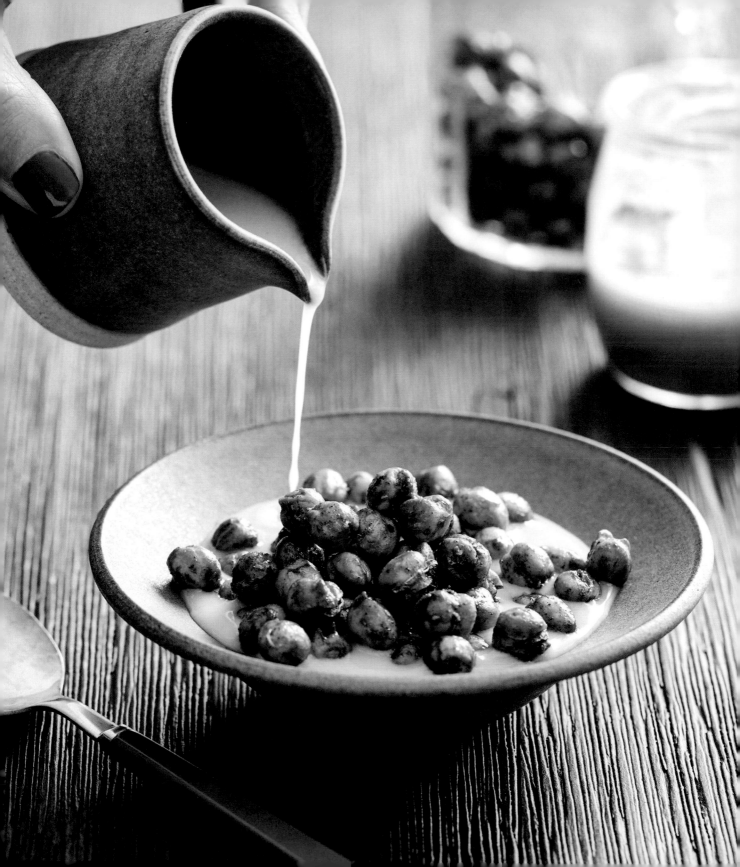

CINNAMON TOAST CEREAL

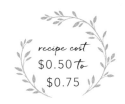

recipe cost
$0.50 to
$0.75

We stopped buying cereal a while back upon discovering that most cereal has been fortified or enriched with folic acid, which is a big "no" for my family. (You can read more about that on InstantLoss.com.) My kids still enjoy it, though, so I set out to develop a cheap and tasty cereal for them. This is such a yummy little number. Make it once and if you enjoy it, I highly recommend tripling the recipe, as it keeps in the pantry for quite a while!

SERVES 2

1 cup canned chickpeas, rinsed and drained

1 tablespoon raw honey, plus more for drizzling

1 teaspoon extra-virgin olive oil

½ teaspoon ground cinnamon, plus more for sprinkling

¼ teaspoon fine sea salt

½ cup Oat Milk (page 288) or other milk

1. Place the chickpeas in a 5.3-quart air-fryer basket and bake at 400°F for 10 minutes.

2. Transfer the chickpeas to a medium bowl. Add the honey, olive oil, cinnamon, and salt. Stir well to coat.

3. Transfer the chickpeas back to the air-fryer basket and bake at 300°F for 10 minutes.

4. Let cool completely.

5. To serve, divide the chickpeas between two medium bowls. Top with oat milk, a drizzle of honey, and a sprinkle of cinnamon. Serve immediately.

6. Store in an airtight container in the pantry for up to 1 month.

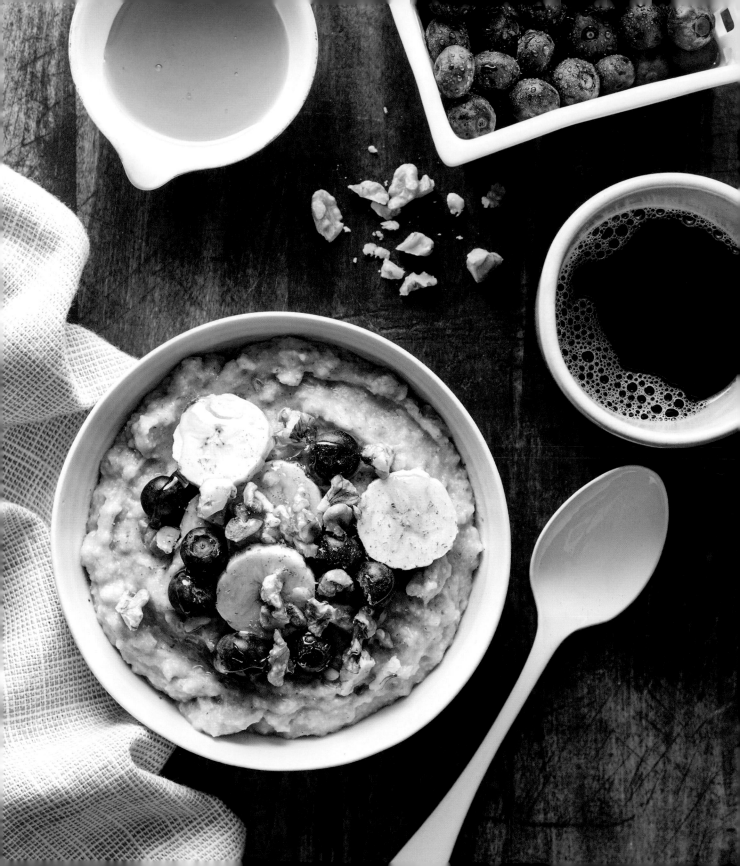

BLUEBERRY-BANANA CREAM *of* OAT

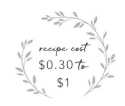

I highly recommend that everyone make their own oat flour at home. It's so much more cost-effective than purchasing it in the grocery store. Simply take 1 cup of gluten free old fashioned rolled oats and blend on high in a high-powered blender until smooth. If you would rather have more of an oatmeal than a cream of oat, you can swap out the oat flour for rolled oats 1:1.

SERVES 2

1 cup oat flour

1 tablespoon raw honey, plus more for drizzling

½ teaspoon ground cinnamon, plus more for sprinkling

⅛ teaspoon fine sea salt

2 cups water

½ medium ripe banana, peeled and sliced

½ cup blueberries (optional)

2 tablespoons chopped raw walnuts (optional)

1. In an electric pressure cooker, combine the flour, honey, cinnamon, salt, and water. Stir well to combine.

2. Place the lid on the cooker and make sure the vent valve is in the SEALING position. Using the display panel, select the MANUAL/PRESSURE COOK function and HIGH PRESSURE. Use the +/− buttons until the display reads 8 minutes.

3. When the cooker beeps, switch the vent valve from the SEALING to the VENTING position, administering a quick release. Use caution while the steam escapes.

4. Divide the oatmeal between two bowls. Top with banana, a drizzle of honey, and a sprinkle of cinnamon. If desired, add blueberries and walnuts.

FRENCH TOAST RICE PORRIDGE

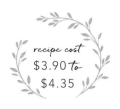

recipe cost
$3.90 to
$4.35

Adults and children alike will love this dish! It's reminiscent of arroz con leche, Mexican rice pudding. My mom used to make something similar with leftover white rice for dessert, but this is just a little healthier! Add sliced strawberries for a nice burst of freshness.

SERVES 6

1½ cups canned full-fat coconut milk or other milk (see page 288)

1 cup water

½ cup brown rice

¼ cup 100 percent pure maple syrup

1 large egg, beaten

¼ teaspoon fine sea salt

¼ teaspoon ground cinnamon, plus more for sprinkling

1. In an electric pressure cooker, combine the coconut milk, water, rice, maple syrup, egg, salt, and cinnamon.

2. Place the lid on the cooker and make sure the vent valve is in the SEALING position. Using the display panel, select the MANUAL/PRESSURE COOK function and HIGH PRESSURE. Use the +/− buttons until the display reads 46 minutes. (Yes, this a long cook time, but it takes that long for the rice to get tender.)

3. When the cooker beeps, let it naturally release the pressure until the display reads LO:05. Switch the vent valve from the SEALING to the VENTING position. Use caution while the steam escapes.

4. Transfer the rice to a large bowl and cover. Chill for a minimum of 3 hours before serving. Serve with a sprinkle of cinnamon.

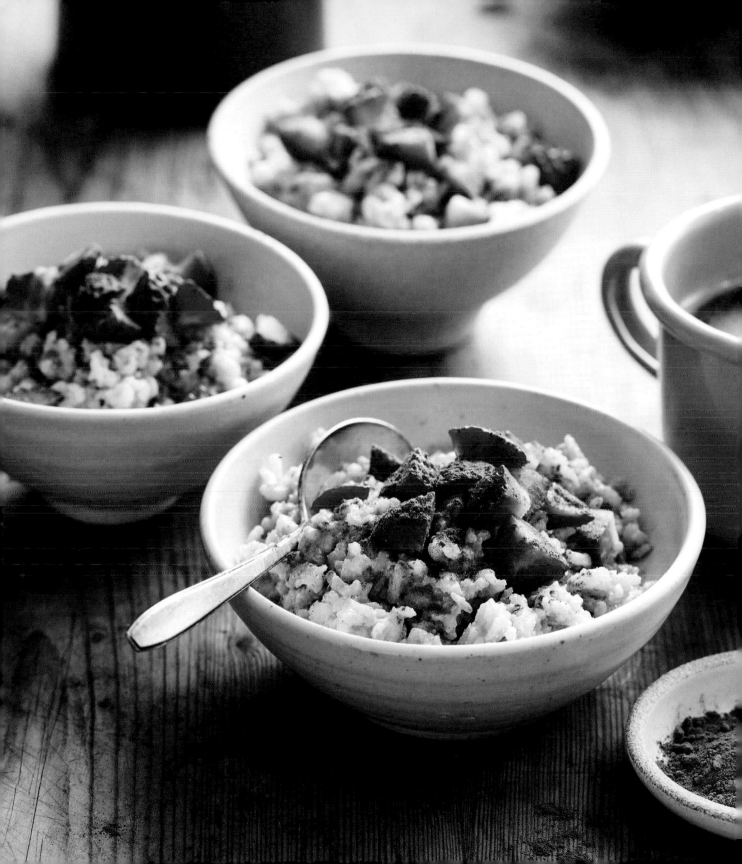

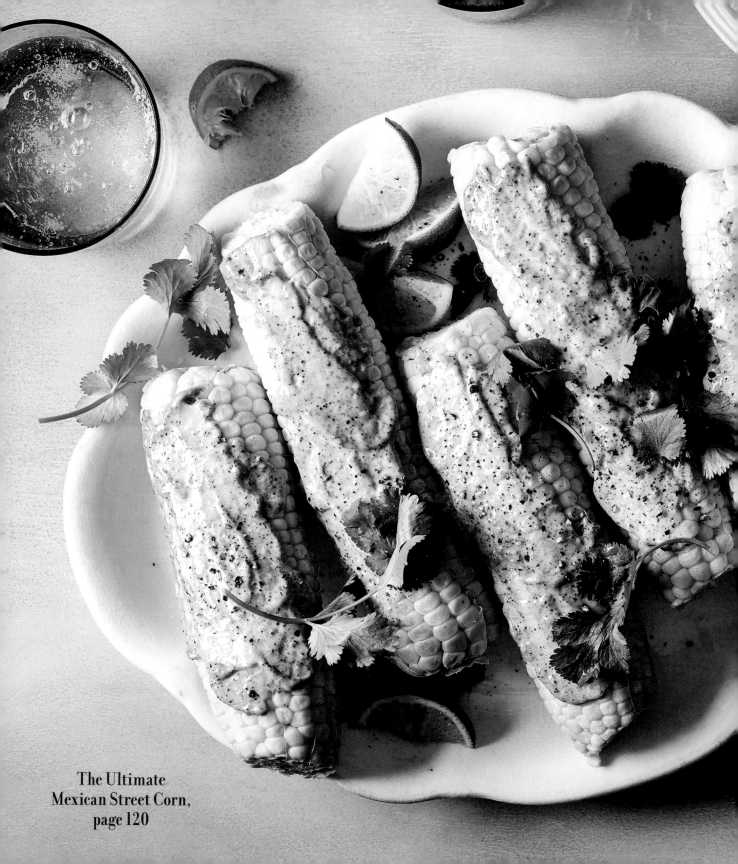

The Ultimate
Mexican Street Corn,
page 120

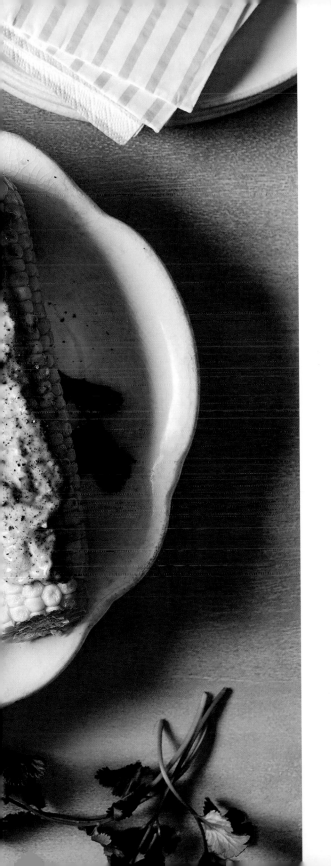

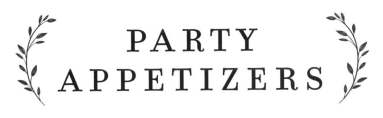

PARTY APPETIZERS

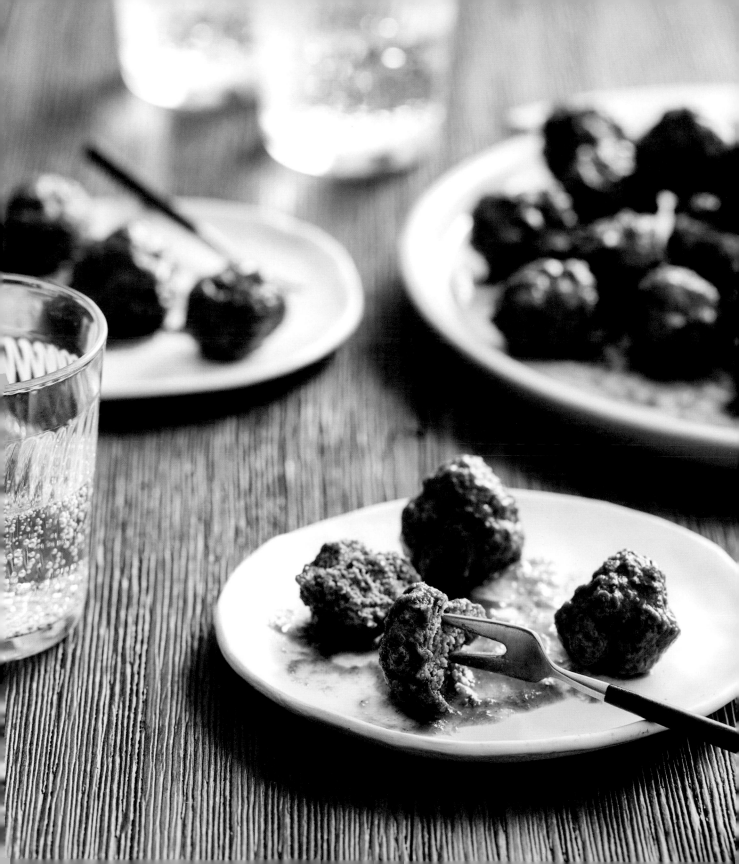

COCKTAIL MEATBALLS

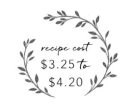

recipe cost
$3.25 to
$4.20

A lot of store-bought barbecue sauce contains high-fructose corn syrup, artificial sweeteners, and thickeners, so I stopped buying it a few years ago. It's so easy to whip it up at home, and it's just delicious in this easy party recipe!

SERVES 4 TO 6

1 pound lean (80/20) ground beef

2 teaspoons garlic powder

1 teaspoon fine sea salt

½ teaspoon ground black pepper

1½ cups Tangy Barbecue Sauce (page 324)

1. Roll the ground beef into ½-inch balls. Arrange the meatballs in the bottom of an electric pressure cooker in a single layer. (It's okay for them to touch.)

2. Sprinkle the meatballs with the garlic powder, salt, and black pepper. Pour the barbecue sauce over the meatballs.

3. Place the lid on the cooker and make sure the vent valve is in the SEALING position. Using the display panel, select the MANUAL/PRESSURE COOK function and HIGH PRESSURE. Use the +/− buttons until the display reads 4 minutes.

4. When the cooker beeps, switch the vent valve from the SEALING to the VENTING position, administering a quick release. Use caution while the steam escapes.

5. Serve hot.

POPPIN' JALAPEÑO POPPERS *with* CILANTRO-LIME AIOLI

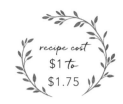

recipe cost $1 *to* $1.75

Dairy-free jalapeño poppers? Y'all. Y'all. Y'all! These are revolutionary. Oftentimes when something is vegan, we use the disclaimer, "Well, for a vegan dish this is pretty good." No. For any dish, this one is pretty freaking spectacular. High in protein, healthy fats, and with just the right amount of spice, this is an appetizer you can proudly serve, and you don't even have to tell anyone it's healthy!

MAKES 12 POPPERS

FOR THE JALAPEÑO POPPERS
¼ cup raw cashews
¼ cup water
1 tablespoon canned green chiles
1½ teaspoons nutritional yeast
2 teaspoons Taco Seasoning (page 325)
½ teaspoon fine sea salt
6 medium jalapeños, halved lengthwise and seeded
1 tablespoon crushed tortilla chips

FOR THE CILANTRO-LIME AIOLI
1 tablespoon Homemade Mayo (page 330) or store-bought
1 teaspoon roughly chopped fresh cilantro, plus more for sprinkling (optional)
½ teaspoon fresh lime juice

1. **MAKE THE POPPERS:** Place the cashews, water, chiles, nutritional yeast, taco seasoning, and salt in a small high-powered blender container. Blend on high until the mixture warms and thickens, 3 to 5 minutes. (If your blender is unable to warm the mixture, transfer to a small saucepan and heat over medium-high heat until the mixture thickens, about 1 minute.)

2. Carefully spoon the mixture into the jalapeño halves and top with the crushed tortilla chips. Arrange the stuffed jalapeño halves in a 5.3-quart air-fryer basket and bake at 380°F for 10 minutes.

3. **MAKE THE AIOLI:** While the jalapeños cook, in a small bowl, combine the mayonnaise, cilantro, and lime juice. Stir well to combine. Transfer the mixture to a plastic sandwich bag and push it down into one corner.

4. When the air fryer beeps, use tongs to transfer the jalapeños from the basket to a plate. Cut a ¼-inch hole corner in the corner of the bag and pipe the aioli onto the peppers. Sprinkle with additional with cilantro, if desired.

NOTE: If you do not have an air fryer, the jalapeños can be baked in a conventional oven at 400°F for 15 minutes.

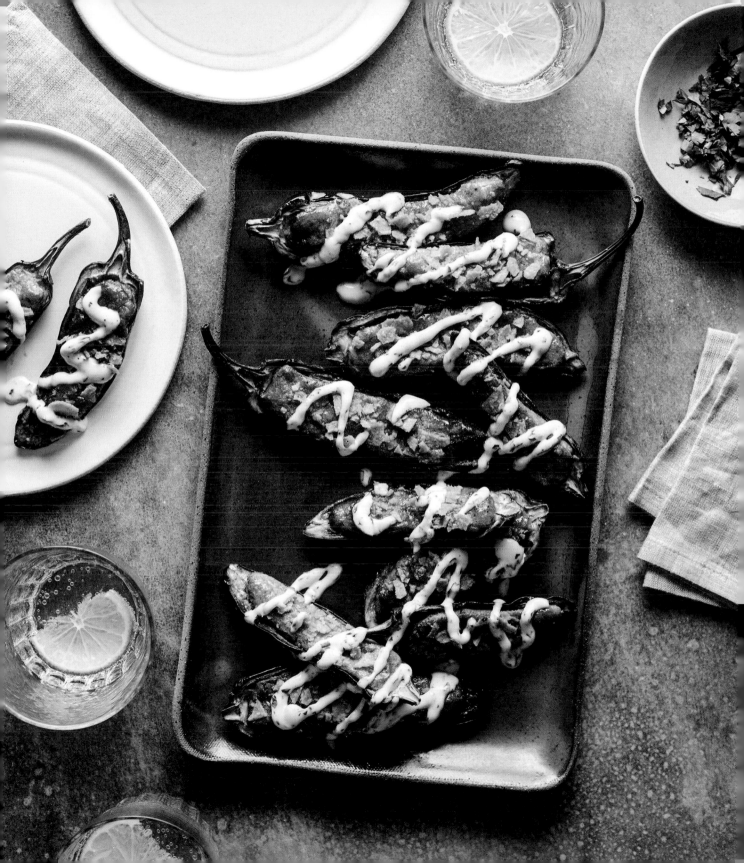

SPICY BUFFALO CAULIFLOWER *with* CREAMY RANCH DRESSING

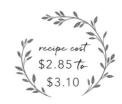

Cassava flour is made out of yucca root. It has become more popular, but at times can still be difficult to source in a traditional grocery store, especially if you live in a rural area. Look for Anthony's or Otto's brand on Amazon or Thrive Market for a great price! It's worth sourcing some to make this spicy buffalo cauliflower—all the flavor of your favorite wings, but without the bad-for-you ingredients!

SERVES 4

1 cup water

1 large head cauliflower, cored and cut into florets

½ cup sriracha

⅓ cup Oat Milk (page 288) or other milk

2 tablespoons extra-virgin olive oil

2 tablespoons raw honey

¼ cup cassava flour

1½ teaspoons fine sea salt

½ teaspoon garlic powder

Creamy Ranch Dressing (page 110)

4 stalks of celery, cut into 3-inch pieces

1. Pour the water into an electric pressure cooker and place a trivet inside. Set the cauliflower on the trivet.

2. Place the lid on the cooker and make sure the vent valve is in the SEALING position. Using the display panel, select the STEAM function and HIGH PRESSURE. Use the +/− buttons until the display reads 1 minute.

3. In a large bowl, combine the sriracha, oat milk, olive oil, and honey. Stir well to combine. Add the flour, salt, and garlic powder and stir well.

4. When the cooker beeps, switch the vent valve from the SEALING to the VENTING position, administering a quick release. Use caution while the steam escapes.

5. Preheat the broiler on high. Carefully transfer the cauliflower from the cooker to the bowl and toss to coat. Place the cauliflower on a baking sheet and broil until the sauce thickens and the cauliflower crisps, about 5 minutes.

6. Serve the cauliflower with Creamy Ranch Dressing and celery sticks.

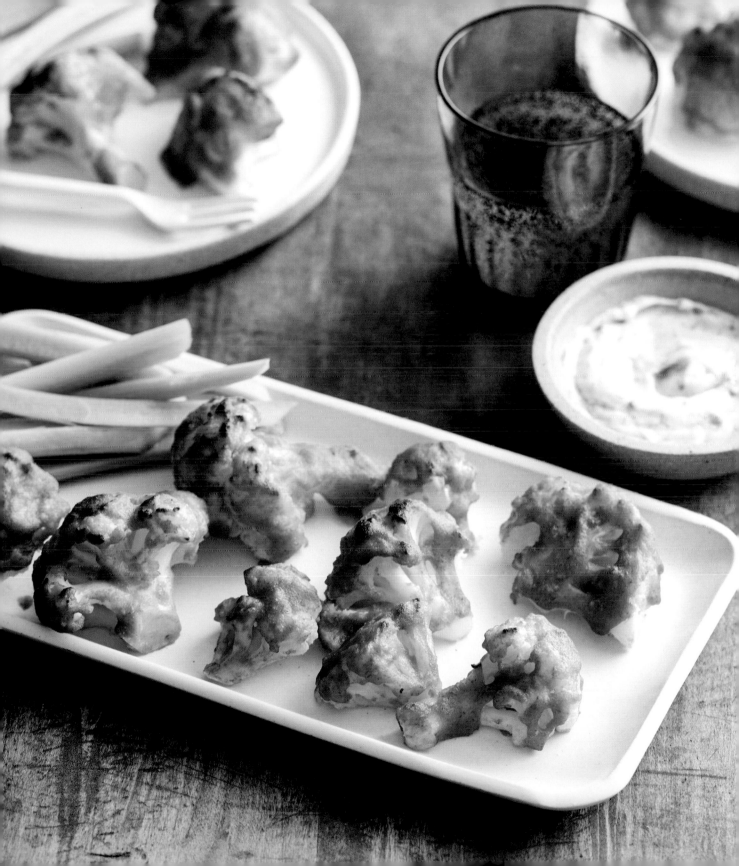

CREAMY RANCH DRESSING

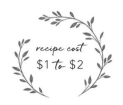

recipe cost
$1 to $2

Ranch lovers, this one's for you. This recipe has all the flavor of the original with none of the processed junk. If you do not have an immersion blender, you can stir the ingredients together in a bowl. I like to blend them because sometimes spices can be gritty—blending ensures they smooth out. But it still tastes great if you mix it by hand!

MAKES ¾ CUP

¾ cup Homemade Mayo (page 330) or store-bought
1 teaspoon apple cider vinegar
1 teaspoon dried parsley flakes
½ teaspoon garlic powder
½ teaspoon onion powder
½ teaspoon dried dill (optional)
¼ teaspoon fine sea salt

In a wide-mouth jar, combine the mayonnaise, vinegar, parsley, garlic powder, onion powder, dill (if using), and salt. Blend until smooth with an immersion blender.

Store in an airtight container in the refrigerator for up to 1 week.

CAJUN POPCORN SHRIMP

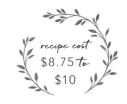

recipe cost
$8.75 *to*
$10

Take it to the next level and serve these tasty shrimp with lemon wedges and parsley for added freshness! I highly recommend using my homemade Cajun Seasoning; store-bought seasonings can have added sugar and a lot more salt.

SERVES 4

¾ cup cassava flour

1 tablespoon plus 1 teaspoon Cajun Seasoning (page 328) or store-bought (see Note)

½ teaspoon fine sea salt

½ teaspoon ground black pepper

1 large egg

4½ teaspoons water

1 pound shrimp (36/40 count), peeled and deveined

Cooking oil spray (see Note)

1. In a shallow bowl, combine the flour, the 1 tablespoon Cajun seasoning, salt, and black pepper. Stir well to combine.

2. In a second bowl, whisk the egg, water, and the 1 teaspoon Cajun seasoning.

3. Working in batches, add a few shrimp to the flour and toss to coat. Shake off any excess flour and add to the bowl with the egg mixture. Coat the shrimp on all sides with egg, then transfer back to the bowl with the flour. Using a dry hand, roll the shrimp around until thoroughly coated, then set on a large plate. Repeat until all of the shrimp have been coated.

4. Coat the bottom of the air-fryer basket with cooking oil spray. Place half of the shrimp in the basket and spray the tops with cooking oil spray. (Do not skip this step, as this is what makes the shrimp crispy.) Bake at 370°F for 8 minutes, or until golden, flipping the shrimp halfway through the cooking time. Repeat for the second batch (see Note).

5. Serve warm.

NOTE: If you use a store-bought seasoning, you may need to reduce the salt in the recipe.

NOTE: If you do not have cooking oil spray, use a silicone brush to brush oil on the shrimp.

NOTE: You can bake the shrimp in a conventional oven. Preheat the oven to 350°F and set a metal cooling rack on a rimmed baking sheet. Arrange all of the coated shrimp on the rack and coat with cooking oil spray. Bake for 12 minutes or until golden, flipping the shrimp and coating with more cooking oil spray halfway through the cooking time.

SHREDDED BEEF TAQUITOS

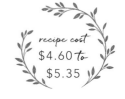

recipe cost
$4.60 to
$5.35

I love to serve taquitos over a bed of lettuce, topped with tomatoes or pico de gallo. You can use the same method for rolling taquitos with any filling—chicken, rice and beans, or even leftover taco soup!

SERVES 4

1½ teaspoons extra-virgin olive oil

8 ounces beef stew meat

1 tablespoon Taco Seasoning (page 325)

½ teaspoon ground black pepper

¼ cup low-sodium beef broth or Bone Broth (page 331)

¼ cup extra-virgin coconut oil, plus more if needed

8 to 10 corn tortillas

1 medium head romaine lettuce, shredded

1 Roma tomato, cored and diced

½ cup No-Queso Queso (page 121)

1. Preheat an electric pressure cooker using the SAUTÉ function and adjust the heat to MORE (see Note page 95). When the display panel reads HOT, add the olive oil, stew meat, taco seasoning, and black pepper. Cook, stirring occasionally, until the meat is lightly browned on all sides. Add the broth.

2. Place the lid on the cooker and make sure the vent valve is in the SEALING position. Using the display panel, select the MANUAL/PRESSURE COOK function and HIGH PRESSURE. Use the +/− buttons until the display reads 35 minutes.

3. When the cooker beeps, let it naturally release the pressure until the display reads LO:10. Switch the vent valve from the SEALING to the VENTING position. Use caution while the steam escapes.

4. Remove the lid and shred the beef into the juices using two forks.

5. Heat a 10-inch pan over medium-high heat. Add the coconut oil and let it warm. Working quickly, use tongs to place one tortilla in the oil, flip it immediately, then place it on a paper towel–lined plate. Repeat until and the tortillas are warmed, stacking each tortilla on top of the one before.

6. Place a generous tablespoon of the shredded beef on each tortilla and gently roll up. Arrange a few of the rolled tortillas in the pan and cook for 2 to 3 minutes on each side, or until browned and crisp. Repeat with remaining rolled tortillas, adding more oil if necessary.

7. Place the finished taquitos back on the paper towel–lined plate to absorb any excess oil.

8. Serve each taquito with shredded lettuce, tomatoes, and a drizzle of No-Queso Queso.

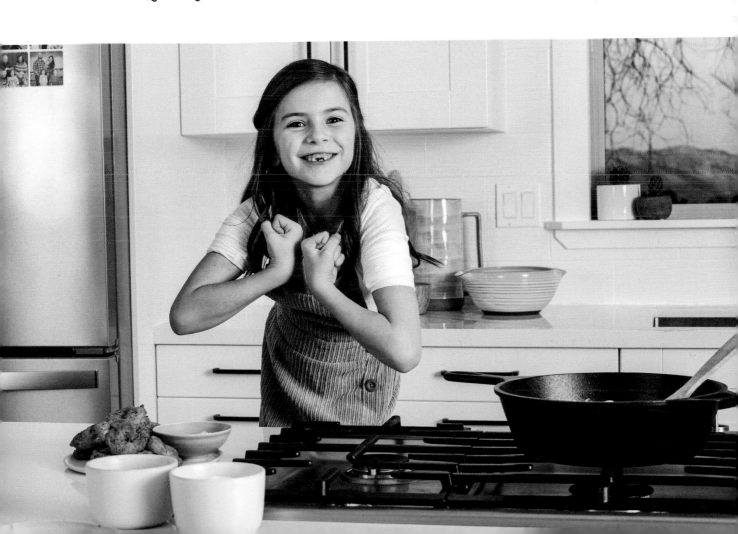

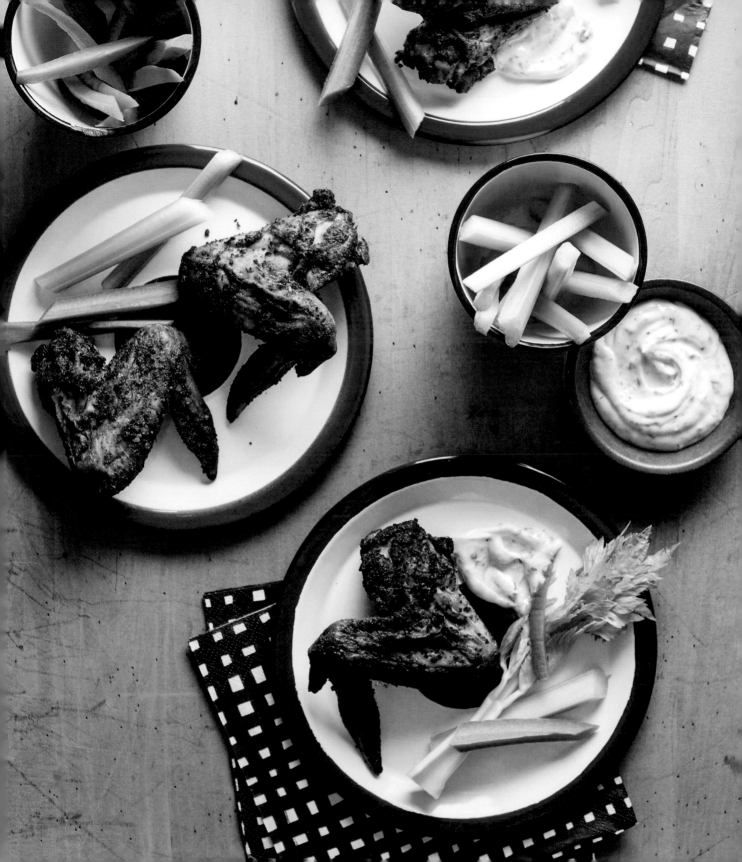

DRY-RUBBED CHILI CHICKEN WINGS

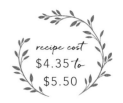

recipe cost
$4.35 to
$5.50

The benefit of cooking with your air fryer is that less oil is required. However, these wings are a scientific marvel because they don't require any oil at all for cooking! I use a secret ingredient—baking powder—to mimic the crispiness you get from deep-frying chicken skin. Same great taste, less fat!

SERVES 4 TO 6

1 pound chicken wings

1 teaspoon baking powder

½ teaspoon cayenne pepper

½ teaspoon chili powder

¼ teaspoon garlic powder

½ teaspoon fine sea salt

¼ teaspoon ground black pepper

1 tablespoon ghee or extra-virgin olive oil

1 cup Creamy Ranch Dressing (page 110)

8 celery sticks

8 carrot sticks

1. Place the chicken wings in a large bowl and sprinkle with the baking powder, cayenne, chili powder, and garlic powder. Toss well, making sure the wings are evenly and thoroughly coated. Cover and transfer the bowl to the refrigerator. Chill for at least 1 hour or up to overnight.

2. Season the wings with the salt and pepper and place inside a 5.3-quart air-fryer basket, standing them upright. Bake at 400°F until cooked through and crispy, about 20 minutes.

3. Transfer the wings to a bowl and toss with the ghee.

4. Arrange the wings on a platter and serve with the ranch dressing, celery sticks, and carrot sticks.

SWEET HEAT CRUNCHY CHICKPEAS

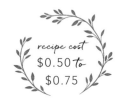

recipe cost
$0.50 to
$0.75

Did you ever eat corn nuts growing up? They were one of my favorite snacks in middle school. This is a much healthier version. They're great for parties or as a grain-free crouton for a salad!

MAKES 1 CUP

1 cup canned chickpeas, rinsed and drained

1 teaspoon extra-virgin olive oil

½ teaspoon coconut sugar

¼ teaspoon chili powder

¼ teaspoon fine sea salt

⅛ teaspoon ground black pepper

⅛ teaspoon smoked paprika

1. Place the chickpeas in a 5.3-quart air-fryer basket and bake at 310°F for 10 minutes.

2. While the chickpeas cook, in a small bowl, combine the olive oil, coconut sugar, chili powder, salt, black pepper, and paprika and stir well.

3. Transfer the chickpeas from the cooker to a second bowl. Drizzle the olive oil seasoning over the chickpeas and toss to coat. Place the chickpeas back inside the air-fryer basket and bake at 300°F for 10 minutes.

4. Let cool completely before serving.

5. Store in an airtight container for up to 3 weeks.

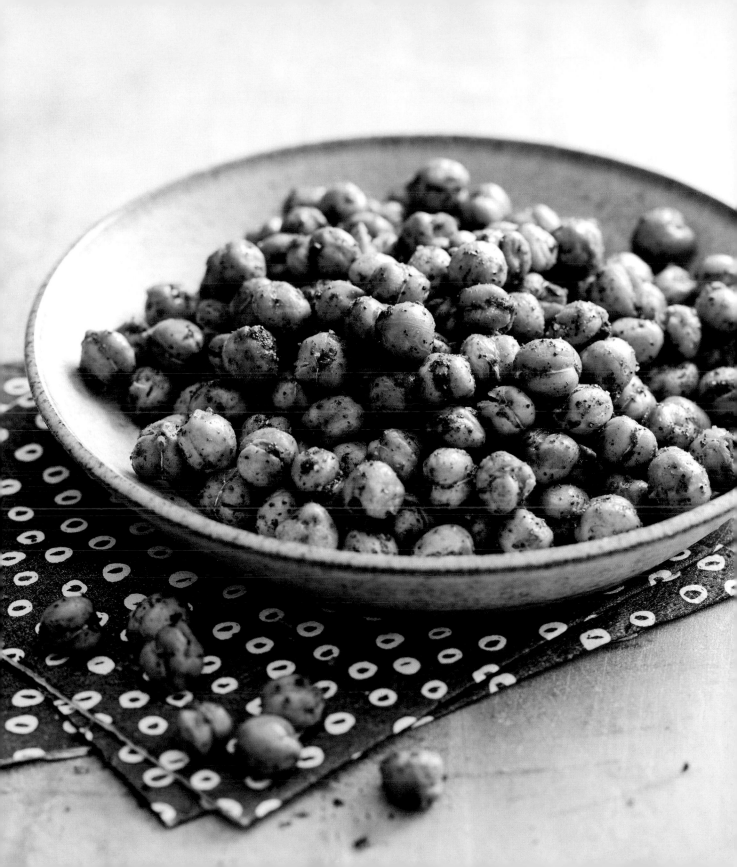

THE ULTIMATE MEXICAN STREET CORN

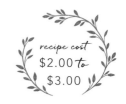

recipe cost
$2.00 *to*
$3.00

Holy moly! You truly haven't lived until you've tried this corn. Last year, I went 100 percent dairy-free after discovering I have a lactose allergy. Traditionally, this corn would be made with a white cheese, but believe me when I tell you that with all of this glorious seasoning, you will not miss the cheese one bit. If you're looking for a side dish to impress your neighbors, this is the one. You will be hailed a flavor genius!

SERVES 4

1 cup water

4 ears corn, husked

2 tablespoons Homemade Mayo (page 330) or store-bought

2 tablespoons fresh lime juice

1 teaspoon fine sea salt

½ teaspoon garlic powder

½ teaspoon chili powder

⅛ teaspoon cayenne pepper

2 tablespoons roughly chopped fresh cilantro

1. Pour the water into an electric pressure cooker and place a trivet inside. Set the corn on the trivet.

2. Place the lid on the cooker and make sure the vent valve is in the SEALING position. Use the display panel, select the MANUAL/PRESSURE COOK function and HIGH PRESSURE. Use the +/− buttons until the display reads 2 minutes.

3. While the corn is cooking, on a large plate, combine the mayonnaise, lime juice, salt, garlic powder, chili powder, cayenne. Blend thoroughly with a fork.

4. When the cooker beeps, switch the vent valve from the SEALING to the VENTING position, administering a quick release. Use caution while the steam escapes.

5. Carefully remove the corn from the pressure cooker and roll each cob in the mixture on the plate, coating evenly. Sprinkle with cilantro and serve immediately.

(This recipe is pictured on page 102.)

NO-QUESO QUESO

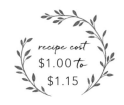

recipe cost
$1.00 to $1.15

When my family moved to Texas, we were introduced to queso—a party dip commonly made with Velveeta cheese and Ro*Tel canned tomatoes with green chilies. After going dairy-free, I decided to get creative and try my hand at making cheese-free queso, and I feel that even the biggest cheese lover will agree that it's pretty great!

MAKES 1 CUP

½ cup raw cashews or unsalted raw shelled sunflower seeds

½ cup sugar-free salsa

2 tablespoons water

1 tablespoon unfortified nutritional yeast

2 teaspoons Taco Seasoning (page 325)

¼ teaspoon fine sea salt

1. In a high-powered blender, combine the cashews, salsa, water, nutritional yeast, taco seasoning, and salt. Blend on high until well combined and the sauce has warmed and thickened, about 5 minutes.

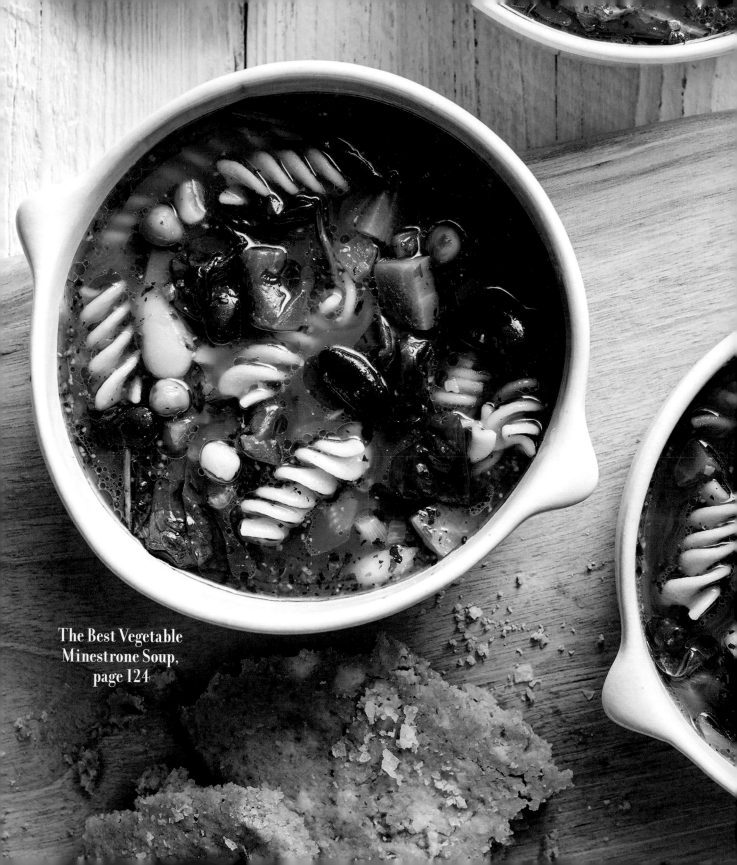

The Best Vegetable
Minestrone Soup,
page 124

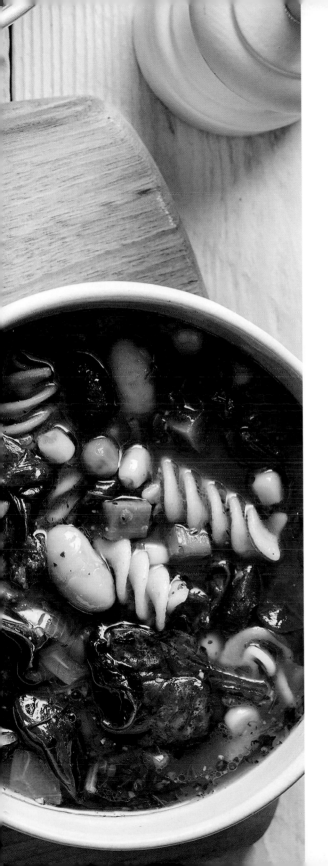

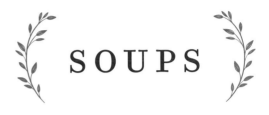

SOUPS

THE BEST VEGETABLE MINESTRONE SOUP

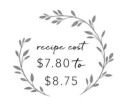

recipe cost
$7.80 *to*
$8.75

Y'all. This is absolutely, hands down, the best minestrone soup I have ever consumed, ever! I use Jovial gluten-free fusilli pasta, but you can use any pasta of your choosing.

SERVES 6

1 medium yellow onion, diced

4 stalks celery, chopped

2 cups frozen mixed vegetables

1 (15-ounce) can diced tomatoes

1 (15-ounce) can red kidney beans, rinsed and drained (see Note)

1 (15-ounce) can cannellini beans, rinsed and drained (see Note)

1 cup Vegetable Broth (page 332) or store-bought

1 cup gluten-free fusilli pasta

¼ cup chopped sun-dried tomatoes

2 tablespoons unfortified nutritional yeast

2 tablespoons tomato paste

2 tablespoons dried minced onion

1 tablespoon garlic powder

2½ teaspoons fine sea salt

2 teaspoons dried basil

2 teaspoons dried oregano

2 teaspoons dried parsley flakes

¼ teaspoon ground black pepper

4 cups water

4 cups baby spinach

1. Preheat an electric pressure cooker using the SAUTÉ function and adjust the heat to MORE (see Note page 95). When the display panel reads HOT, add the yellow onion and celery. Cook, stirring infrequently, until the onion softens and begins to become translucent, about 3 minutes.

2. Add the mixed vegetables, diced tomatoes, kidney beans, cannellini beans, broth, pasta, sun-dried tomatoes, nutritional yeast, tomato paste, dried onion, garlic powder, salt, basil, oregano, parsley, black pepper, and water.

3. Place the lid on the cooker and make sure the vent valve is in the SEALING position. Using the display panel, press the CANCEL button to turn off the SAUTÉ function, then select the MANUAL/PRESSURE COOK function and HIGH PRESSURE. Use the +/− buttons until the display reads 6 minutes.

4. When the cooker beeps, let it naturally release the pressure until the display reads LO:05. Switch the vent valve from the SEALING to the VENTING position. Use caution while the steam escapes.

5. Remove the lid and stir in the spinach.

NOTE: If you prefer to use dried beans in this recipe, simply substitute ½ cup dried beans for each 15-ounce can of beans. After sautéing the onion and the celery, add all of the ingredients to electric pressure cooker except for the pasta, frozen vegetables, and spinach. Select the BEAN/CHILI function on the cooker and HIGH PRESSURE, and cook for 45 minutes. When the cooker beeps, carefully release the pressure immediately, and add the pasta and frozen vegetables. Seal the lid again, select the MANUAL/HIGH PRESSURE function and cook for 6 minutes. Let the cooker naturally release the pressure for 5 minutes before releasing the pressure. Stir in the spinach and serve.

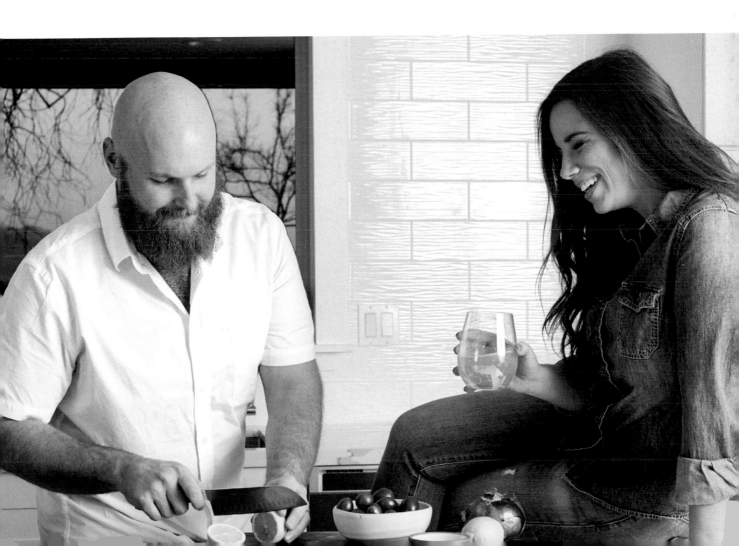

HERB *and* SPINACH LENTIL SOUP

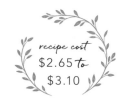

recipe cost
$2.65 *to*
$3.10

Why do some pressure-cooker recipes require a natural release while other call for a quick release? What's inside the cooker greatly dictates how long you need to let the pressure release. Generally, soups can be quick-released, but sometimes things can spit, leading to a mess. If you quick-release this soup, for instance, it will sputter because of the reaction between the lentils and tomato. To save you from red splatter on your cupboards, it's best to let the cooker naturally release the pressure for ten minutes before opening the vent valve.

SERVES 4

3 cups low-sodium beef broth or Bone Broth (page 331)

2 cups water

2 cups frozen chopped spinach

⅔ cup brown lentils

1 (6-ounce) can tomato paste

1 medium yellow onion, diced

1 large carrot, peeled and diced (see Note)

1 tablespoon dried parsley flakes

1 tablespoon red wine vinegar

1 teaspoon garlic powder

½ teaspoon dried thyme

½ teaspoon fine sea salt

¼ teaspoon dried dill weed

¼ teaspoon ground black pepper

1. In an electric pressure cooker, combine the broth, water, spinach, lentils, tomato paste, onion, carrot, parsley, vinegar, garlic powder, thyme, salt, dill weed, and black pepper and stir well.

2. Place the lid on the cooker and make sure the vent valve is in the SEALING position. Using the display panel, select the MANUAL/PRESSURE COOK function and HIGH PRESSURE. Use the +/− buttons until the display reads 15 minutes.

3. When the cooker beeps, let it naturally release the pressure until the display reads LO:10. Switch the vent valve from the SEALING to the VENTING position. Use caution while the steam escapes.

NOTE: If I use organic carrots, I do not peel them as there is a lot of nutrient value in the skin. I do wash them well to remove any dirt or debris. The peel of carrots treated with pesticides holds the majority of the chemical, so I do peel those.

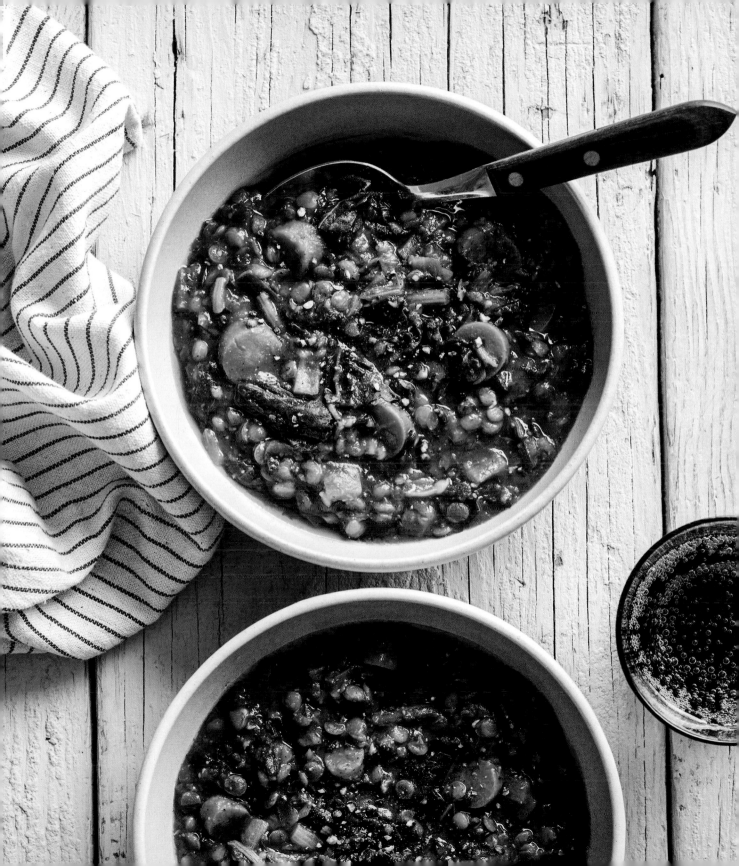

SUMMER VEGETABLE RATATOUILLE

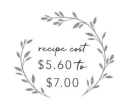

recipe cost
$5.60 to
$7.00

When the garden is bursting with fresh produce and your kitchen is overflowing, there is ratatouille—a delicious French dish whose name means "motley stew." It's packed full of flavor!

SERVES 6

1. In an electric pressure cooker, combine the chickpeas, tomatoes, rice, celery, carrots, kale, water, broth, olive oil, basil, oregano, dried onion, garlic powder, salt, and pepper and stir.

2. Place the lid on the cooker and make sure the vent valve is in the SEALING position. Using the display panel, select the MANUAL/PRESSURE COOK function and HIGH PRESSURE. Use the +/− buttons until the display reads 15 minutes.

3. When the cooker beeps, let it naturally release the pressure until the display reads LO:05. Switch the vent valve from the SEALING to the VENTING position. Use caution while the steam escapes.

4. Remove the lid and stir in the squash, zucchini, corn, and peas. Place the lid back on the cooker and allow the vegetables to cook in the residual heat until tender, about 5 minutes.

5. Serve warm with lemon wedges and fresh herbs, if desired.

- 2 cups canned chickpeas, rinsed and drained
- 1 (15-ounce) can diced tomatoes
- ½ cup cooked brown rice
- 4 stalks celery, diced
- 2 large carrots, peeled and chopped (see Note page 51)
- 1 cup chopped kale (ribs removed)
- 1 cup water
- 4 cups Vegetable Broth (page 332) or store-bought
- 1 tablespoon extra-virgin olive oil
- 2 teaspoons dried basil
- 2 teaspoons dried oregano
- 1 tablespoon dried minced onion
- 1 teaspoon garlic powder
- 2½ teaspoons fine sea salt
- ½ teaspoon ground black pepper
- 1 medium yellow squash, sliced
- 1 medium zucchini, sliced
- 2 cups frozen yellow corn
- 1 cup frozen peas
- Lemon wedges
- Fresh herbs such as parsley, basil, tarragon, and/or dill (optional)

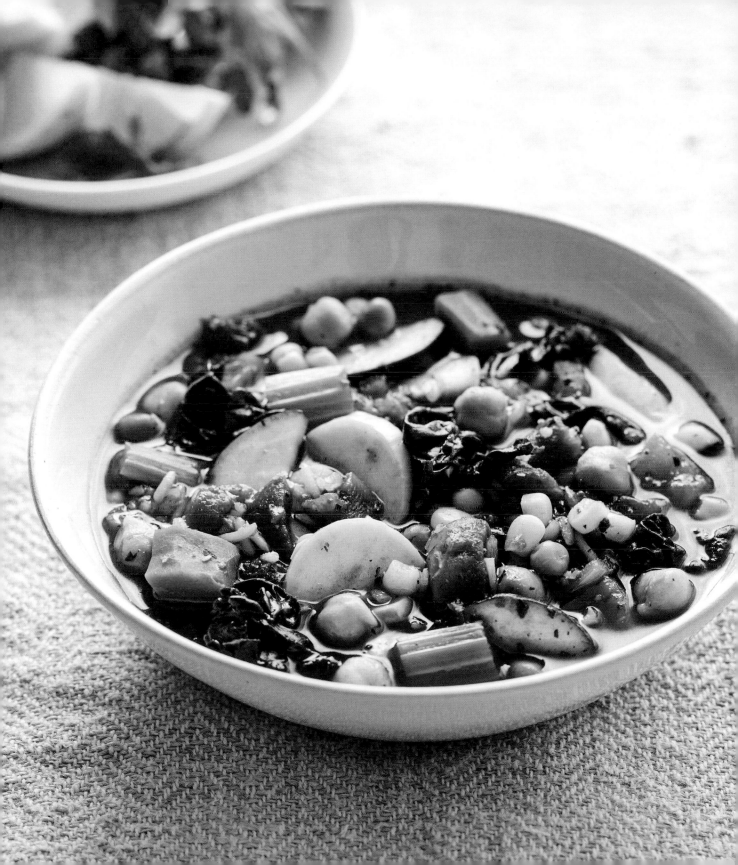

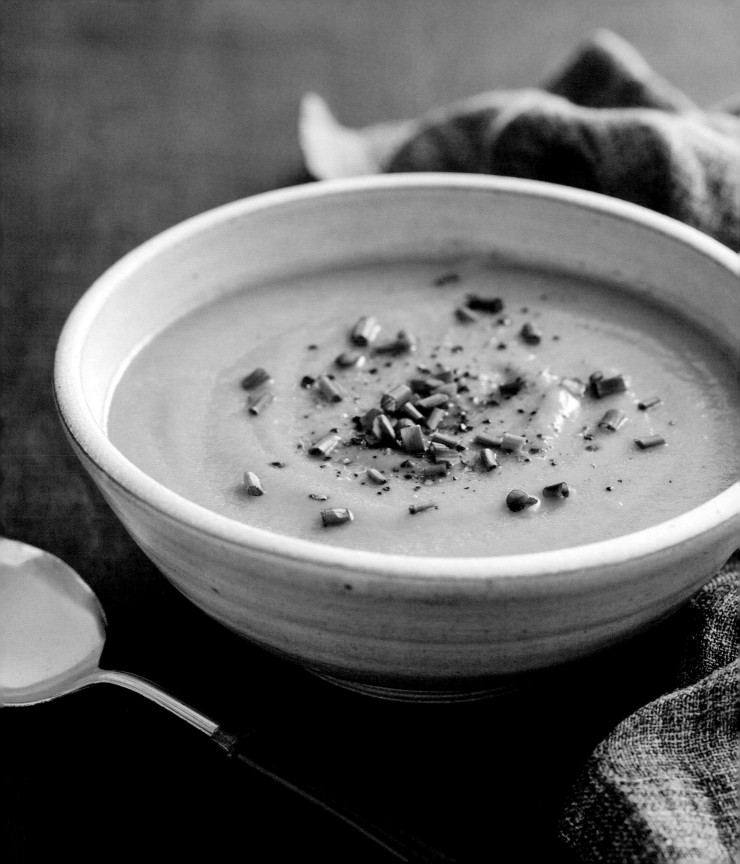

CARROT-GINGER SOUP

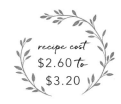

recipe cost
$2.60 *to*
$3.20

Lightly sweet with a classic ginger bite, this warm soup is mild and comforting. Perfect for the days when you may not want to indulge in a heavy meal but need something to take the edge off of your hunger. I love pureed soups. This pairs beautifully with a salad and the Olive Oil and Herb Focaccia on page 67.

SERVES 4

- 1 tablespoon extra-virgin olive oil
- 1 pound large carrots, peeled and diced (see Note page 51)
- 1 large yellow onion, diced
- 2½ cups Vegetable Broth (page 332) or store-bought
- ½ cup canned full-fat coconut milk
- 1 tablespoon grated fresh ginger
- ½ teaspoon fine sea salt
- ¼ teaspoon ground black pepper
- 2 tablespoons fresh chives or green onions, for serving (optional)

1. Preheat an electric pressure cooker using the SAUTÉ function and adjust the heat to MORE (see Note page 95). When the display panel reads HOT, add the olive oil, carrots, and onion. Cook, stirring infrequently, until the carrots get a little color and the onions soften, about 5 minutes.

2. Add the broth, coconut milk, ginger, salt, and black pepper.

3. Place the lid on the cooker and make sure the vent valve is in the SEALING position. Using the display panel, press the CANCEL button to turn off the SAUTÉ function, then select the MANUAL/PRESSURE COOK function and HIGH PRESSURE. Use the +/− buttons until the display reads 10 minutes.

4. When the cooker beeps, let it naturally release the pressure until the display reads LO:05. Switch the vent valve from the SEALING to the VENTING position. Use caution while the steam escapes.

5. Remove the lid and, using an immersion blender, carefully puree the soup. Serve warm topped with chives, if desired.

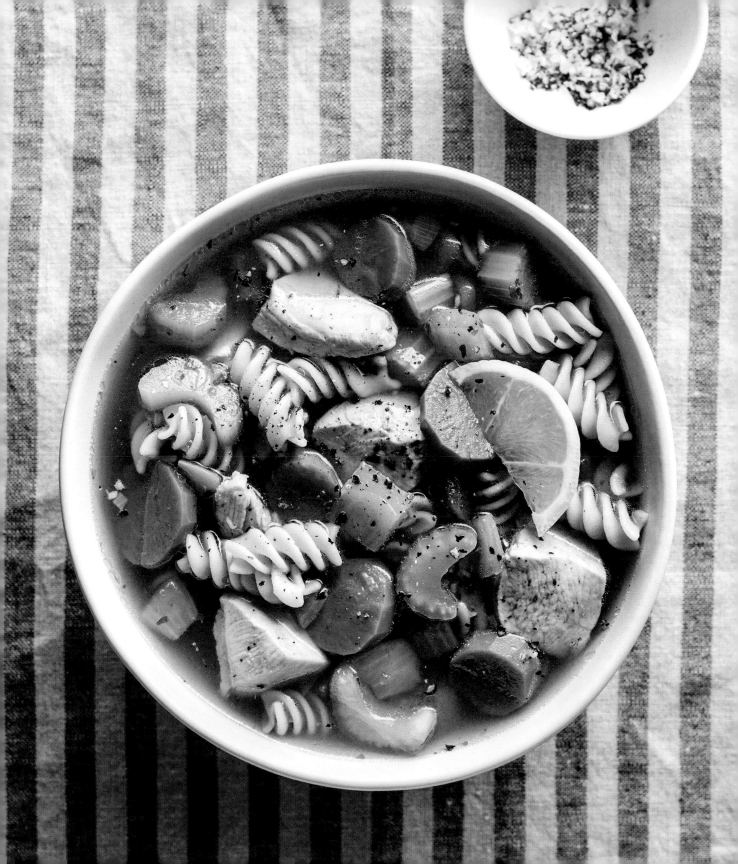

GREEK LEMON-CHICKEN SOUP

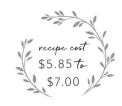

We call this "Cheer-You-Up Chicken Soup" at my house. It's my go-to sick-day soup, perfectly mild for tummy bugs, fevers, and colds. Every home needs a go-to chicken soup recipe and I hope this one brings your family the same happiness it brings mine.

1. Preheat an electric pressure cooker using the SAUTÉ function and adjust the heat to MORE (see Note page 95). When the display panel reads HOT, add the olive oil, chicken, onion, celery, carrots, garlic, dried onion, parsley, salt, oregano, and black pepper. Cook, stirring occasionally, until the chicken gets a little color and the onions soften, about 6 minutes.

2. Add the water, broth, lemon zest, lemon juice, and pasta. Stir well to combine.

3. Place the lid on the cooker and make sure the vent valve is in the SEALING position. Using the display panel, press the CANCEL button to turn off the SAUTÉ function, then select the MANUAL/PRESSURE COOK function and HIGH PRESSURE. Use the +/− buttons until the display reads 6 minutes.

4. When the cooker beeps, let it naturally release the pressure until the display reads LO:10. Switch the vent valve from the SEALING to the VENTING position. Use caution while the steam escapes.

SERVES 4

- 1 tablespoon extra-virgin olive oil
- 1 pound boneless, skinless chicken breasts, cut into bite-size pieces
- ½ medium yellow onion, diced
- 4 stalks celery, diced
- 2 large carrots, peeled and diced (see Note page 51)
- 3 cloves garlic, minced
- 1 tablespoon dried minced onion
- 2 teaspoons dried parsley flakes
- 1 teaspoon dried oregano
- 1½ teaspoons fine sea salt
- ½ teaspoon ground black pepper
- 2 cups water
- 1½ cups low-sodium chicken broth or Bone Broth (page 331)
- 1½ teaspoons freshly grated lemon zest
- 1 tablespoon fresh lemon juice
- 4 ounces gluten-free fusilli pasta

CAULIFLOWER CHEESE BISQUE

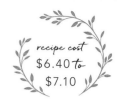

recipe cost
$6.40 to
$7.10

This is one of my favorite soups in this book. I love when I can get something to taste cheesy when it doesn't have any cheese in it at all! If you do not have any cauliflower on hand, this dish will work with broccoli as a 1:1 sub, or you can do a mixture of the two!

SERVES 4

4 cups cauliflower florets

2 cups Vegetable Broth (page 332) or store-bought

1 cup raw cashews or unsalted sunflower seeds

1 cup water

½ cup unfortified nutritional yeast

¼ cup Oat Milk (page 288) or other milk

1 large carrot, peeled and diced (see Note page 51)

½ medium yellow onion, diced

1 tablespoon extra-virgin olive oil

1 tablespoon fresh lemon juice

1½ teaspoons minced garlic

1½ teaspoons fine sea salt

1 teaspoon mustard powder

1 teaspoon paprika

¼ teaspoon ground black pepper

⅛ teaspoon cayenne pepper

1. In an electric pressure cooker, combine the cauliflower, broth, cashews, water, nutritional yeast, oat milk, carrot, onion, olive oil, lemon juice, garlic, salt, mustard powder, paprika, black pepper, and cayenne and stir well.

2. Place the lid on the cooker and make sure the vent valve is in the SEALING position. Using the display panel, select the MANUAL/PRESSURE COOK function and HIGH PRESSURE. Use the +/− buttons until the display reads 10 minutes.

3. When the cooker beeps, let it naturally release the pressure until the display reads LO:05. Switch the vent valve from the SEALING to the VENTING position. Use caution while the steam escapes.

4. Remove the lid and using an immersion blender, carefully puree the soup until it reaches the desired consistency.

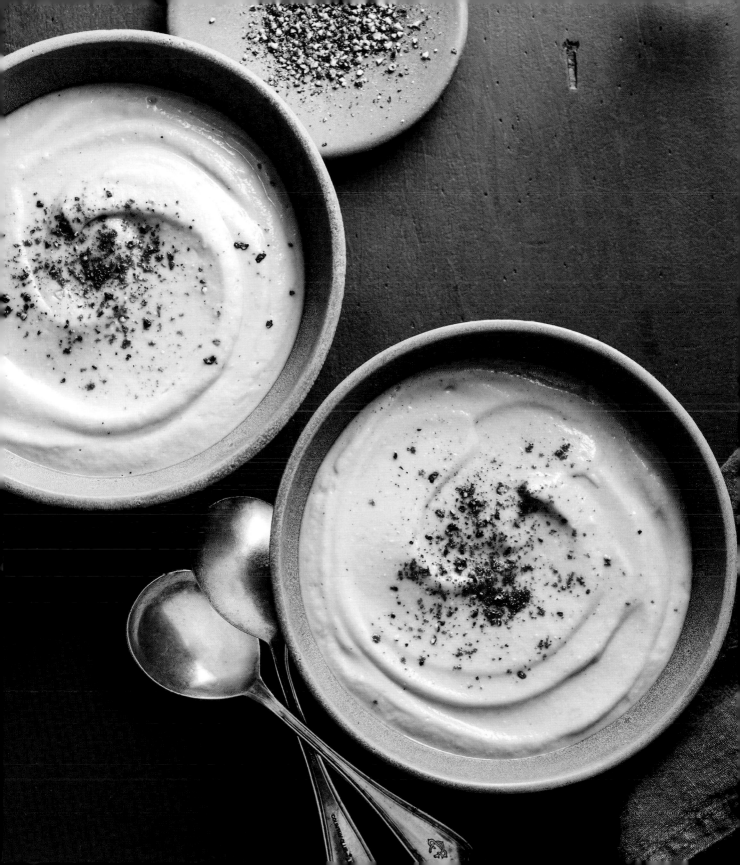

LASAGNA SOUP *with* CASHEW RICOTTA CHEESE

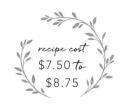

recipe cost
$7.50 *to*
$8.75

My mother is a great many things, but the kitchen has never been her happy place. The dishes she does prepare, though, she does with excellence. Growing up, her lasagna was loved by the entire family and it was something I made for my own family quite often. It, however, was not a dish we could keep around once we discovered our food intolerances. It's not easy finding cost-effective gluten-free lasagna noodles! Last year I decided to take a new approach to lasagna—and turned it into a healthier soup! This Lasagna Soup gives you all the flavors of a most beloved dish and it's gluten- and dairy-free!

SERVES 4

FOR THE LASAGNA SOUP

1 pound lean ground beef

½ yellow onion, diced

1 cup sliced fresh kale (ribs removed)

½ cup fresh basil, plus more for sprinkling

1 tablespoon dried minced onion

1 teaspoon fine sea salt

½ teaspoon red pepper flakes

½ teaspoon dried basil

2 cups low-sodium chicken broth or Bone Broth (page 331)

2 cups water

1 (15-ounce) can diced tomatoes

4 ounces brown rice macaroni noodles

1 tablespoon tomato paste

1. MAKE THE SOUP: Preheat an electric pressure cooker using the SAUTÉ function and adjust the heat to MORE (see Note page 95). When the display panel reads HOT, add the ground beef and yellow onion. Cook, stirring occasionally, until the onion is translucent, about 5 minutes.

2. Stir in the kale, fresh basil, dried onion, salt, red pepper flakes, and dried basil. Cook for about 1 minute. Add the broth, water, tomatoes, macaroni noodles, and tomato paste. Do not stir.

3. Place the lid on the cooker and make sure the vent valve is in the SEALING position. Using the display panel, press the CANCEL button, then select the MANUAL/PRESSURE COOK function and HIGH PRESSURE. Use the +/− buttons until the display reads 6 minutes.

4. MAKE THE CHEESE: In a high-powered blender, combine the cashews, water, olive oil, lemon juice, and salt. Blend on high until the cheese resembles ricotta, about 10 seconds.

5. When the cooker beeps, switch the vent valve from the SEALING to the VENTING position, administering a quick release. Use caution while the steam escapes.

6. Ladle the soup into four bowls. Top with the cashew ricotta cheese and additional fresh basil.

NOTE: If you are not dairy-free, you can use 1 cup dairy ricotta cheese.

FOR THE CASHEW RICOTTA CHEESE (SEE NOTE)

1 cup raw cashews or unsalted sunflower seeds if you are nut free

3 tablespoons water

1 tablespoon extra-virgin olive oil

1 tablespoon fresh lemon juice

½ teaspoon fine sea salt

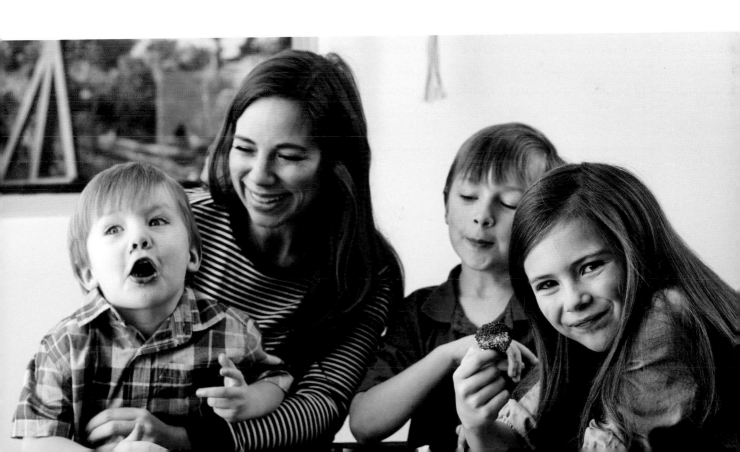

SOUTHWEST CHICKEN FAJITA SOUP

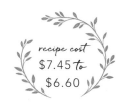

recipe cost
$7.45 *to*
$6.60

Bell peppers aren't cheap, especially if you invest in organic produce. I love to wait until bell peppers go on sale at my local store. I stock up, cut them into strips, and freeze them so that when they're at a premium I don't have to buy them. If you can't find them on sale, big-box stores like Costco usually have large packs for a decent price.

SERVES 4 TO 6

1 large yellow onion, thinly sliced

1 medium red bell pepper, seeded and thinly sliced

1 medium yellow bell pepper, seeded and thinly sliced

1 small jalapeño, seeded and thinly sliced

1 pound boneless, skinless chicken breasts, cut into bite-size pieces

2 teaspoons chili powder

1 teaspoon paprika

1 teaspoon fine sea salt

½ teaspoon garlic powder

½ teaspoon onion powder

½ teaspoon cumin

1 (15-ounce) can fire-roasted tomatoes

2 cups cooked black beans

2 cups low-sodium chicken broth or Bone Broth (page 331)

1 tablespoon arrowroot powder

1 tablespoon hot sauce

½ cup chopped fresh cilantro leaves (optional)

1. Preheat an electric pressure cooker using the SAUTÉ function and adjust the heat to MORE (see Note page 95). When the display panel reads HOT, add the onion, bell peppers, and jalapeño. Cook, stirring occasionally, until the peppers soften and the onion is translucent, about 10 minutes.

2. Add the chicken, chili powder, paprika, salt, garlic powder, onion powder, and cumin and stir to combine. Let the chicken cook for 6 minutes, stirring occasionally. Add the tomatoes, beans, broth, arrowroot powder, and hot sauce and stir well.

3. Place the lid on the cooker and make sure the vent valve is in the SEALING position. Using the display panel, press the CANCEL button to turn off the SAUTÉ function, then select the MANUAL/PRESSURE COOK function and HIGH PRESSURE. Use the +/− buttons until the display reads 10 minutes.

4. When the cooker beeps, let it naturally release the pressure until the display reads LO:05. Switch the vent valve from the SEALING to the VENTING position. Use caution while the steam escapes.

5. Top with cilantro, if desired.

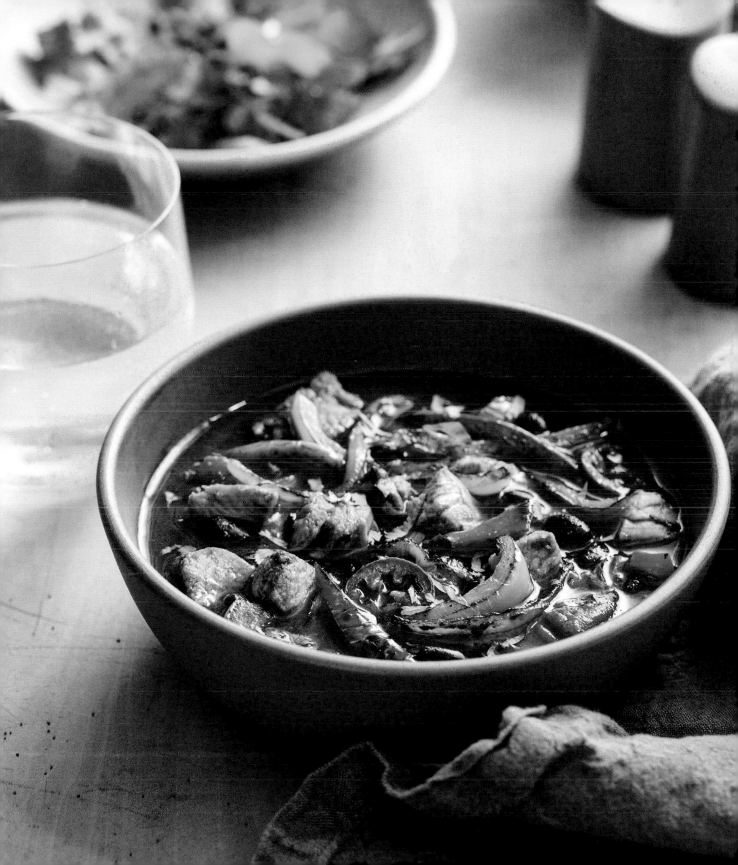

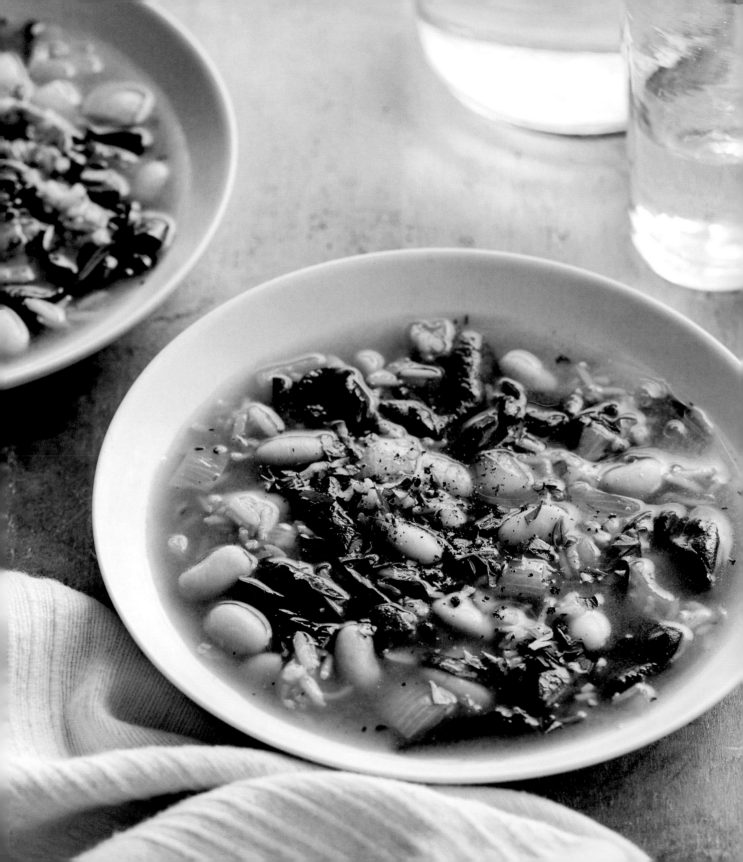

SPINACH—WHITE BEAN SOUP

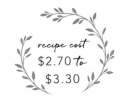

This simple "dump meal" is a perfect lunchtime or weeknight soup. If you cannot find dried cannellini beans, any white beans—such as navy beans or great northern beans—will work in this tasty soup!

SERVES 4

4 cups Vegetable Broth (page 332) or store-bought

1 cup dried cannellini beans

¼ cup brown rice

½ large yellow onion, diced

Juice of 1 medium lemon

2 tablespoons chopped fresh parsley (optional)

1 tablespoon extra-virgin olive oil

2 cloves garlic, minced

1 teaspoon dried thyme

1 teaspoon dried basil

1 teaspoon fine sea salt

½ teaspoon ground black pepper

2 bay leaves

2 cups baby spinach

1. In an electric pressure cooker, combine the broth, beans, rice, onion, lemon juice, parsley, olive oil, garlic, thyme, basil, salt, black pepper, and bay leaves and stir well.

2. Place the lid on the cooker and make sure the vent valve is in the SEALING position. Using the display panel, select the MANUAL/PRESSURE COOK function and HIGH PRESSURE. Use the +/− buttons until the display reads 1 hour.

3. When the cooker beeps, let it naturally release the pressure until the display reads LO:05. Switch the vent valve from the SEALING to the VENTING position. Use caution while the steam escapes.

4. Remove the lid, discard the bay leaves, and stir in the spinach.

5. Serve hot.

NO-POTATO POTATO SOUP

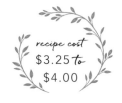

recipe cost
$3.25 *to*
$4.00

In the weight-loss community there is a general fear of potatoes, which is silly, because potatoes don't make you fat. Eating an overabundance of any food or food group can cause you to gain weight. But I digress. Knowing that many who are trying to lose weight omit potatoes from their diets, I wanted to develop a soup that tasted just like potato soup without the potatoes! If you have a hankering for a warm potato soup, this is your huckleberry. You won't even miss the bacon or cheese!

SERVES 4

3 cups water

1 cup red lentils, rinsed and drained

¼ cup hemp hearts

½ medium yellow onion, diced

1 tablespoon extra-virgin olive oil

1 bunch chives

1 sprig fresh basil

1½ teaspoons fine sea salt, plus more to taste

½ teaspoon ground black pepper

1. In an electric pressure cooker, combine the water, lentils, hemp hearts, onion, olive oil, chives, basil, salt, and black pepper.

2. Place the lid on the cooker and make sure the vent valve is in the SEALING position. Using the display panel, select the MANUAL/PRESSURE COOK function and HIGH PRESSURE. Use the +/− buttons until the display reads 6 minutes.

3. When the cooker beeps, let it naturally release the pressure until the display reads LO:05. Switch the vent valve from the SEALING to the VENTING position. Use caution while the steam escapes.

4. Remove the lid and, using an immersion blender, carefully puree the soup until it reaches the desired consistency. Season with salt to taste.

CLAM CHOWDER

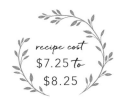

Thick and decadent, this chowder is a treat for seafood lovers and nonlovers alike! Bumble Bee makes canned minced clams that are wild caught! (You can find them at Walmart next to the tuna fish.) Sugar is listed in the ingredients, but it couldn't be more than a trace amount because the clams actually have zero grams of sugar.

SERVES 4

- 1 tablespoon extra-virgin olive oil
- 4 strips nitrate-free bacon, chopped
- ½ cup diced yellow onion
- ½ cup diced celery
- 4 cloves garlic, minced
- ¾ teaspoon fine sea salt
- ½ teaspoon dried thyme
- ¼ teaspoon ground black pepper
- 2 tablespoons chickpea flour
- 1 tablespoon arrowroot powder
- 2¼ cups unsweetened almond milk or soy milk (see Note)
- 2 (6.5-ounce) cans minced clams, with the juice
- 8 ounces potatoes, peeled and diced
- 1 tablespoon chopped fresh parsley

1. Preheat an electric pressure cooker using the SAUTÉ function and adjust the heat to MORE (see Note page 95).

2. When the display panel reads HOT, add the olive oil, bacon, onion, celery, garlic, salt, thyme, and black pepper. Cook, stirring infrequently, until the vegetables soften, about 5 minutes.

3. Add the chickpea flour and arrowroot powder and stir to combine. Pour in the almond milk, clams with juice, and potatoes and stir well.

4. Place the lid on the cooker and make sure the vent valve is in the SEALING position. Using the display panel, select the CANCEL button to turn off the SAUTÉ function, then select the MANUAL/PRESSURE COOK function and LOW PRESSURE. Use the +/− buttons until the display reads 8 minutes.

5. When the cooker beeps, let it naturally release the pressure until the display reads LO:10. Switch the vent valve from the SEALING to the VENTING position. Use caution while the steam escapes.

6. Remove the lid, give the soup a good stir, and ladle into four bowls. Sprinkle with parsley and serve.

NOTE: This recipe was tested using almond and soy milk. Oat milk will not work in this recipe—it will cause the bottom of the cooker to scorch and the cooker will not come to pressure.

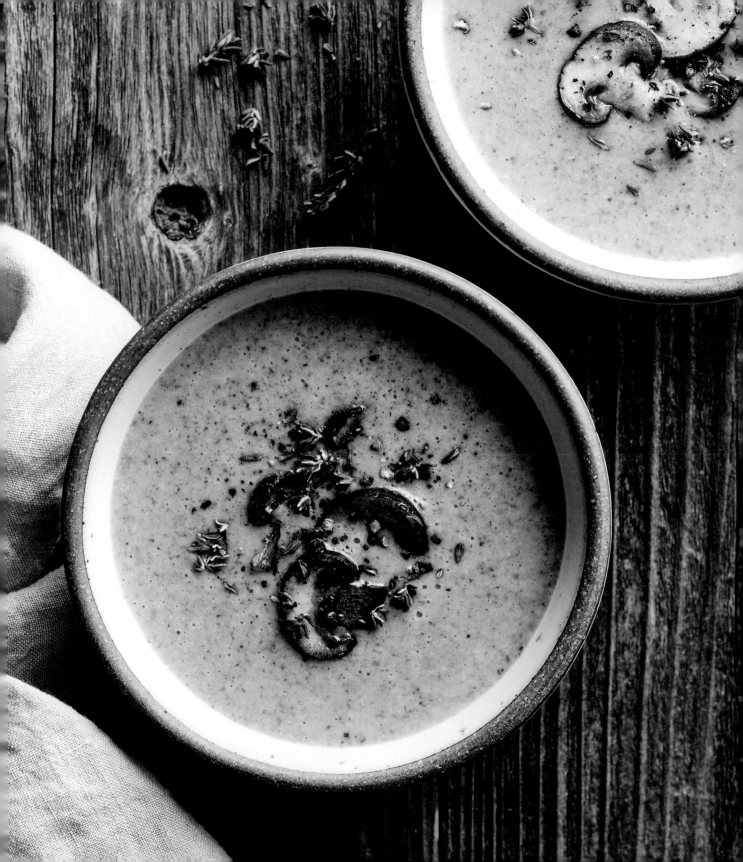

CREAM *of* MUSHROOM SOUP BASE

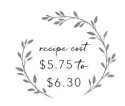

recipe cost
$5.75 *to*
$6.30

This is a thick condensed soup designed to replace canned store-bought condensed cream of mushroom soup, so you can continue to make all of your family's favorite casseroles without worrying about what's actually in the food you're consuming! Use this to replace canned condensed soup 1:1. The base will freeze well for up to twelve months. You can measure it out and freeze in a muffin tin, then pop out the pucks and store them in an airtight container or freezer bag, removing portions as you need them.

SERVES 4

2 tablespoons extra-virgin olive oil

16 ounces cremini or button mushrooms, wiped clean and chopped

1 cup diced yellow onion

4 cloves garlic, minced

1⅛ teaspoons fine sea salt

½ teaspoon dried thyme

¼ teaspoon ground black pepper

2 tablespoons arrowroot powder

2½ cups unsweetened almond milk or soy milk (see Note)

1. Preheat an electric pressure cooker using the SAUTÉ function and adjust the heat to MORE (see Note page 95). When the display panel reads HOT, add the olive oil, mushrooms, onion, garlic, salt, thyme, and black pepper. Cook, stirring infrequently, until the mushrooms wilt and soften, about 10 minutes. Add the arrowroot powder and stir to combine. Stir in the almond milk.

2. Place the lid on the cooker and make sure the vent valve is in the SEALING position. Using the display panel, press the CANCEL button to turn off the SAUTÉ function, then select the MANUAL/PRESSURE COOK function and LOW PRESSURE. Use the +/− buttons until the display reads 5 minutes.

3. When the cooker beeps, let it naturally release the pressure until the display reads LO:10. Switch the vent valve from the SEALING to the VENTING position. Use caution while the steam escapes.

4. Remove the lid and using an immersion blender or blender, carefully puree the soup until smooth. This is ready to use in recipes in place of condensed soup, or thin with milk of choice to serve as soup.

NOTE: This recipe was tested using almond and soy milk. Oat milk will not work in this recipe—it will cause the bottom of the cooker to scorch and the cooker will not come to pressure.

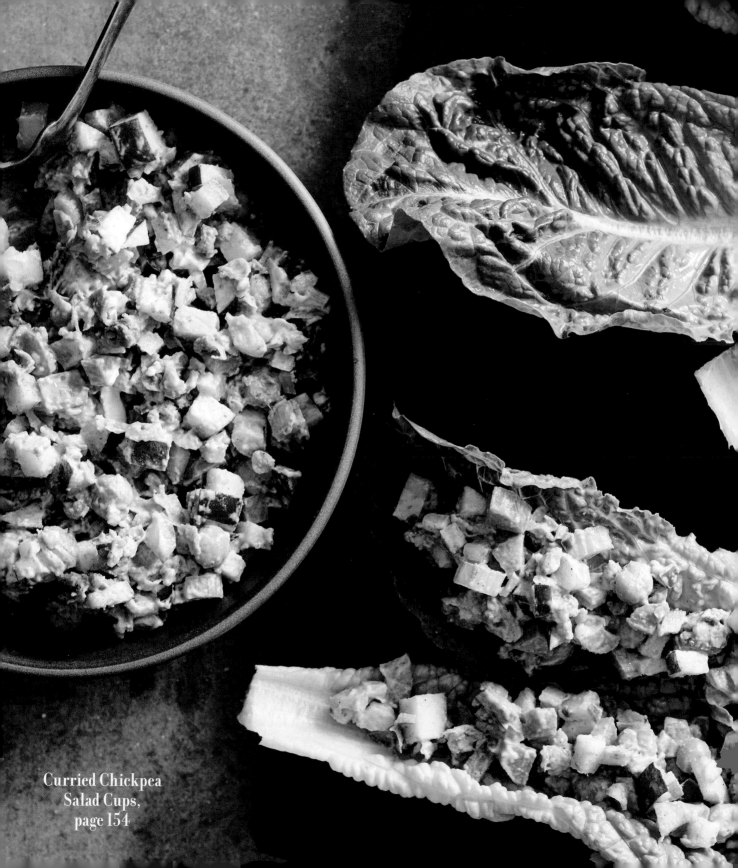

Curried Chickpea
Salad Cups,
page 154

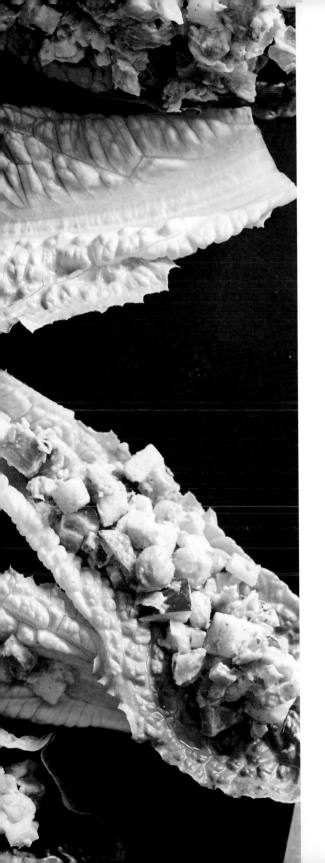

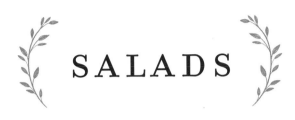

SALADS

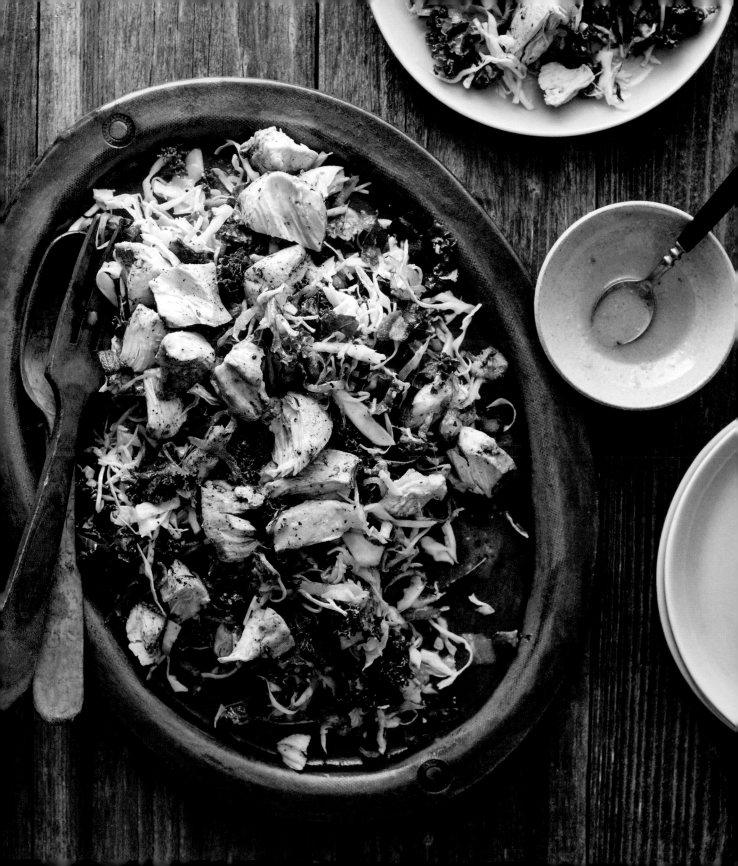

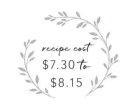

recipe cost
$7.30 to
$8.15

KALE *and* CABBAGE CHICKEN–BACON SALAD

Be prepared to be blown away—this delicious, no-waste salad is so cost friendly because instead of using extra oil to make a vinaigrette, I use the leftover pan juices from the delicious cooked chicken and bacon! Not only does that lend itself to making a tastier dish because the flavor profile has been layered, but it's at a cost savings to you! From now on, before throwing out your pan juices, see if you might be able to repurpose them in a dressing or soup!

1. MAKE THE SALAD: Preheat an electric pressure cooker using the SAUTÉ function and adjust the heat to MORE (see Note page 95). When the display panel reads HOT, add the 1 teaspoon olive oil, bacon, onion, and ¼ teaspoon of the salt. Cook, stirring occasionally, until the bacon is crispy and the onions caramelize, 15 to 20 minutes. Transfer the onion mixture to a large bowl.

2. In a large bowl, toss the chicken in the remaining 1 tablespoon olive oil, remaining 1 teaspoon salt, and black pepper.

3. Add the broth to the cooker and scrape up any browned bits. Add the chicken and stir to coat.

4. Place the lid on the cooker and make sure the vent valve is in the SEALING position. Using the display panel, press the CANCEL button to turn off the SAUTÉ function, then select the MANUAL/PRESS COOK function and HIGH PRESSURE. Use the +/− buttons until the display reads 5 minutes.

5. While the chicken is cooking, add the kale and cabbage to the onion mixture in the large bowl and mix together.

SERVES 4

FOR THE SALAD

1 tablespoon plus 1 teaspoon extra-virgin olive oil

4 strips nitrate-free bacon, diced

1 medium yellow onion, thinly sliced

1¼ teaspoons fine sea salt

1 pound boneless, skinless chicken breasts, cut into 1½-inch cubes

½ teaspoon ground black pepper

¼ cup low-sodium chicken broth or water

4 cups chopped fresh kale (ribs removed)

2 cups shredded green cabbage

(recipe continues)

6. **MAKE THE VINAIGRETTE:** In a small bowl, whisk together the vinegar, maple syrup, mustard, garlic powder, salt, and black pepper.

7. When the cooker beeps, switch the vent valve from the SEALING to the VENTING position, administering a quick release. Use caution while the steam escapes. Carefully remove the liner of the cooker and measure out ¼ cup of chicken pan juices. Add the juices to the vinaigrette and stir to combine.

8. Add the vinaigrette to the salad and toss. Top with the chicken and serve immediately.

FOR THE TANGY MUSTARD VINAIGRETTE

- 2 tablespoons apple cider vinegar
- 1 tablespoon 100 percent pure maple syrup
- 1 tablespoon Dijon mustard
- ¼ teaspoon garlic powder
- ¼ teaspoon fine sea salt
- ¼ teaspoon ground black pepper

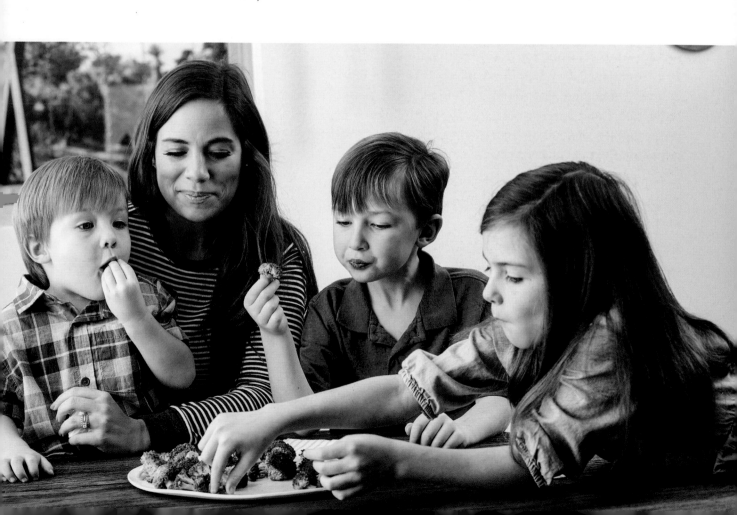

CHICKEN WALDORF SALAD

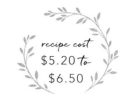
recipe cost
$5.20 *to*
$6.50

Waldorf is just a fancy name for a salad made primarily out of fruits and nuts. It's perfect served over lettuce as an appetizer or light meal. In order to make this dish nut-allergy friendly, I use sunflower seeds instead of nuts. If you do not have an allergy, pecans or walnuts are great in lieu of the sunflower seeds.

SERVES 4

1 pound boneless, skinless chicken breasts

½ teaspoon fine sea salt

¼ teaspoon garlic powder

¼ teaspoon ground black pepper

1 tablespoon extra-virgin olive oil

¼ cup water or chicken broth

1 cup quartered purple seedless grapes

1 cup diced celery

½ small Gala apple, cored and chopped

¾ cup Homemade Mayo (page 330) or store-bought

½ cup shelled sunflower seeds

2 large heads romaine lettuce, chopped

1. Preheat an electric pressure cooker using the SAUTÉ function and adjust the heat to MORE (see Note page 95). In a large bowl, combine the chicken breasts, salt, garlic powder, and black pepper and massage to coat. When the display panel reads HOT, add the olive oil and let it warm. Arrange the chicken on the bottom of the cooker in a single layer and cook for 5 minutes on each side.

2. Add the water, then place the lid on the pressure cooker and make sure the vent valve is in the SEALING position. Using the display panel, select the MANUAL/PRESSURE COOK function and HIGH PRESSURE. Use the +/− buttons until the display reads 6 minutes.

3. When the cooker beeps, let it naturally release the pressure until the display reads LO:05. Switch the vent valve from the SEALING to the VENTING position. Use caution while the steam escapes.

4. Carefully transfer the chicken breasts from the cooker to a large bowl. Shred the chicken using two forks. Add the grapes, celery, apple, mayonnaise, and sunflower seeds and stir to combine.

5. Cover and let chill for a minimum of 2 hours before serving. Serve over romaine lettuce.

ASIAN CHICKEN SALAD

recipe cost
$7.00 *to*
$8.20

I could eat this salad every day, it's that dang good. My kids go wild for it, too. It's so beautiful and vibrant, it just makes you feel good to see a bowl with that many colors in it! If you have a peanut allergy, you can use tahini or sunflower butter instead of peanut or almond and sub your favorite seeds for the almonds.

1. **MAKE THE CHICKEN:** In an electric pressure cooker, combine the chicken, garlic, coconut aminos, sesame oil, ginger, salt, black pepper, mandarin orange, and green onion.

2. Place the lid on the pressure cooker and make sure the vent valve is in the SEALING position. Select the MANUAL/PRESSURE COOK function and HIGH PRESSURE. Use the +/− buttons until the display reads 6 minutes.

3. **MAKE THE DRESSING:** In a wide-mouth jar, combine the orange juice, avocado oil, coconut aminos, vinegar, almond butter, ginger, sesame oil, and salt. Blend using an immersion blender until smooth.

4. **MAKE THE SALAD:** In a large bowl, combine the romaine, cabbage, carrot, almonds, and green onion.

5. When the cooker beeps, let it naturally release the pressure until the display reads LO:05. Switch the vent valve from the SEALING to the VENTING position. Use caution while the steam escapes.

6. Transfer the chicken and juices to a food processor and pulse three times to shred the chicken. (If you do not have a food processor, you can shred the chicken into the juices by hand or use a hand mixer.)

7. Top the salad with the chicken and drizzle with the dressing. Toss to combine and serve.

SERVES 4

FOR THE CHICKEN
1 pound boneless, skinless chicken breasts

6 cloves garlic, minced

1 tablespoon coconut aminos

2 teaspoons toasted sesame oil

1 teaspoon grated fresh ginger

½ teaspoon fine sea salt

¼ teaspoon ground black pepper

1 mandarin orange, peeled and sectioned

1 green onion, thinly sliced

FOR THE DRESSING
¼ cup fresh orange juice

3 tablespoons avocado oil

1 tablespoon coconut aminos

1 tablespoon rice vinegar

1 tablespoon raw almond butter or organic peanut butter

2 teaspoons grated fresh ginger

1 teaspoon toasted sesame oil

⅛ teaspoon fine sea salt

FOR THE SALAD
1 large head romaine lettuce, thinly sliced

2 cups finely shredded red cabbage

1 large carrot, peeled and shredded (see Note page 51)

2 tablespoons slivered almonds

1 green onion, thinly sliced

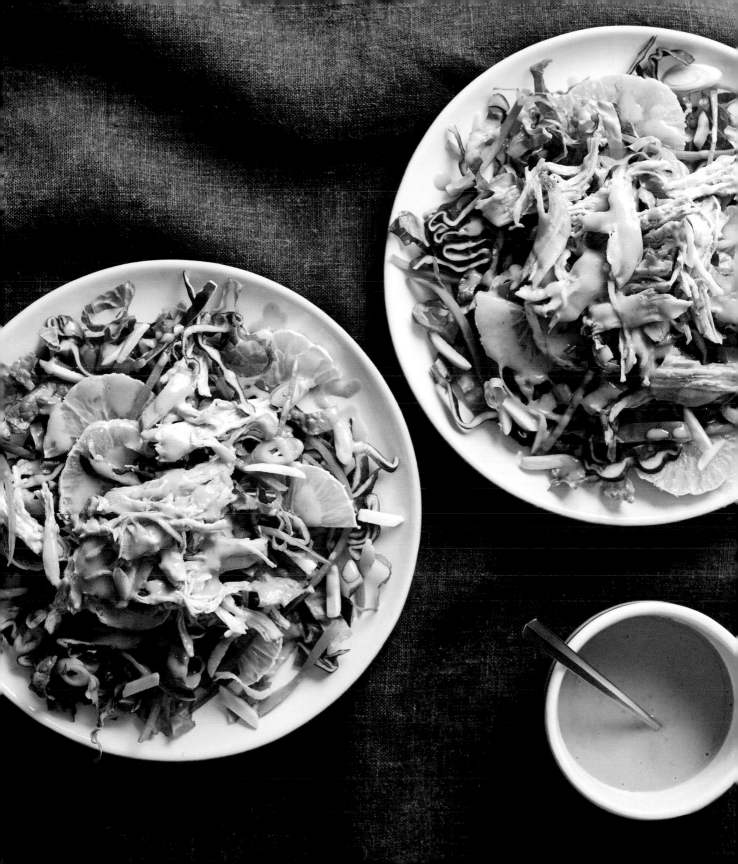

CURRIED CHICKPEA SALAD CUPS

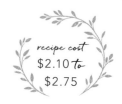

recipe cost
$2.10 *to*
$2.75

This is a great weekday lunch—it comes together in under ten minutes and keeps well in the refrigerator for up to five days. The curry is very mild. If you cannot consume legumes, shredded cooked boneless chicken breasts or thighs work well as a 1:1 replacement for chickpeas. See the Cook Time Cheat Sheet on page 25 for how to cook chickpeas or chicken breast in your pressure cooker.

1. In a large bowl, combine the chickpeas, lime juice, curry powder, tahini, and salt. Mash with a potato masher until the chickpeas are broken up. Add the onion, celery, apple, carrot, jalapeño, and mayonnaise. Stir well to combine.

2. Serve in the romaine lettuce cups. Top with cilantro, if desired.

SERVES 4

- 2½ cups cooked chickpeas
- 1 tablespoon fresh lime juice
- 2 teaspoons curry powder
- 1 teaspoon Homemade Tahini (page 329) or store-bought
- ½ teaspoon fine sea salt
- ⅓ cup chopped red onion
- 2 stalks celery, diced
- ½ small Gala apple, cored and diced
- ⅓ cup diced carrot (see Note page 51)
- ½ small jalapeño, seeded and diced
- ¼ cup Homemade Mayo (page 330) or store-bought
- 1 large head romaine lettuce, leaves separated, rinsed, and patted dry
- 2 tablespoons fresh cilantro leaves (optional)

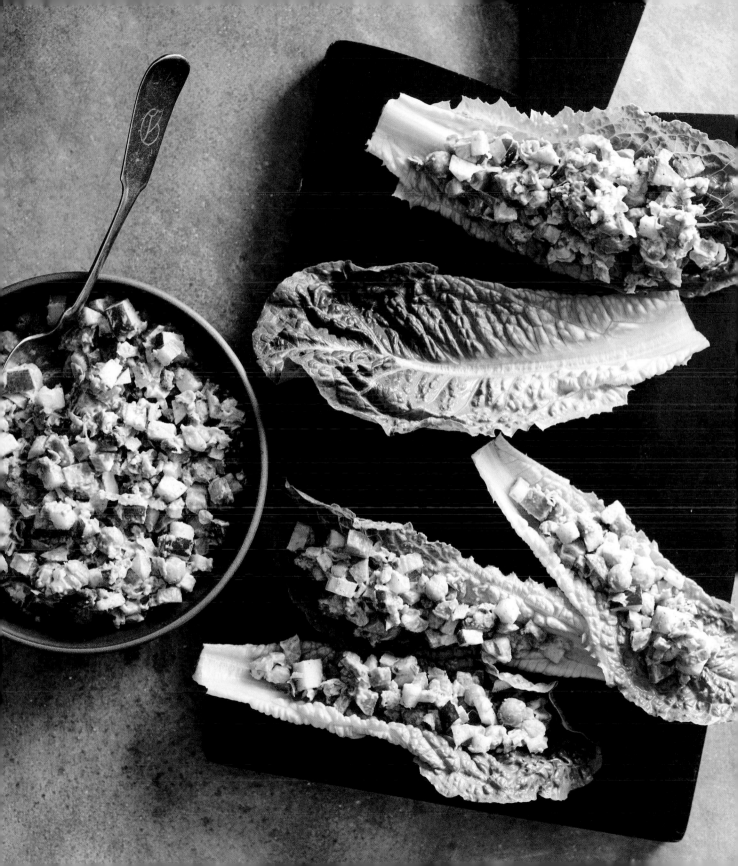

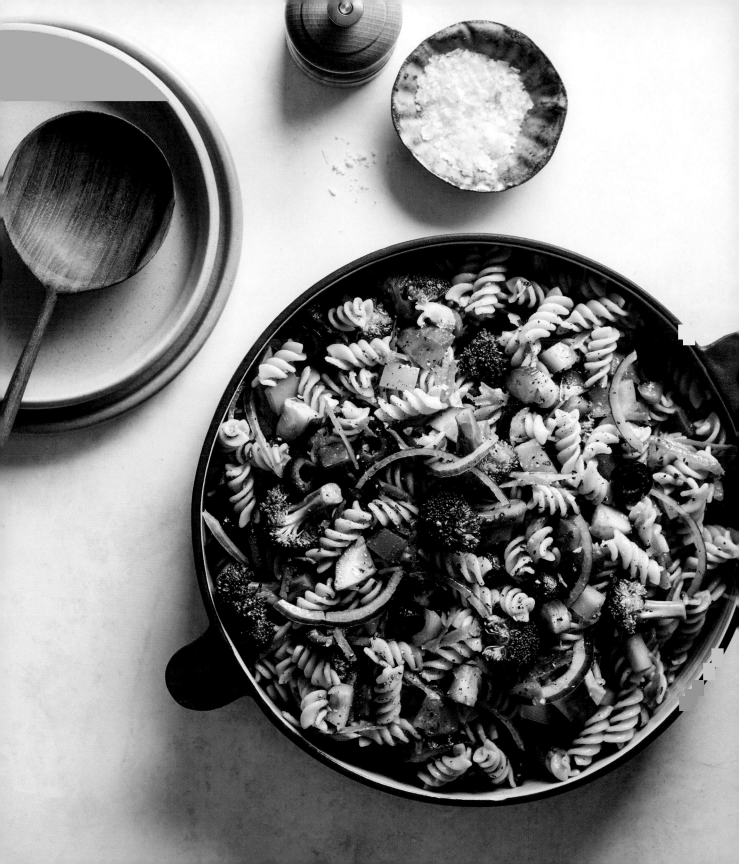

ITALIAN PASTA SALAD

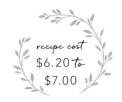

recipe cost
$6.20 to
$7.00

I love salads that double as a fabulous side dish for a party or a light, tasty lunch! This is such a colorful salad, it's the perfect companion for a summer party or to keep in the refrigerator to pull out for lunches throughout the week.

SERVES 4 TO 6

1 (12-ounce) box brown rice fusilli pasta

6 cups water

½ teaspoon fine sea salt

2 Roma tomatoes, cored and diced

1½ cups diced broccoli florets

1 cup diced cucumber

1 medium yellow bell pepper, seeded and diced

¾ cup shredded carrots (see Note page 51)

½ cup chopped black olives

⅓ cup diced red onion

1 cup Italian Dressing (page 158)

1. In an electric pressure cooker, combine the pasta, water, and salt. Stir well to combine.

2. Place the lid on the cooker and make sure the vent valve is in the SEALING position. Using the display panel, select the MANUAL/PRESSURE COOK function and HIGH PRESSURE. Use the +/− buttons until the display reads 6 minutes.

3. When the cooker beeps, switch the vent valve from the SEALING to the VENTING position, administering a quick release. Use caution while the steam escapes.

4. Drain the pasta, rinse under cool water, and drain again. Transfer to a large bowl. Add the tomatoes, broccoli, cucumber, bell pepper, carrots, black olives, onion, and Italian dressing. Toss to coat.

ITALIAN DRESSING

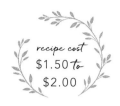

recipe cost
$1.50 to
$2.00

I have such a struggle in the dressing aisle at the store. The stuff that's affordable is full of processed sugars, hydrogenated oils, and tons of preservatives. The stuff with great ingredients can be $6+ a bottle. The budget-minded mama in me is always at war with the price tag of the good stuff. This prompted me to begin making my own dressings. It's easier than you'd think, usually only requiring a spoon/whisk and a bowl. Or if you like a little more emulsion, a cheap immersion blender always yields beautiful results! This recipe only costs $1.50 to $2.00 to make from home. All the benefits of the expensive stuff and none of the drawbacks!

MAKES 1 CUP

¾ cup extra-virgin olive oil

3 tablespoons red wine vinegar

1 teaspoon 100 percent maple syrup

1 teaspoon dried minced onion

1 teaspoon dried oregano

1 teaspoon fine sea salt

½ teaspoon garlic powder

½ teaspoon dried parsley flakes

¼ teaspoon dried basil

¼ teaspoon ground black pepper

⅛ teaspoon dried thyme

1. In a wide-mouth jar, combine the olive oil, vinegar, maple syrup, onion, oregano, garlic powder, parsley, basil, black pepper and thyme. Blend using an immersion blender until smooth.

2. Store in an airtight container in the refrigerator for up to 2 weeks. Shake well before using.

MEDITERRANEAN EGG SALAD

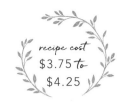

recipe cost
$3.75 to
$4.25

I don't know about you, but I never have toasted sesame seeds or pine nuts on hand—but I do always have their raw counterparts. To toast your own, simply warm a pan over medium heat on the stovetop and toss the seeds or nuts with a little oil. Toast until lightly brown and fragrant. It only takes a minute or two and it really adds a special something to this salad!

SERVES 4

1 cup water

8 large eggs

½ cup pitted and chopped green olives

¼ cup extra-virgin olive oil

¼ cup toasted pine nuts

2 tablespoons coarsely chopped fresh cilantro leaves

1 tablespoon chopped red onion

1 teaspoon freshly grated lemon zest

2 teaspoons fresh lemon juice

1½ teaspoons minced fresh thyme

1½ teaspoons toasted sesame seeds

¼ teaspoon fine sea salt

¼ teaspoon ground black pepper

1. Pour the water into an electric pressure cooker and place a trivet or steamer basket inside. Set the eggs on the trivet or in the basket.

2. Place the lid on the cooker and make sure the vent valve is in the SEALING position. Using the display panel, select the MANUAL/PRESSURE COOK function and HIGH PRESSURE. Use the +/– buttons until the display reads 5 minutes. While the eggs cook, prepare an ice bath for when they're finished cooking.

3. When the cooker beeps, let it naturally release the pressure until the display reads LO:05. Switch the vent valve from the SEALING to the VENTING position. Use caution while the steam escapes.

4. Immediately plunge the eggs into the ice bath. Let chill for 5 minutes before peeling.

5. In a large bowl, combine the olives, olive oil, pine nuts, cilantro, onion, lemon zest, lemon juice, thyme, sesame seeds, salt, and black pepper.

6. Peel and chop the eggs. Add the eggs to the bowl, and stir gently. Serve immediately or store covered in the refrigerator until ready to serve.

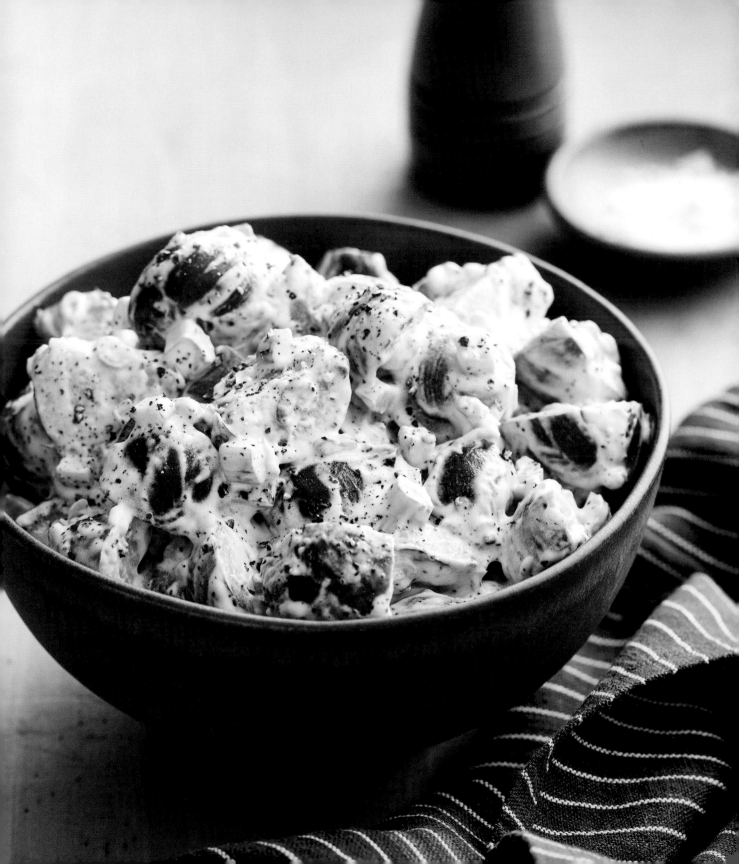

RUSTIC POTATO SALAD

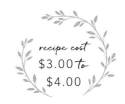

recipe cost
$3.00 to
$4.00

Who doesn't love potato salad? Growing up, my parents would buy those *huge* containers of it from Costco or Sam's and man, I could eat that stuff day and night. The fact is, though, that there are many ingredients in the store-bought stuff that can be left out if you make it at home! It's about $10 at the supermarket for a large container, but you can serve four to six with this recipe and it costs less than $4.00!

SERVES 4 TO 6

1½ pounds small red potatoes, quartered

⅓ cup water

½ cup Homemade Mayo (page 330) or store-bought

3 stalks celery, diced

2 green onions, thinly sliced

1 tablespoon sweet relish

1½ teaspoons yellow mustard

1 teaspoon apple cider vinegar

1 teaspoon celery seed

¼ to ½ teaspoon fine sea salt

⅛ teaspoon ground black pepper

1. Combine the potatoes and water into an electric pressure cooker.

2. Place the lid on the cooker and make sure the vent valve is in the SEALING position. Using the display panel, select the MANUAL/PRESSURE COOK function and LOW PRESSURE. Use the +/− buttons until the display reads 8 minutes.

3. When the cooker beeps, switch the vent valve from the SEALING to the VENTING position, administering a quick release. Use caution while the steam escapes.

4. Using a slotted spoon, carefully transfer the potatoes from the cooker to a large bowl. Add the mayonnaise, celery, green onions, relish, yellow mustard, vinegar, celery seed, salt to taste, and black pepper. Stir gently to combine.

5. Cover and chill for a minimum of 2 hours before serving.

CRUNCHY CHICKPEA CAESAR SALAD

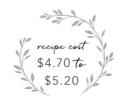

recipe cost
$4.70 *to*
$5.20

This vegetarian take on a classic salad packs a great crunch without traditional croutons, has a tasty umami flavor, and is made without dairy. Add grilled chicken if you are not vegetarian and would like an extra protein punch.

SERVES 4

FOR THE CHICKPEA CROUTONS
1 cup cooked chickpeas
1 teaspoon extra-virgin olive oil
¼ teaspoon fine sea salt
¼ teaspoon garlic powder
⅛ teaspoon chili powder

FOR THE CAESAR DRESSING
¼ cup Homemade Mayo (page 330) or store-bought
2 tablespoons extra-virgin olive oil
½ teaspoon reduced-sodium Worcestershire sauce
¼ teaspoon Dijon mustard
⅛ teaspoon garlic powder
⅛ teaspoon fine sea salt
⅛ teaspoon ground black pepper

FOR THE SALAD
1 small bunch kale (ribs removed), chopped
1 large head romaine lettuce, chopped
⅓ cup hemp hearts

1. **MAKE THE CROUTONS:** Place the chickpeas in a 5.3-quart air-fryer basket and bake at 400°F for 10 minutes. Transfer to a medium bowl. Add the olive oil, salt, garlic powder, and chili powder. Stir well to combine.

2. Return the chickpeas to the air-fryer basket and bake at 300°F for 10 minutes. Let cool completely.

3. **MAKE THE DRESSING:** In a medium bowl, combine the mayonnaise, olive oil, Worcestershire sauce, mustard, garlic powder, salt, and pepper. Whisk until smooth.

4. **MAKE THE SALAD:** In a large bowl, toss together the kale and romaine. Add the dressing and hemp hearts and toss to combine. Top with the crunchy chickpeas.

NOTE: If you do not have an air fryer, you can bake the chickpeas on a rimmed baking sheet in a conventional oven. Bake at 400°F for 20 minutes, then toss with the olive oil and seasonings and bake for an additional 15 minutes.

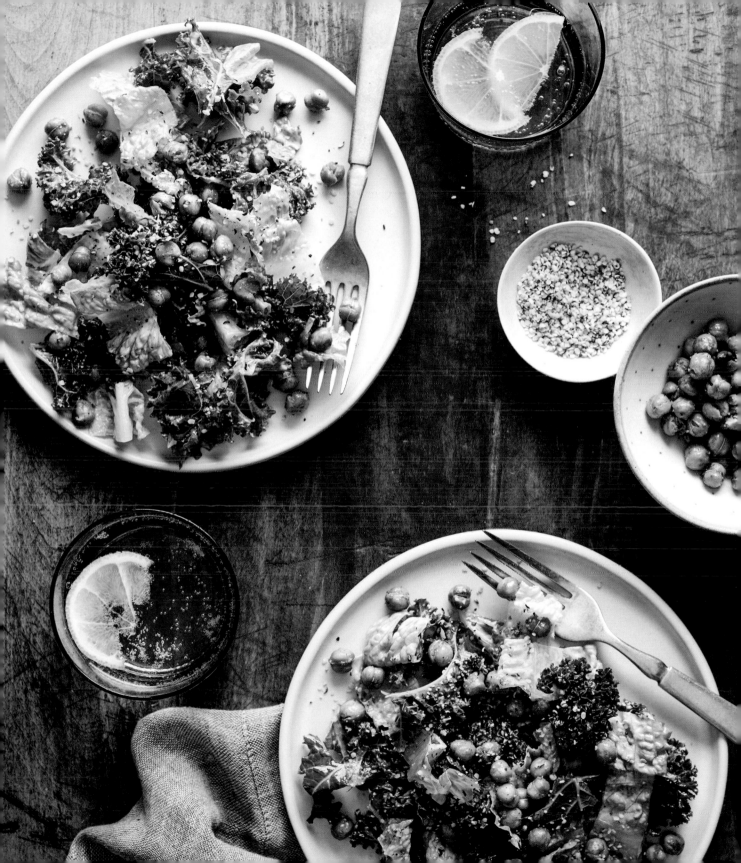

CILANTRO-LIME QUINOA SALAD

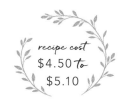

recipe cost
$4.50 *to*
$5.10

This mild, refreshing little salad is perfect for sharing or serving at a summer barbecue. My favorite sugar-free hot sauce is El Pato. My mom's family used it when she was growing up and now it's a staple in my home. It adds the perfect little oomph to this salad. We can get it for $0.30 a can here in Southern California. I know that might not be the case everywhere, so use your favorite low-cost mild hot sauce.

SERVES 4

1 cup quinoa, rinsed and drained

1½ cups water or Vegetable Broth (page 332)

1 tablespoon fresh lime juice

2 cups frozen peas, thawed

½ cup frozen yellow corn, thawed

½ small red onion, diced

½ cup chopped fresh cilantro leaves

4 cups mixed greens

¼ cup avocado oil

2 tablespoons sugar-free mild hot sauce

½ teaspoon ground cumin

¼ teaspoon chili powder

¼ teaspoon fine sea salt

1. In an electric pressure cooker, combine the quinoa, water, and lime juice.

2. Place the lid on the cooker and make sure the vent valve is in the SEALING position. Using the display panel, select the MANUAL/PRESSURE COOK function and HIGH PRESSURE. Use the +/− buttons until the display reads 1 minute.

3. When the cooker beeps, let it naturally release the pressure until the display reads LO:10. Switch the vent valve from the SEALING to the VENTING position. Use caution while the steam escapes.

4. Remove the lid and stir in the peas, corn, onion, and cilantro. Transfer to a large bowl and allow to cool. Toss with the mixed greens.

5. In a small bowl, stir together the avocado oil, hot sauce, cumin, chili powder, and salt. Drizzle over the salad and toss to combine.

6. Store in an airtight container in the refrigerator for up to 2 days.

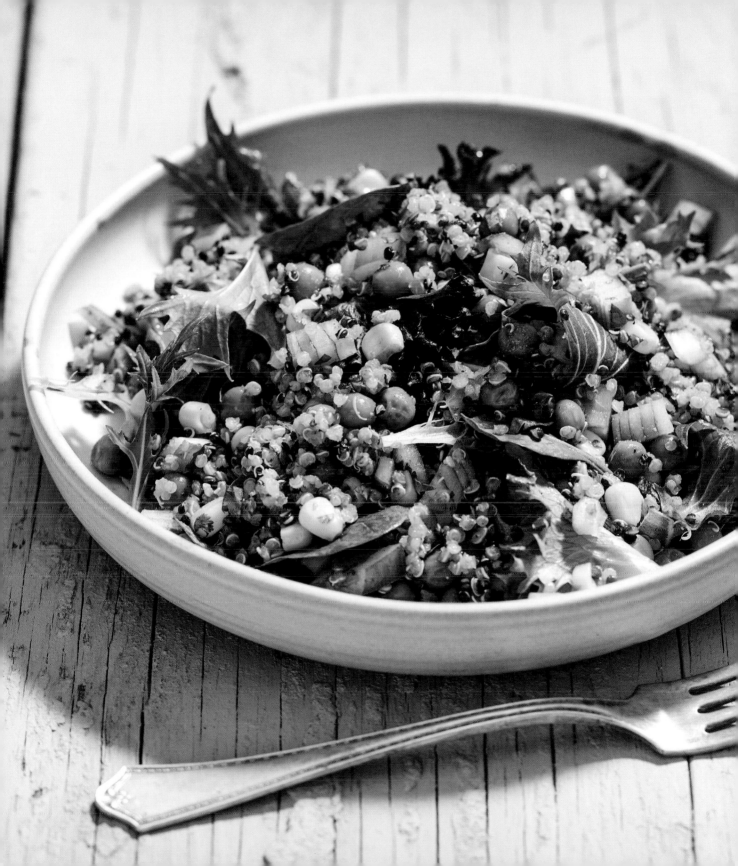

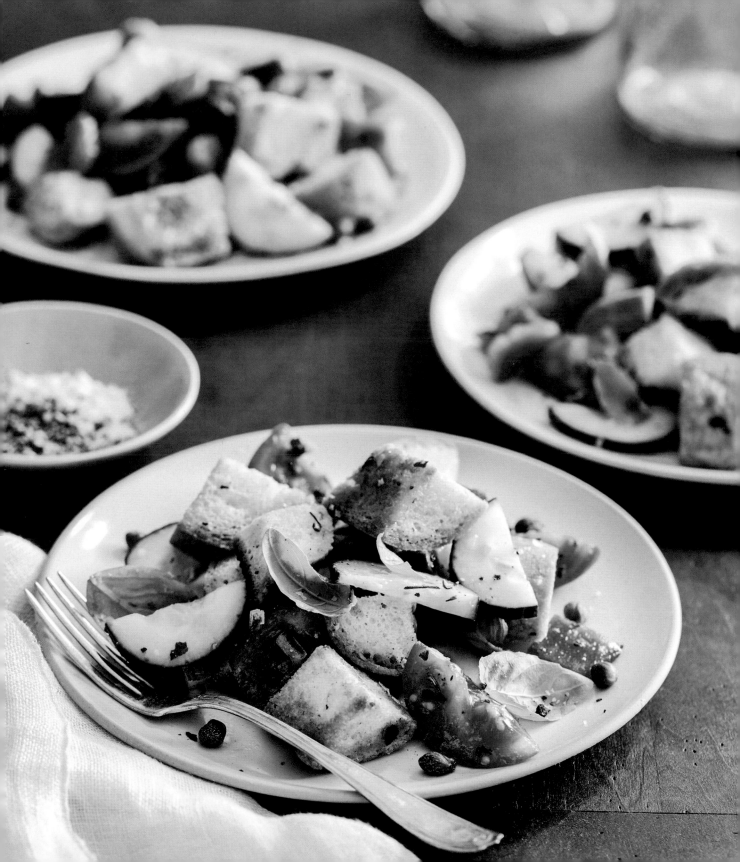

PANZANELLA

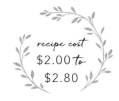

recipe cost
$2.00 *to*
$2.80

Panzanella is a Tuscan chopped salad that's very popular in the summertime in Italy! It is bread-based and accompanied by onions, tomatoes, and cucumbers. It's usually made with stale or old bread that's toasted in oil to revitalize it. It's perfect made with my Olive Oil and Herb Focaccia or a yummy French bread.

SERVES 4

1 tablespoon extra-virgin olive oil

1½ cups 1-inch cubes Olive Oil and Herb Focaccia (page 67) or French-style bread

Fine sea salt

1 medium ripe tomato, cut into 1-inch cubes

½ medium cucumber, sliced ½ inch thick

¼ cup diced red bell pepper

2 tablespoons diced red onion

¼ cup coarsely chopped fresh basil

1 tablespoon capers, drained

¼ cup Italian Dressing (page 158)

Ground black pepper

1. Heat a skillet over medium-high heat. Add the olive oil and let it warm. Add the bread to the pan and sprinkle with ¼ teaspoon salt. Toast the bread in the hot oil, stirring frequently, until nicely browned, about 8 minutes.

2. In a large bowl, combine the tomato, cucumber, bell pepper, onion, basil, and capers. Add the toasted bread. Drizzle with the Italian dressing. Season to taste with additional salt and black pepper. Toss to coat.

3. Allow the salad to marinate for an hour at room temperature before serving.

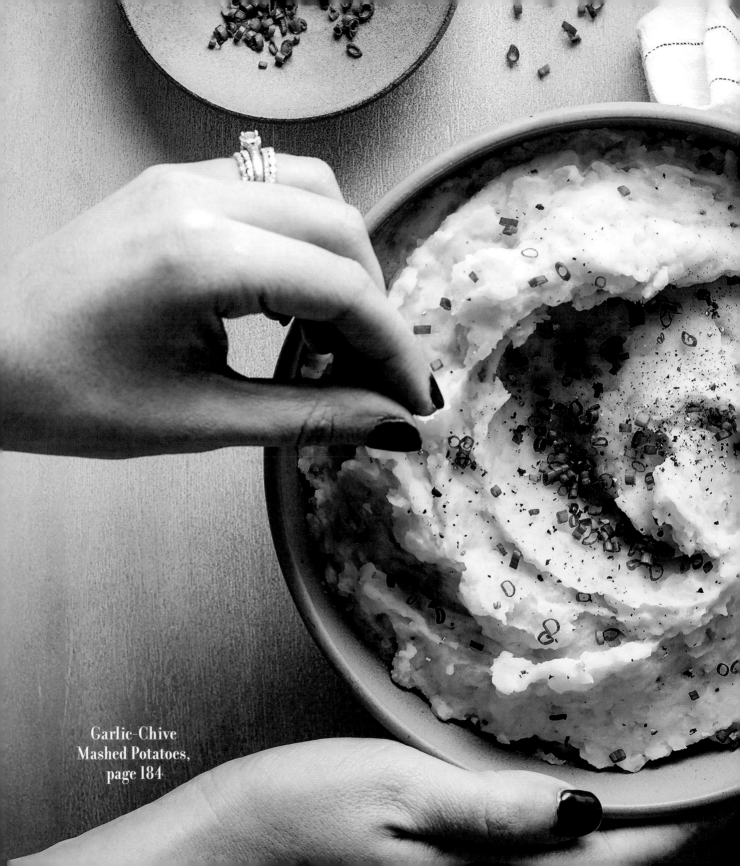

Garlic-Chive
Mashed Potatoes,
page 184

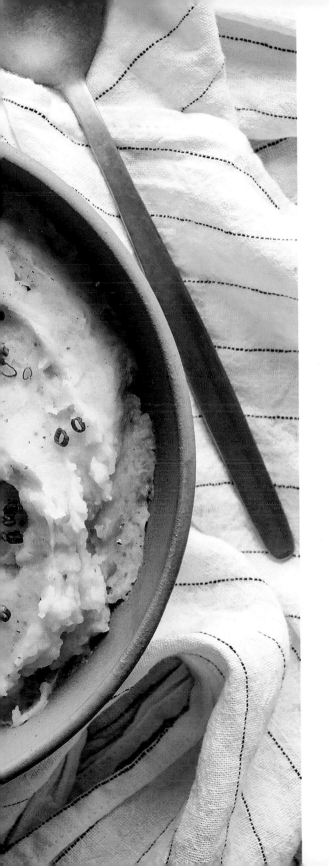

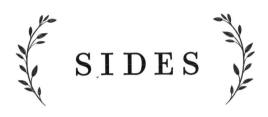

SIDES

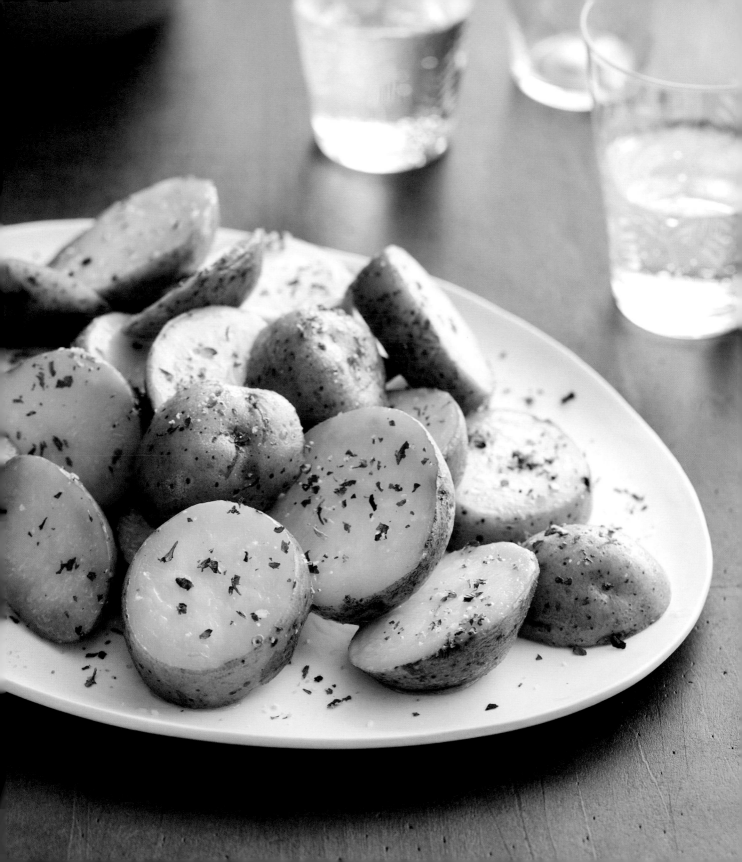

GARLIC *and* HERB DINNER POTATOES

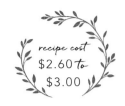

recipe cost
$2.60 to
$3.00

Best. Potatoes. Ever. You may want to double the recipe because (I'm warning you) these are going to make you a dinner superstar! If you don't like a tiny hint of spice, omit the red pepper flakes.

1. In an electric pressure cooker, combine the potatoes and bacon grease. Stir to coat. Add the water.

2. Place the lid on the cooker and make sure the vent valve is in the SEALING position. Using the display panel, select the MANUAL/PRESSURE COOK function and LOW PRESSURE. Use the +/− buttons until the display reads 8 minutes.

3. When the cooker beeps, switch the vent valve from the SEALING to the VENTING position, administering a quick release. Use caution while the steam escapes.

4. Using a slotted spoon, transfer the potatoes from the cooker to a medium bowl. Add the salt, parsley, garlic powder, and red pepper flakes, if desired. Toss to coat and serve hot.

SERVES 4

6 medium gold potatoes, cut in thirds

1 tablespoon bacon grease or extra-virgin olive oil

⅓ cup water

1 teaspoon fine sea salt

½ teaspoon dried parsley flakes

½ teaspoon garlic powder

⅛ teaspoon red pepper flakes (optional)

BARBECUE BEEF *and* BEANS

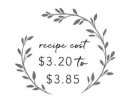

recipe cost
$3.20 *to*
$3.85

Remember those cans of Bush's baked beans that you used to microwave for dinner—or was that just my family? Anyway, this is super reminiscent but about fifteen times more delicious, with the added bonus that it's actually good for you! This is a fabulous side to bring to a work potluck. It keeps well in the refrigerator for about five days.

SERVES 4 TO 6

4 ounces lean ground beef

½ yellow onion, diced

½ cup diced green bell pepper

4 cups shredded green cabbage

1 cup dried pinto beans

½ cup Tangy Barbecue Sauce (page 324)

2 cups water

¾ cup canned diced tomatoes with juice

½ teaspoon fine sea salt

⅛ teaspoon ground black pepper

1. Preheat an electric pressure cooker using the SAUTÉ function and adjust the heat to MORE (see Note page 95). When the display reads HOT, add the ground beef, onion, and bell pepper. Cook, stirring occasionally, until the onion softens and is translucent, about 3 minutes.

2. Stir in the cabbage, beans, barbecue sauce, water, tomatoes, salt, and black pepper.

3. Place the lid on the cooker and make sure the vent valve is in the SEALING position. Using the display panel, press the CANCEL button to turn off the SAUTÉ function, then select the MANUAL/PRESSURE COOK function and HIGH PRESSURE. Use the +/− buttons until the display reads 1 hour 15 minutes.

4. When the cooker beeps, switch the vent valve from the SEALING to the VENTING position, administering a quick release. Use caution while the steam escapes.

5. Let cool for 15 minutes before serving.

CASAMIENTO

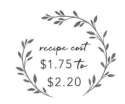

recipe cost
$1.75 to
$2.20

Casamiento—"marriage" in Spanish—is reference to the perfect blending of rice and beans. Although it's a traditional dish, there are many variations. Depending on the household, it is made with red or black beans. *Fríjol de seda*, red silk bean, is the traditional red bean. You can find these beans in the Hispanic section of your local market, or you could use red kidney beans. Many cooks add tomatoes, bell peppers, yellow onion, and cumin. I decided to simplify and make this a dump recipe, no real knife skills required. Depending on the salsa you use, the amount of salt will vary. Make sure to salt to taste before serving.

SERVES 6

1 cup dried red kidney beans

1 cup brown rice

1 cup sugar-free salsa

½ bunch fresh cilantro, stems and leaves separated, roughly chopped

2 tablespoons dried minced onion

5 cups water

Fine sea salt

1. In an electric pressure cooker, combine the beans, rice, salsa, cilantro stems, dried onion, and water. Stir to combine.

2. Place the lid on the cooker and make sure the vent valve is in the SEALING position. Using the display panel, select the MANUAL/PRESSURE COOK function and HIGH PRESSURE. Use the +/− buttons until the display reads 1 hour 15 minutes.

3. When the cooker beeps, let it naturally release the pressure until the display reads LO:10. Switch the vent valve from the SEALING to the VENTING position. Use caution while the steam escapes.

4. Let stand 10 minutes. Add salt to taste and stir, then top with cilantro leaves.

MAPLE-CHILI MASHED SWEET POTATOES

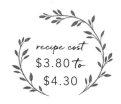

Maple and sweet potatoes: Could this *be* any more "Fall-licious"? I highly recommend getting yourself a steamer basket for steaming things like vegetables and eggs—it will save you so much headache. (The trivet is great for cooking in the cooker, but leaves something to be desired in the steaming capacity.)

SERVES 4 TO 6

1 cup water

2 pounds sweet potatoes, peeled and cut into 1-inch pieces

3 tablespoons 100 percent pure maple syrup

1 tablespoon extra-virgin olive oil

½ teaspoon fine sea salt

½ teaspoon chili powder

½ teaspoon ground cinnamon

¼ teaspoon cayenne pepper

½ cup chopped raw pecans

1. Pour the water into an electric pressure cooker and place a trivet or steamer basket inside.

2. Set the sweet potatoes on the trivet or steamer basket.

3. Place the lid on the cooker and make sure the vent valve is in the SEALING position. Using the display panel, select the STEAM function and HIGH PRESSURE. Use the +/− buttons until the display reads 5 minutes.

4. When the cooker beeps, switch the vent valve from the SEALING to the VENTING position, administering a quick release. Use caution while the steam escapes.

5. Using a slotted spoon, transfer the sweet potatoes from the cooker to a large bowl. Add the maple syrup, olive oil, salt, chili powder, cinnamon, and cayenne. Using a potato masher, mash the potatoes until smooth.

6. Top with pecans and serve hot.

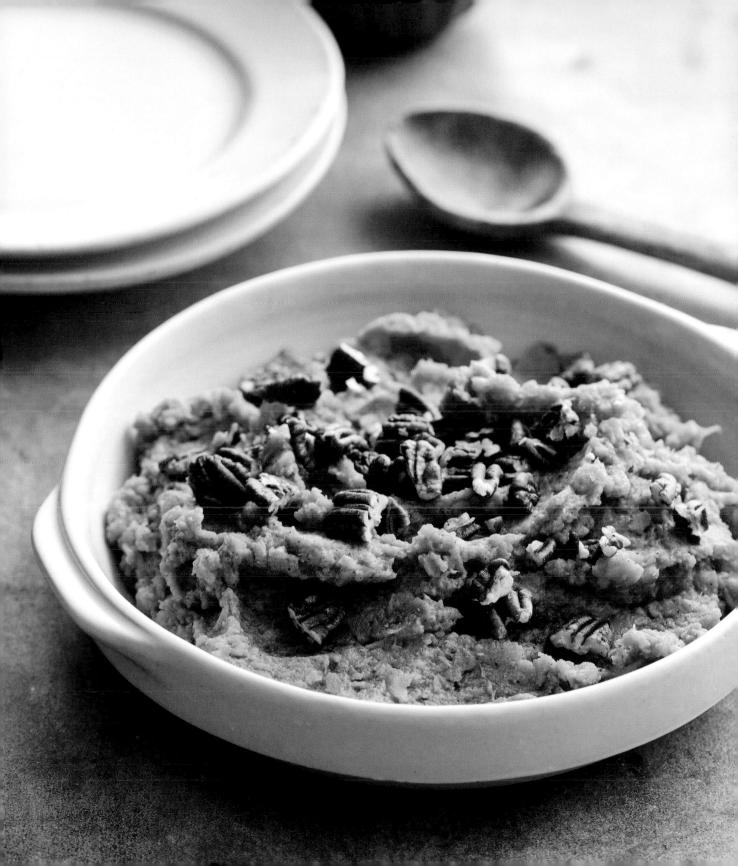

CITRUS-GLAZED CARROTS *with* CHIVES

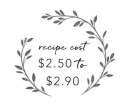

recipe cost $2.50 *to* $2.90

These simple glazed carrots make the perfect addition to any weeknight dinner.

1. In an electric pressure cooker, combine the carrots, orange juice, olive oil, and salt.

2. Place the lid on the cooker and make sure the vent valve is in the SEALING position. Using the display panel, select the MANUAL/PRESSURE COOK function and HIGH PRESSURE. Use the +/− buttons until the display reads 2 minutes.

3. When the cooker beeps, switch the vent valve from the SEALING to the VENTING position, administering a quick release. Use caution while the steam escapes.

4. Remove the lid and using the display panel, press the CANCEL button, then select the SAUTÉ function. Cook, stirring occasionally, allowing the carrots to caramelize, about 5 minutes.

5. Transfer the carrots to a serving dish. Season with additional salt to taste, if desired.

6. Top with walnuts and chives.

SERVES 4

1 pound carrots, peeled, halved, and cut into 2-inch pieces (see Note page 51)

2 tablespoons fresh orange juice

4½ teaspoons extra-virgin olive oil

¼ teaspoon fine sea salt, plus more to taste

½ cup chopped raw walnuts

2 tablespoons finely chopped fresh chives

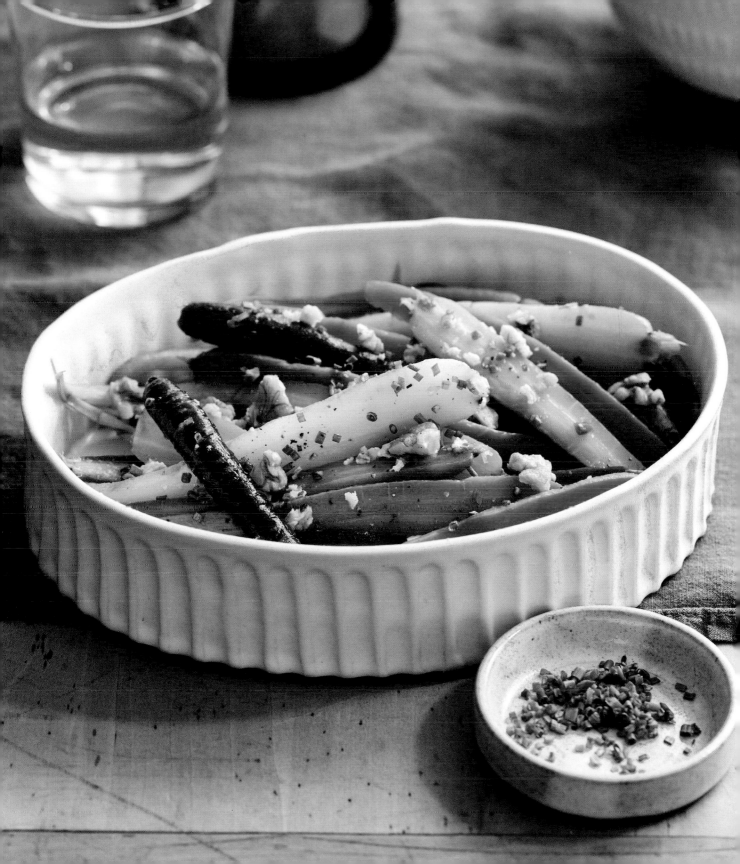

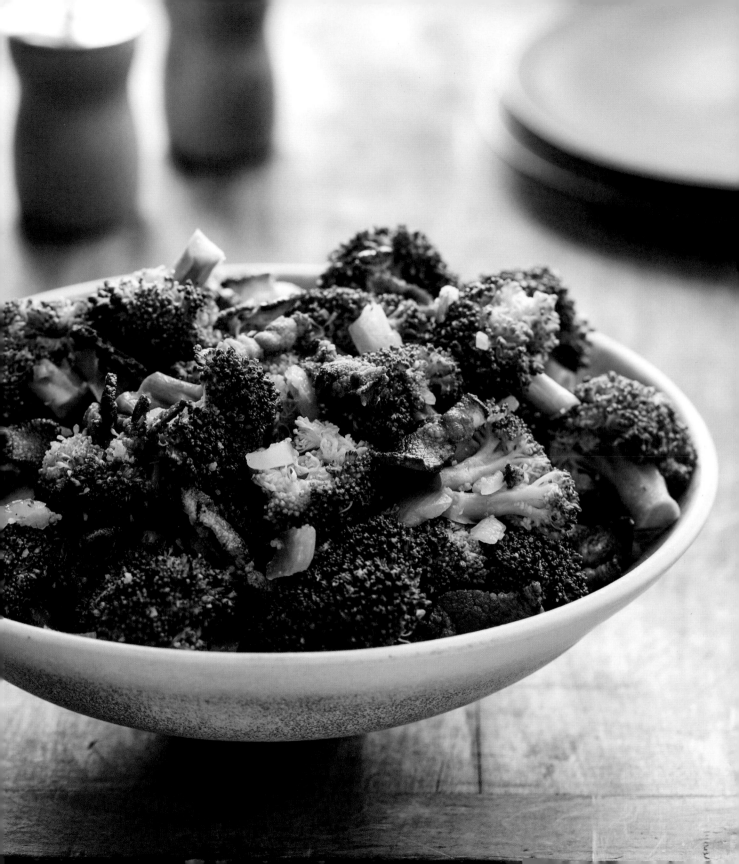

BACON *and* BROCCOLI

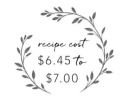

recipe cost $6.45 *to* $7.00

Do I even need to explain this one? I feel like anything with bacon in the title is an automatic home run. Might as well call this "World Series Champ Broccoli"!

SERVES 4

1½ teaspoons extra-virgin olive oil

4 strips nitrate-free bacon, diced

½ yellow onion, diced

1 pound fresh or frozen broccoli florets

¼ cup water

1 tablespoon dried minced onion

1 teaspoon fine sea salt

½ teaspoon garlic powder

½ teaspoon onion powder

1. Preheat an electric pressure cooker using the SAUTÉ function and adjust the heat to MORE (see Note page 95). When the display reads HOT, add the olive oil, bacon, and yellow onion. Cook, stirring occasionally, until the bacon is crisp, about 10 minutes. Transfer the bacon to a paper towel–lined plate.

2. Add the broccoli, water, dried onion, salt, garlic powder, and onion powder. Stir to combine.

3. Place the lid on the cooker and make sure the vent valve is in the SEALING position. Using the display panel, press the CANCEL button to turn off the SAUTÉ function, then select the STEAM function and LOW PRESSURE. Use the +/− buttons until the display reads 1 minute.

4. When the cooker beeps, switch the vent valve from the SEALING to the VENTING position. Use caution while the steam escapes.

5. Using a slotted spoon, remove the broccoli from the cooker. Top with bacon.

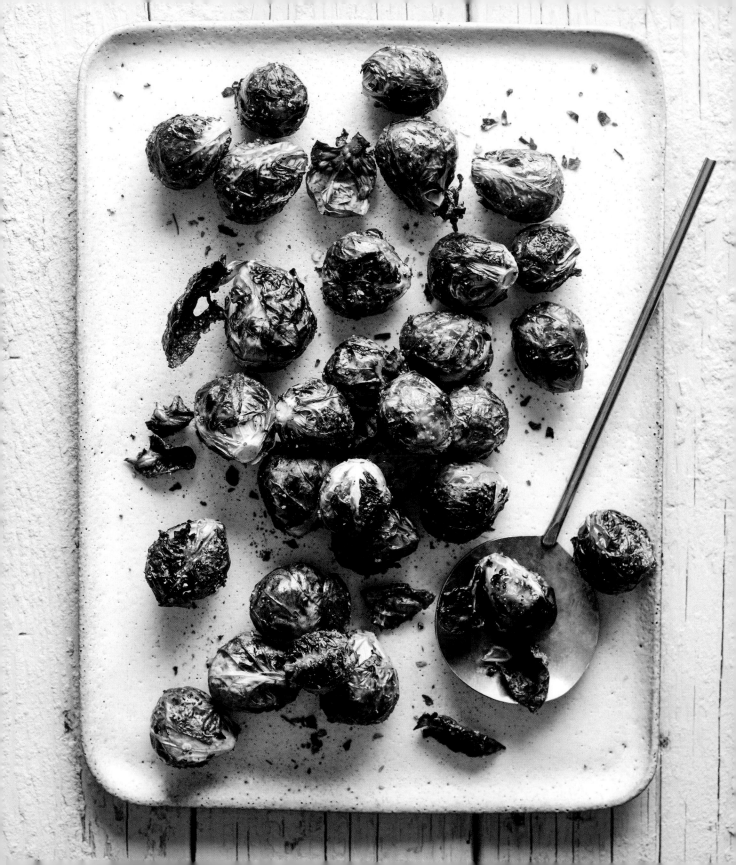

ZESTY ITALIAN BRUSSELS SPROUTS

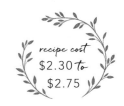

recipe cost
$2.30 *to*
$2.75

Four years ago, there was no vegetable I hated more than Brussels sprouts. It didn't matter how they were prepared, they always tasted overwhelmingly bitter to me. Thank the Lord for regenerating taste buds, though, because over the course of a year—while changing my diet—I fell in love with Brussels sprouts. They remain one of my favorite greens today.

SERVES 4

1 pound frozen Brussels sprouts

1 tablespoon extra-virgin olive oil

1 tablespoon Italian seasoning

1 teaspoon fresh lemon juice

½ teaspoon fine sea salt

½ teaspoon garlic powder

¼ teaspoon ground black pepper

1. In a large bowl, combine the Brussels sprouts, olive oil, Italian seasoning, lemon juice, salt, garlic powder, and black pepper. Stir well to coat.

2. Arrange the Brussels sprouts in a 5.3-quart air-fryer basket and bake at 370°F for 15 minutes.

NOTE: If you do not have an air fryer, these can be baked in a conventional oven at 400°F for 30 minutes, tossing every 10 minutes. Serve hot.

THE SIMPLEST COLLARD GREENS

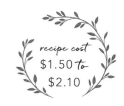

recipe cost
$1.50 to
$2.10

Collard greens are a giant in the healthy greens category, with 18 percent more calcium per serving than kale and double the amount of protein and iron. This is definitely a leafy green you want to incorporate into your diet! If you can't find collard greens in the grocery store, you can sub them 1:1 with kale in this recipe.

SERVES 4

1 large bunch collard greens (about 10 ounces), stems and ribs removed

2 teaspoons extra-virgin olive oil

½ cup low-sodium chicken broth or Vegetable Broth (page 332)

1 teaspoon fine sea salt

1 tablespoon fresh lemon juice

¼ teaspoon red pepper flakes

1. Stack the collard greens, roll them up, and thinly slice.

2. Preheat an electric pressure cooker using the SAUTÉ function and adjust the heat to NORMAL (see Note).

3. When the display reads HOT, add the olive oil and collard greens. Cook, stirring frequently, until the greens begin to wilt, about 3 minutes. Stir in the broth, salt, lemon juice, and red pepper flakes.

4. Place the lid on your pressure cooker and make sure the vent valve is in the SEALING position.

5. Using the display panel, press the CANCEL button to turn off the SAUTÉ function, then select the MANUAL/PRESSURE COOK function and HIGH PRESSURE. Use the +/− buttons until the display reads 5 minutes.

6. When the cooker beeps, switch the vent valve from the SEALING to the VENTING position, administering a quick release. Use caution while the steam escapes.

NOTE: Your cooker might not have and ADJUST button; if that is the case, just press the SAUTÉ button until NORMAL is highlighted.

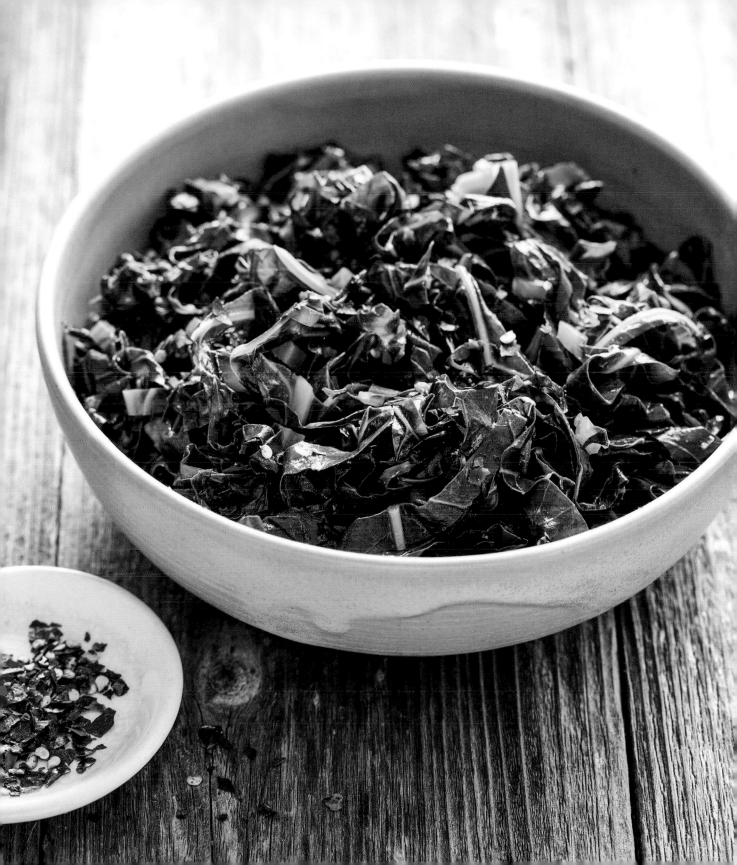

GARLIC-CHIVE MASHED POTATOES

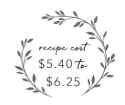

I don't believe potatoes should be done anywhere but in an electric pressure cooker. You won't believe how perfectly creamy they are! I'm sure we've all experienced Thanksgiving dinners where we're lassoed to the stove for hours watching an insane amount of potatoes come to boil. Let me help simplify your life and save you some time: Just make them in your pressure cooker!

SERVES 4 TO 6

1 cup water

2 pounds russet potatoes, peeled and cut into 1-inch pieces

½ cup Oat Milk (page 288) or other milk

3 tablespoons ghee or extra-virgin olive oil

1 teaspoon fine sea salt

½ teaspoon garlic powder

½ teaspoon ground black pepper

3 tablespoons finely chopped fresh chives

1. Pour the water into an electric pressure cooker and place a trivet or steamer basket inside.

2. Set the potatoes on the trivet or steamer basket.

3. Place the lid on the cooker and make sure the vent valve is in the SEALING position. Using the display panel, select the STEAM function and HIGH PRESSURE. Use the +/− buttons until the display reads 8 minutes.

4. When the cooker beeps, switch the vent valve from the SEALING to the VENTING position, administering a quick release. Use caution while the steam escapes.

5. Using a slotted spoon, transfer the potatoes from the cooker to a large bowl. Add the oat milk, ghee, salt, garlic powder, and black pepper. Using a potato masher, mash the potatoes until smooth.

6. Top with chives and serve hot.

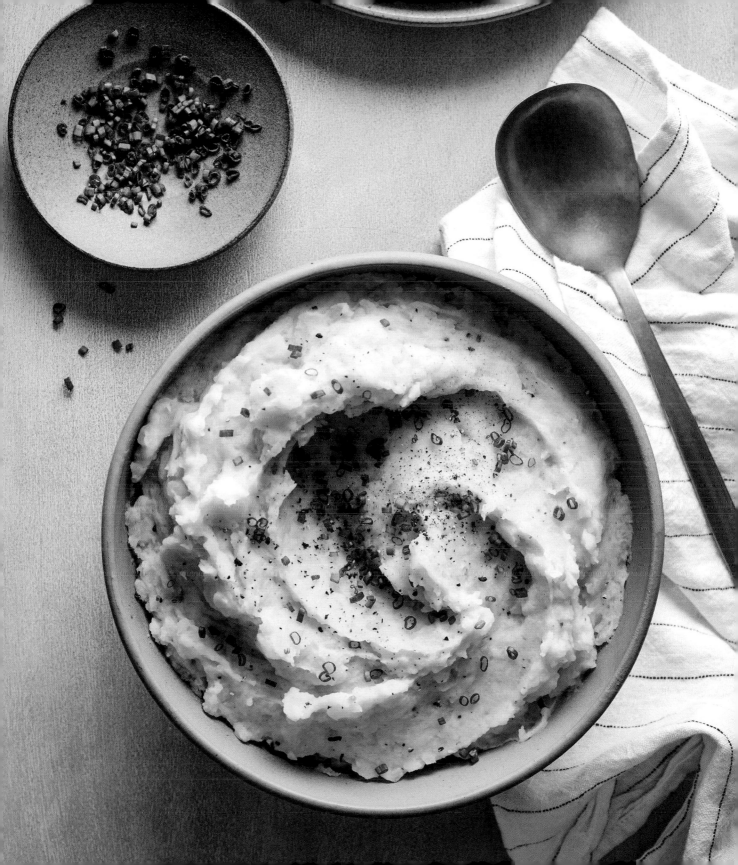

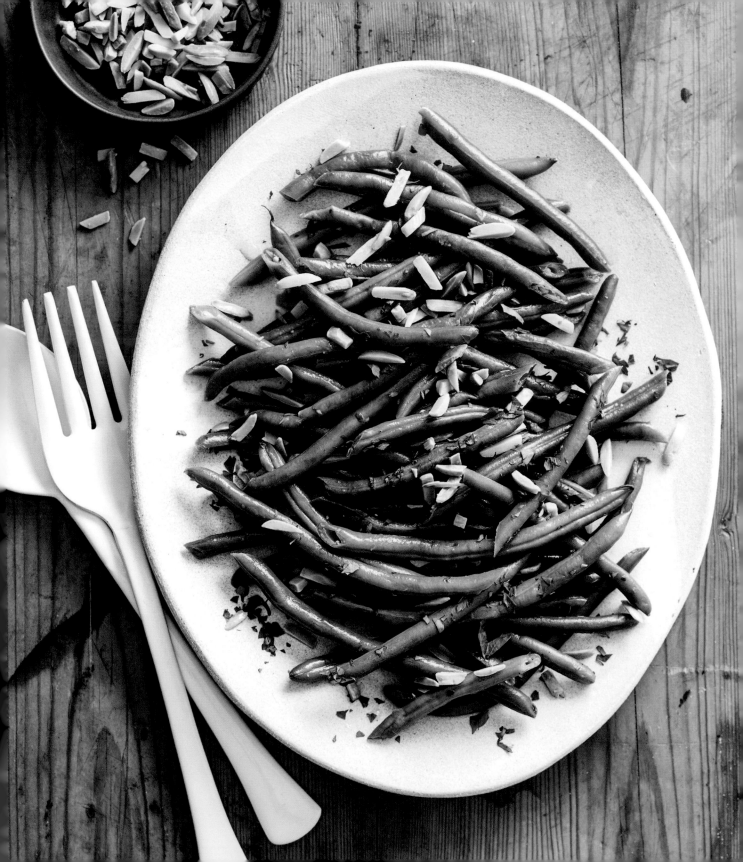

GREEN BEANS AMANDINE

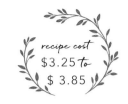

This side is light and fresh, yielding perfectly tender green beans. *Amandine* is a French culinary term that means garnished with almonds. The toasted almonds certainly elevate the beans, but if you have a nut allergy, you can omit them or use toasted pumpkin seeds or Toasted Acorn Squash Seeds (page 272) for a little crunch!

SERVES 4 TO 6

2 tablespoons extra-virgin olive oil

½ cup slivered almonds

¼ cup low-sodium chicken broth or Vegetable Broth (page 332)

1 pound green beans, trimmed

2 teaspoons fresh lemon juice

¾ teaspoon fine sea salt

¼ teaspoon ground black pepper

2 tablespoons chopped fresh parsley leaves

1. Preheat an electric pressure cooker using the SAUTÉ function and adjust the heat to NORMAL (see Note page 182).

2. When the display reads HOT, add the olive oil and slivered almonds. Toast the almonds, stirring frequently, until they begin to turn golden, about 3 minutes. Using a slotted spoon, transfer the almonds from the cooker to a paper towel–lined plate.

3. Using the display panel, select the CANCEL button to turn off the SAUTÉ function. Add the broth, green beans, lemon juice, salt, and black pepper.

4. Place the lid on the cooker and make sure the vent valve is in the SEALING position. Using the display panel, select the MANUAL/PRESSURE COOK function and HIGH PRESSURE. Use the +/− buttons until the display reads 5 minutes.

5. When the cooker beeps, switch the vent valve from the SEALING to the VENTING position, administering a quick release. Use caution while the steam escapes.

6. Remove the lid. Using a slotted spoon, transfer the green beans from the cooker to a serving dish. Sprinkle with the toasted almonds and parsley and serve.

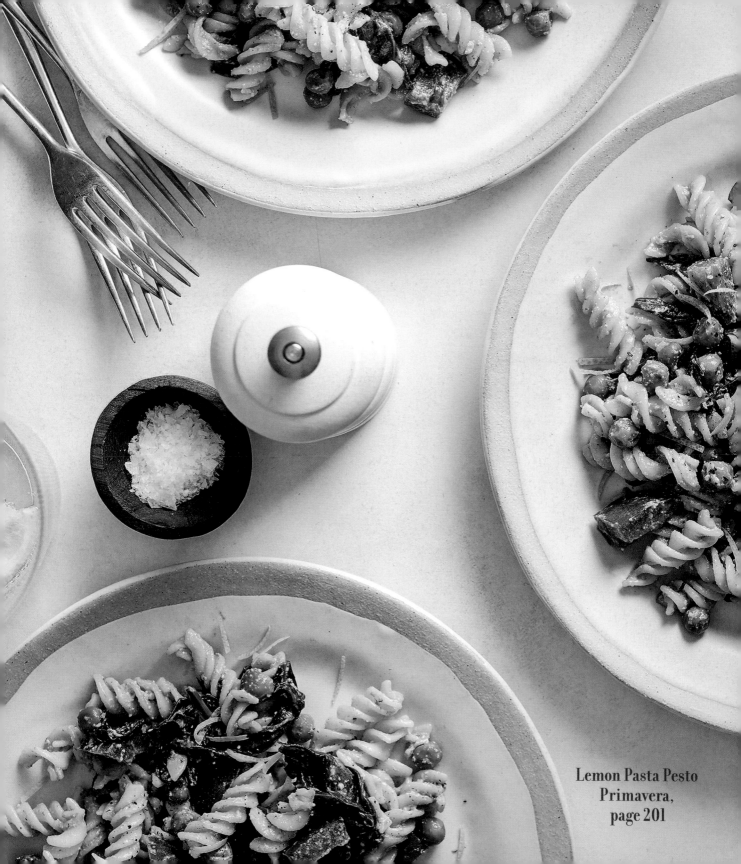

Lemon Pasta Pesto
Primavera,
page 201

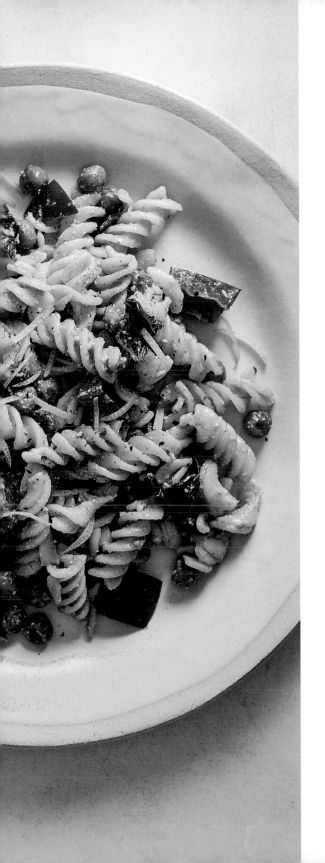

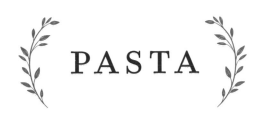

PASTA

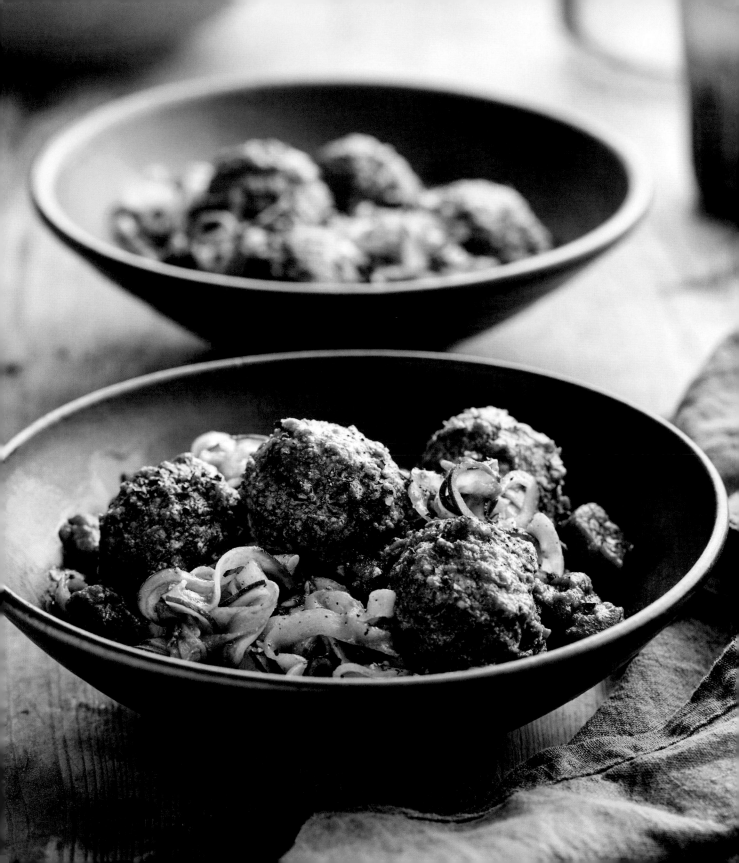

ZUCCHINI SPAGHETTI *with* MEATBALLS

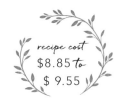

This classic Italian sauce with meatballs is a lightened up take on a family favorite! When cooked, zucchini can release a lot of moisture. If that bothers you, omit the zucchini from the cooker and instead serve the sauce and meatballs over the uncooked zucchini. The warmth from the sauce will cook it just a touch, making it perfectly al dente.

Kid Tip: Cook a little traditional pasta and serve the zucchini, pasta sauce, and meatballs on top so it's not a radical change for children who aren't used to vegetable noodles.

SERVES 4

1 pound lean ground beef

1 large egg

1 teaspoon fine sea salt

¾ teaspoon garlic powder

1¾ teaspoons dried oregano

¼ teaspoon dried rosemary

¼ teaspoon dried thyme

¼ teaspoon ground black pepper

2 (15-ounce) cans crushed tomatoes

½ large yellow onion, diced

2 cloves garlic, minced

1½ teaspoons dried basil

1 teaspoon red pepper flakes (optional)

1 tablespoon extra-virgin olive oil

3 large zucchini, spiralized (see Note)

1. In a large bowl, combine the ground beef, egg, ½ teaspoon of the salt, ¼ teaspoon of the garlic powder, ¼ teaspoon of the oregano, rosemary, thyme, and black pepper. Divide the mixture into 16 equal portions and roll into balls.

2. Preheat an electric pressure cooker using the SAUTÉ function and adjust the heat to MORE (see Note page 95).

3. While the cooker preheats, in a medium bowl, combine the tomatoes, onion, garlic, remaining ½ teaspoon salt, remaining 1½ teaspoons oregano, basil, remaining ½ teaspoon garlic powder, red pepper flakes, if using. Stir to combine.

4. When the display panel reads HOT, add the olive oil and meatballs. Let the bottoms of the meatballs brown, about 3 minutes. Add the zucchini noodles on top of the meatballs, followed by the tomato sauce.

5. Place the lid on the cooker and make sure the vent valve is in the SEALING position. Using the display panel, select the MANUAL/PRESSURE COOK function and HIGH PRESSURE. Use the +/− buttons until the display reads 5 minutes.

6. When the cooker beeps, switch the vent valve from the SEALING to the VENTING position, administering a quick release. Use caution while the steam escapes. Serve immediately.

NOTE: After you spiralize zucchini, you will be left with the long center core—do not throw it away. Just chop it up and mix it in.

CREAMY KALE *and* TOMATO PASTA

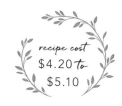

recipe cost
$4.20 *to*
$5.10

Make sure that there are people around to feast with when you make this creamy pasta! It's highly addictive, and only gets better the longer it sits. Gluten-free pasta can be outrageously expensive at health food stores, but Walmart and other markets have started releasing their own brand of gluten-free treats. Look for Walmart's Great Value brown rice gluten-free pasta, or check out their gluten-free section for other budget-friendly brands—Jovial and Ancient Harvest are two of my favorites.

SERVES 4

1 tablespoon extra-virgin olive oil

2 cups shredded kale (ribs removed)

2 cups halved grape tomatoes

½ medium yellow onion, diced

3 cloves garlic, minced

10 ounces gluten-free penne pasta

2 cups Vegetable Broth (page 332) or store-bought

1 cup almond milk or other milk (see page 288)

1 teaspoon fine sea salt

¼ teaspoon garlic powder

¼ teaspoon ground black pepper

1. Preheat an electric pressure cooker using the SAUTÉ function and adjust the heat to MORE (see Note page 95). When the display panel reads HOT, add the olive oil, kale, tomatoes, and onion. Cook, stirring occasionally, until the onion softens and is translucent, about 3 minutes. Stir in the garlic.

2. Add the penne, broth, almond milk, salt, garlic powder, and black pepper and stir to combine. Place the lid on the cooker and make sure the vent valve is in the SEALING position. Using the display panel, press the CANCEL button to turn off the SAUTÉ function, then select the MANUAL/PRESS COOK function and HIGH PRESSURE. Use the +/− buttons until the display reads 6 minutes.

3. When the cooker beeps, switch the vent valve from the SEALING to the VENTING position, administering a quick release. Use caution while the steam escapes.

4. Let stand for 10 minutes before serving to allow the sauce to thicken. Serve warm.

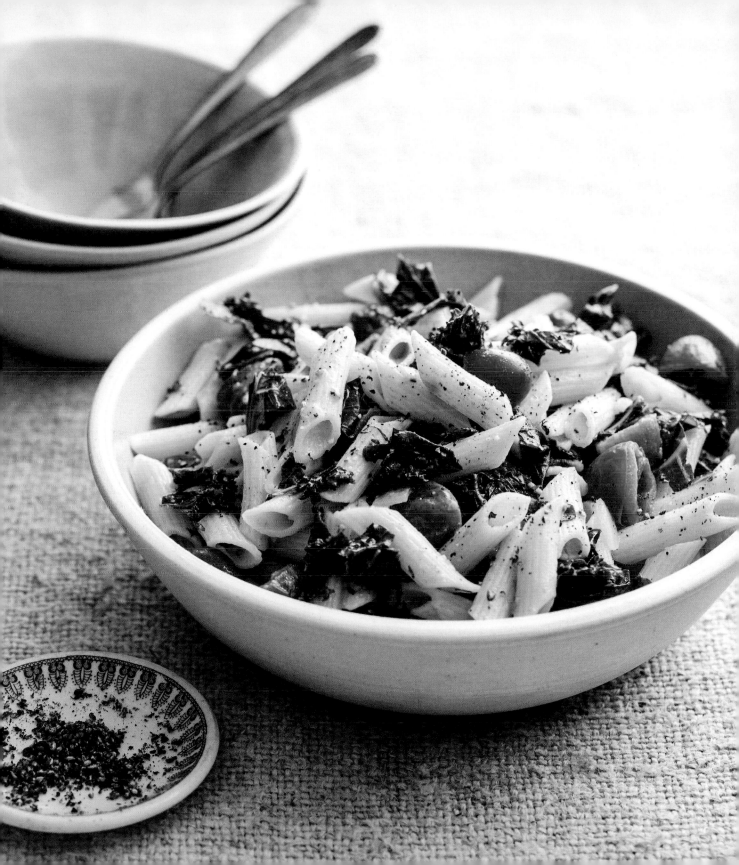

SAUSAGE PIZZA PASTA

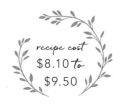

recipe cost
$8.10 *to* $9.50

This recipe came about by unusual means. A friend of mine challenged me to create a new dish for dinner using the meager ingredients I had on hand, and this is what I threw together. (You can watch the full video on the Instant Loss YouTube channel.) Honestly, I was not expecting it to turn out as good as it did. It tastes just like pizza topped with Italian sausage, but in pasta form. This is a fun, family-friendly dish that comes together in a hurry!

SERVES 6

- 1 pound ground Italian-style pork sausage
- 1 large yellow onion, diced
- 2 teaspoons garlic powder
- 2 teaspoons dried minced onion
- 1½ teaspoons fine sea salt
- ¾ teaspoon ground black pepper
- ⅛ teaspoon red pepper flakes
- 12 ounces gluten-free brown rice penne pasta
- 1½ cups water
- 1 (15-ounce) can tomato sauce
- 1 (15-ounce) can diced tomatoes
- ¼ cup chopped fresh basil (optional)

1. Preheat an electric pressure cooker using the SAUTÉ function and adjust the heat to MORE (see Note page 95).

2. When the display panel reads HOT, add the sausage and onion. Cook, stirring occasionally, until the onion is translucent, about 5 minutes. Add the garlic powder, dried onion, salt, black pepper, and red pepper flakes. Stir to combine.

3. Add the pasta, water, tomato sauce, and tomatoes. Do not stir. Place the lid on the cooker and make sure the vent valve is in the SEALING position. Using the display panel, select the MANUAL/PRESSURE COOK function and HIGH PRESSURE. Use the +/− buttons until the display reads 6 minutes.

4. When the cooker beeps, switch the vent valve from the SEALING to the VENTING position, administering a quick release. Use caution while the steam escapes.

5. Stir to combine. Garnish with basil, if desired.

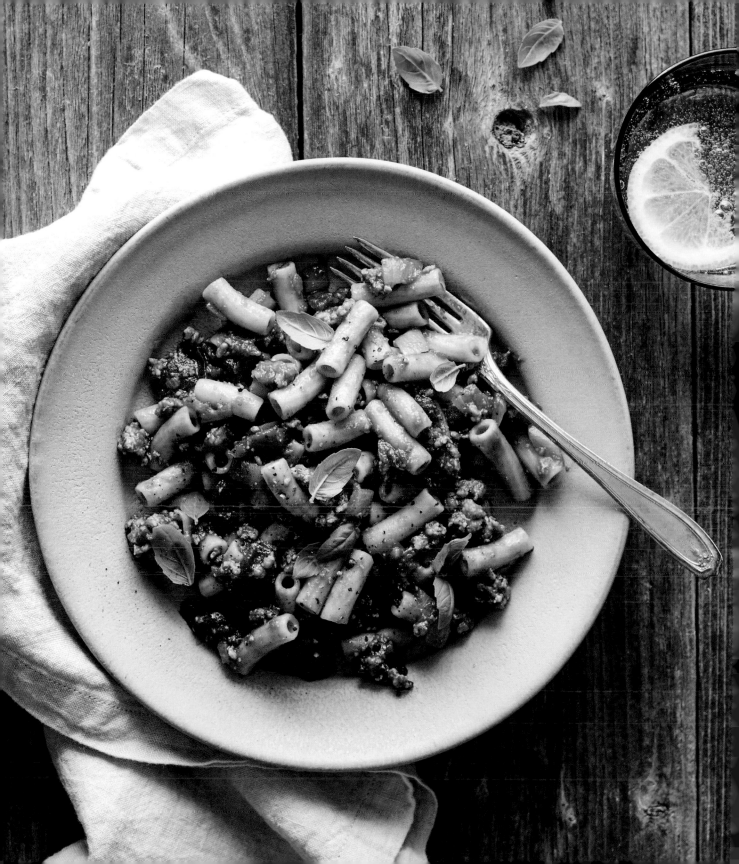

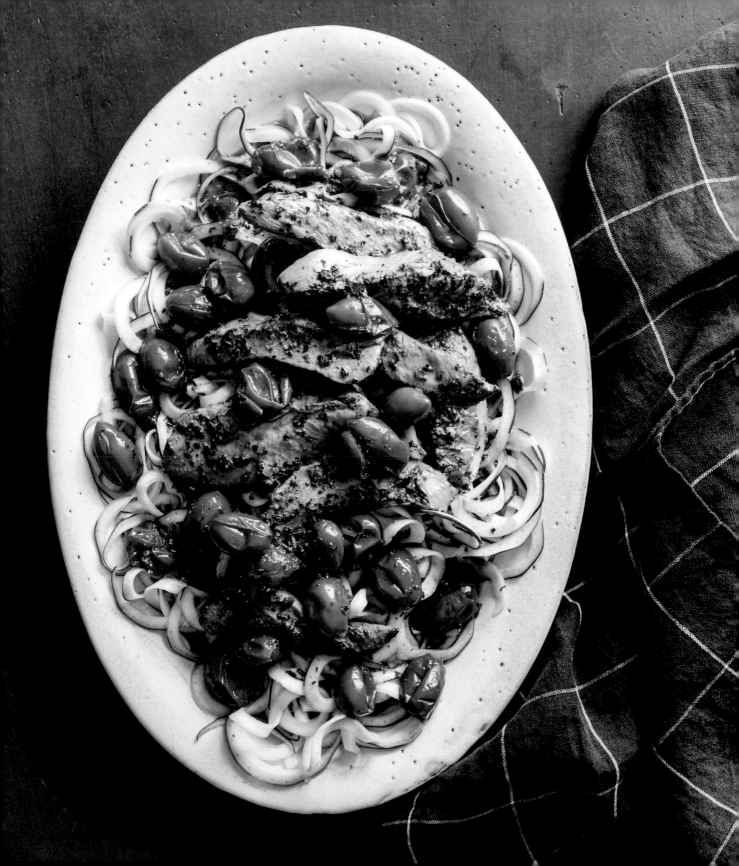

BALSAMIC-DIJON CHICKEN *over* ZUCCHINI NOODLES

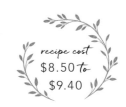

recipe cost
$8.50 *to* $9.40

This is one of my favorite weeknight dinners—rich in tangy herbal flavor, it is one of the most beloved recipes on my website, InstantLoss.com. You can also use boneless chicken breasts or thighs in this recipe. Pick up whatever is on sale this week—you can't go wrong!

SERVES 4

1 pound boneless, skinless chicken tenders

1 tablespoon extra-virgin olive oil

1 tablespoon balsamic vinegar

1 tablespoon Dijon mustard

1 tablespoon dried basil

1 teaspoon fine sea salt

½ teaspoon lemon pepper

½ teaspoon garlic powder

½ teaspoon dried minced onion

2 cups cherry tomatoes

½ cup low-sodium chicken broth or Bone Broth (page 331)

2 large zucchini, spiralized (see Note page 51)

1. Preheat an electric pressure cooker using the SAUTÉ function and adjust the heat to MORE (see Note page 95).

2. In a medium bowl, combine the chicken, olive oil, vinegar, mustard, basil, salt, lemon pepper, garlic powder, and dried onion. Stir well to coat.

3. When the display panel reads HOT, add the chicken and cook for 2 minutes on each side. Stir in the tomatoes and broth.

4. Place the lid on the cooker and make sure the vent valve is in the SEALING position. Using the display panel, select the MANUAL/PRESSURE COOK function and HIGH PRESSURE. Use the +/− buttons until the display reads 5 minutes. Divide the zucchini noodles among four plates.

5. When the cooker beeps, let it naturally release the pressure until the display reads LO:05. Switch the vent valve from the SEALING to the VENTING position. Use caution while the steam escapes.

6. Top the zucchini noodles with the chicken and tomatoes. Spoon the sauce from the cooker over the top. The heat from the sauce will cook the noodles just a touch, making them perfectly al dente.

LEMON-PEPPER CHICKEN *with* ASPARAGUS

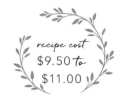

recipe cost
$9.50 *to*
$11.00

The spaghetti squash can be premade and reheated for this recipe so you don't have to cook two things at once—although this is where having two pressure cookers comes in handy!

SERVES 4

1 tablespoon extra-virgin olive oil

1 pound boneless, skinless chicken breasts, cut into bite-size pieces

3 cloves garlic, minced

2 teaspoons lemon pepper

½ teaspoon fine sea salt

¼ teaspoon ground black pepper

⅓ cup low-sodium chicken broth or Bone Broth (page 331)

2 teaspoons freshly grated lemon zest

1 tablespoon fresh lemon juice

12 ounces pencil-thin asparagus, trimmed and cut into thirds

2 teaspoons arrowroot powder

½ recipe Spaghetti Squash (page 333)

2 tablespoons thinly sliced fresh lemongrass (optional)

1. Preheat an electric pressure cooker using the SAUTÉ function and adjust the heat to MORE (see Note page 95).

2. When the display panel reads HOT, add the olive oil, chicken, garlic, lemon pepper, salt, and black pepper. Stir to combine. Cook, stirring infrequently, until the chicken is browned, about 3 minutes. Add the broth, lemon zest, and lemon juice.

3. Place the lid on the cooker and make sure the vent valve is in the SEALING position. Using the display panel, select the MANUAL/PRESSURE COOK function and HIGH PRESSURE. Use the +/− buttons until the display reads 3 minutes.

4. When the cooker beeps, let it naturally release the pressure until the display reads LO:05. Switch the vent valve from the SEALING to the VENTING position. Use caution while the steam escapes.

5. Using the display panel, press the CANCEL button, then select the SAUTÉ function and adjust the heat to MORE (see Note page 95). Stir in the asparagus and arrowroot powder and cook until the asparagus is tender and the sauce thickens, about 5 minutes.

6. Serve warm over spaghetti squash and sprinkle with lemongrass, if desired.

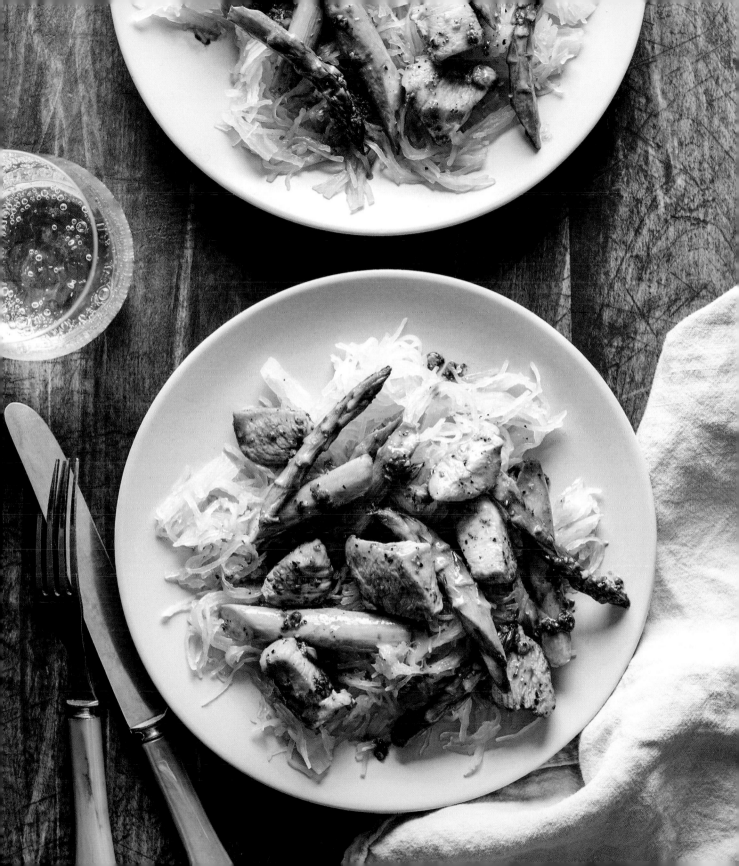

TUNA-NOODLE CASSEROLE

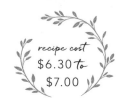

recipe cost
$6.30 *to*
$7.00

This is a magical time-saving dish! Simply toss all of the ingredients together and transfer them to a dish that fits inside your pressure cooker. Make sure the dish is plenty deep—the mixture will fill it all the way to the top. I use a Nordic Ware 7-inch springform pan. It's actually 7½-inches in diameter, including the base, and 3 inches tall.

SERVES 4

2 cups Cream of Mushroom Soup Base (page 145)

1¼ cups low-sodium chicken broth or Bone Broth (page 331)

2 (5-ounce) cans wild-caught solid tuna, drained

8 ounces gluten-free pasta, such as rotini or penne

1 cup frozen peas

1½ teaspoons dried parsley flakes

1½ teaspoons dried minced onion

¾ teaspoon fine sea salt

¼ teaspoon ground black pepper

½ teaspoon garlic powder

1 cup water

½ cup Sweet Heat Crunchy Chickpeas (page 118, optional)

1. In a large bowl, combine the soup base, broth, tuna, pasta, peas, parsley, dried onion, salt, black pepper, and garlic powder. Stir to combine. Transfer the mixture to a deep 7-inch round baking dish. Cover with foil.

2. Pour the water into the cooker. Set the dish on a trivet and carefully lower the trivet and dish into the cooker.

3. Place the lid on the cooker and make sure the vent valve is in the SEALING position. Using the display panel, select the MANUAL/PRESSURE COOK function and HIGH PRESSURE. Use the +/− buttons until the display reads 6 minutes.

4. While the pasta cooks, place the chickpeas in a resealable plastic bag. Using the bottom of a glass, crush the chickpeas until they resemble breadcrumbs.

5. When the cooker beeps, switch the vent valve from the SEALING to the VENTING position, administering a quick release. Use caution while the steam escapes.

6. Remove the foil. Stir the pasta and top with the crushed chickpeas.

LEMON PASTA PESTO PRIMAVERA

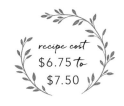

recipe cost
$6.75 *to*
$7.50

The off-brand of sriracha from Trader Joe's is just a little cheaper than traditional sriracha and works just as well with this pasta. Don't let the sriracha keep you from making the recipe. It doesn't make the dish spicy, rather, it adds the perfect little flavor boost.

SERVES 4

FOR THE PASTA

8 ounces gluten-free pasta, such as penne or rotini

3 cups water

¾ teaspoon fine sea salt

2 cups packed baby spinach

1 cup frozen peas

2 Roma tomatoes, cored and diced

1 tablespoon fresh grated lemon zest

1 teaspoon sriracha

FOR THE PESTO

1½ cups tightly packed fresh basil leaves

½ cup raw cashews or pine nuts

½ cup extra-virgin olive oil

2 tablespoons fresh lemon juice

2 tablespoons unfortified nutritional yeast

¼ teaspoon fine sea salt

½ teaspoon garlic powder

¼ teaspoon ground black pepper

1. **MAKE THE PASTA:** In an electric pressure cooker, combine the pasta, water, and ½ teaspoon of the salt.

2. Place the lid on the cooker and make sure the vent valve is in the SEALING position. Using the display panel, select the MANUAL/PRESSURE COOK function and HIGH PRESSURE. Use the +/− buttons until the display reads 6 minutes.

3. **MAKE THE PESTO:** While the pasta cooks, in a high-powered blender or food processor, combine the basil, cashews, olive oil, lemon juice, nutritional yeast, salt, garlic powder, and black pepper. Blend or process until smooth and creamy.

4. When the cooker beeps, switch the vent valve from the SEALING to the VENTING position, administering a quick release. Use caution while the steam escapes.

5. Drain the pasta and return to the cooker. Stir in the pesto, spinach, peas, tomatoes, lemon zest, remaining ¼ teaspoon salt, and sriracha. Place the lid back on the cooker and let warm for 3 minutes before serving.

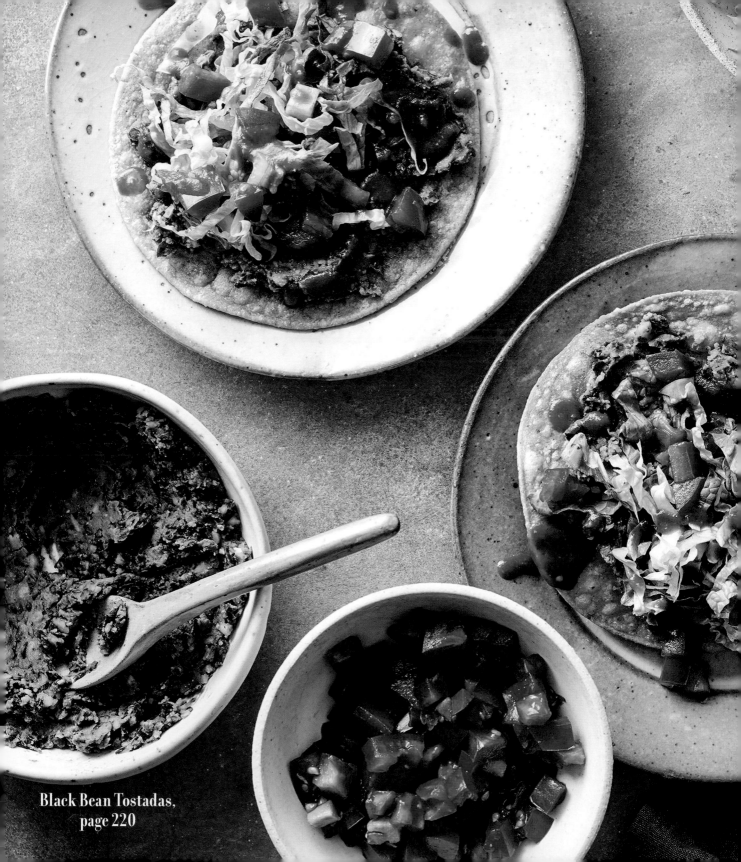

Black Bean Tostadas,
page 220

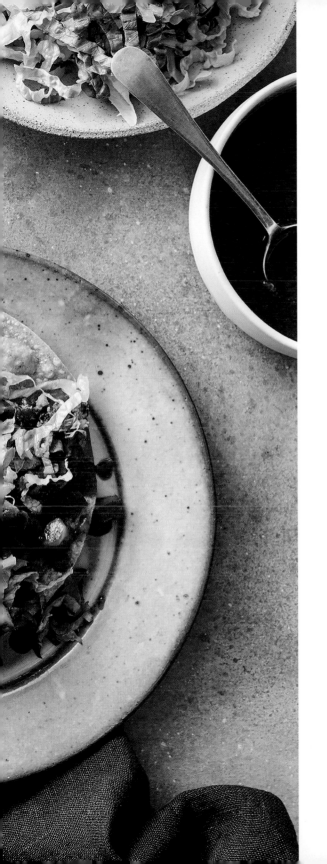

 # RESTAURANT FAVORITES

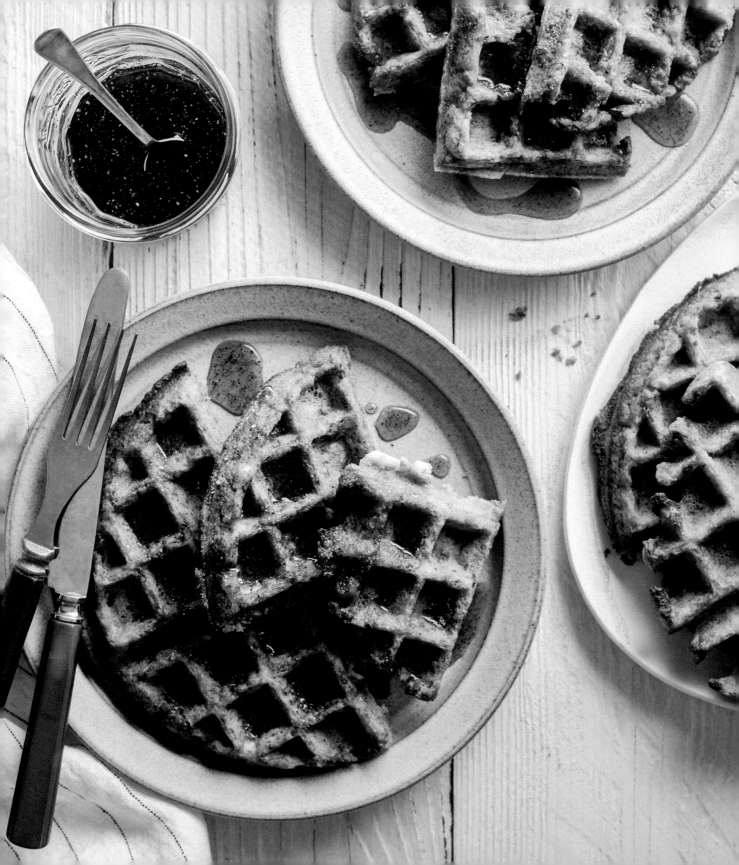

SAVORY GARLIC-HERB CHICKEN WAFFLES *with* MAPLE-CHILI SYRUP

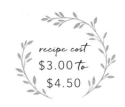

recipe cost
$3.00 *to*
$4.50

I really wanted to include a recipe for chicken and waffles in this book, but I'm not about to invest so much time on breakfast. Dredging the chicken, frying the chicken, making the batter, making the waffles. So. Much. Work. Y'all know I enjoy simplifying things, so I simplified! Instead of making the dishes separately, I combined them! The chicken is *inside* the waffle, making this a chicken waffle! Drizzle it with the Maple-Chili Syrup for a real treat. I use the Dash Mini Maker Waffle Maker, which you can buy for less than $10 from Amazon or Target.

MAKES 12 MINI OR 4 REGULAR-SIZE WAFFLES

FOR THE CHICKEN

1 cup cooked and shredded unseasoned chicken breast

2 teaspoons extra-virgin olive oil

½ teaspoon fine sea salt

½ teaspoon garlic powder

½ teaspoon dried rosemary

FOR THE WAFFLES

1 cup gluten-free old-fashioned rolled oats

½ cup coconut flour

1 large egg

1 tablespoon extra-virgin olive oil

1 teaspoon apple cider vinegar

½ teaspoon baking soda

1½ teaspoons fine sea salt

2 cups water

Cooking oil spray

Maple-Chili Syrup (page 206)

1. **MAKE THE CHICKEN:** In a large bowl, combine the chicken, olive oil, salt, garlic powder, and rosemary. Stir to combine.

2. **MAKE THE WAFFLES:** In a high-powered blender, combine the rolled oats, flour, egg, olive oil, vinegar, baking soda, salt, and water. Blend on high until a smooth batter forms, about 1 minute. Pour the batter over the chicken and stir to combine.

3. Preheat a mini waffle maker according to the manufacturer's instructions. Once the griddle has preheated, spray it with cooking oil spray. Pour 3 tablespoons of the batter into the waffle maker and cook until golden and crispy, about 5 minutes. Repeat until all of the batter is used up.

4. Serve waffles with Maple-Chili Syrup.

5. To store, freeze in an airtight freezer bag for up to 6 months. Reheat in a toaster or toaster oven.

MAPLE-CHILI SYRUP

recipe cost
$0.70 to
$0.85

In a small bowl, combine the maple syrup, chili powder, and garlic powder. Stir to mix well.

MAKES ¼ CUP

¼ cup 100 percent pure maple syrup

¼ teaspoon chili powder

¼ teaspoon garlic powder

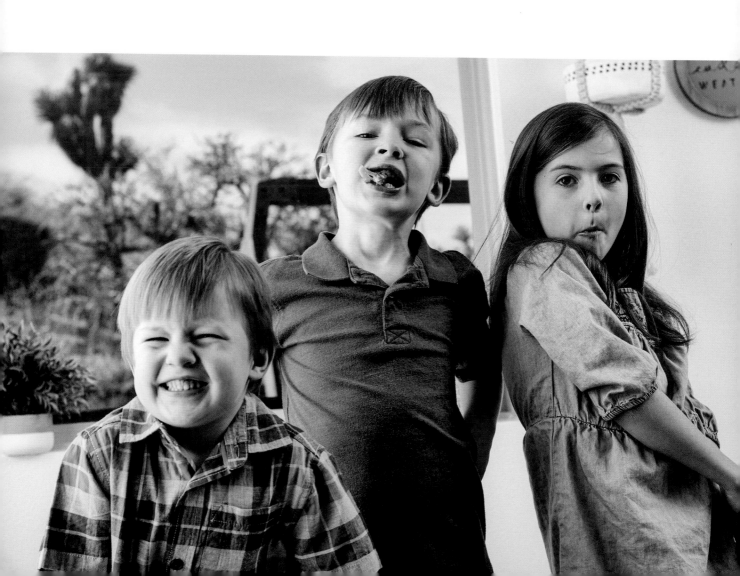

MIGAS

recipe cost
$6.45 *to*
$8.00

Migas—meaning "crumbs" in Spanish—is a dish I ate often while living in Texas. It is traditionally served with black beans, but it is mighty tasty on its own. It's like a breakfast-style tostada all crumbled up so you can eat it with a fork!

SERVES 6

12 large eggs

1 tablespoon unfortified nutritional yeast

1 tablespoon dried minced onion

1 teaspoon garlic powder

1 teaspoon fine sea salt

½ teaspoon paprika

¼ teaspoon ground cumin

¼ teaspoon ground black pepper

⅛ teaspoon turmeric

⅛ teaspoon cayenne pepper

¼ cup extra-virgin olive oil, plus more if needed

4 corn tortillas

1 medium red bell pepper, seeded and diced

1 medium jalapeño, seeded and diced

½ medium red onion, diced

1 large Roma tomato, cored and diced

¼ cup chopped fresh cilantro leaves

1 large avocado, pitted, peeled, and diced

1. In a large bowl, whisk together the eggs, nutritional yeast, dried onion, garlic powder, salt, paprika, cumin, black pepper, turmeric, and cayenne.

2. Heat a 12-inch pan over medium-high heat. Add the olive oil to the pan and let it warm. Working quickly, use tongs to place one corn tortilla in the oil, flip it immediately, then place on a paper towel–lined plate. Repeat until all the corn tortillas are warmed, stacking each tortilla on top of the one before. Cut each of the tortillas into 6 strips, then cut each strip into 6 pieces.

3. Add more oil to the pan, if necessary. Add the bell pepper, jalapeño, and red onion and cook until the vegetables are lightly charred, about 5 minutes. Add the tomato and tortillas and stir to combine.

4. Reduce the heat to low and add the egg mixture. Stir gently to mix with the vegetables and tortillas, gently folding the mixture occasionally, until eggs are cooked through.

5. Stir in the cilantro, top with the avocado, and serve hot.

BRITTANY'S CALIFORNIA BURGERS

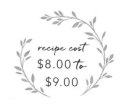

recipe cost
$8.00 to
$9.00

I'm a California girl, born and raised, and I will always have a soft spot for In-N-Out's protein-style burger. This isn't an exact replica, but it's pretty close and it will definitely hit the spot come burger night!

MAKES 8 BURGERS (SERVES 4)

FOR THE SPECIAL SAUCE

½ cup Homemade Mayo (page 330) or store-bought

3 tablespoons naturally sweetened ketchup

2 tablespoons organic sweet relish

1 teaspoon apple cider vinegar

⅛ teaspoon fine sea salt

FOR THE BURGERS

1 pound lean ground beef

1¼ teaspoons fine sea salt

1 teaspoon onion powder

½ teaspoon ground black pepper

5 tablespoons extra-virgin olive oil

1 large yellow onion, thinly sliced

1 large head butterhead lettuce

2 Roma tomatoes, cored and thinly sliced

16 organic sliced pickles, dill or sweet

1. **MAKE THE SAUCE:** In a small bowl, combine the mayonnaise, ketchup, relish, vinegar, and salt. Stir to combine. Chill until ready to serve.

2. **MAKE THE BURGERS:** Heat a cast-iron skillet over medium-high heat.

3. In a medium bowl, combine the ground beef, salt, onion powder, and black pepper. Gently mix the ingredients together; do not overwork the meat or it can become tough.

4. Divide the meat into 8 equal portions. Roll each portion into a ball. Lay a piece of parchment paper on the counter. Using your palm, flatten each ball into a large, very thin patty, about ¼ inch thick.

5. Add 1½ teaspoons olive oil to the skillet. Once the oil is hot, add one patty to the skillet and cook for 3 minutes on each side. Transfer the finished patty to a plate and cook each additional patty in the same fashion.

6. When the patties are cooked, cover and set aside. Add the remaining 1 tablespoon olive oil to the pan along with the onion. Cook the onion, stirring occasionally, until it is light brown in color, about 13 minutes.

7. For each burger, layer two lettuce leaves to form the bottom of the wrap. Place a patty on top and smear with the special sauce, then top with tomato, onion, and pickles. Place one lettuce leaf on top.

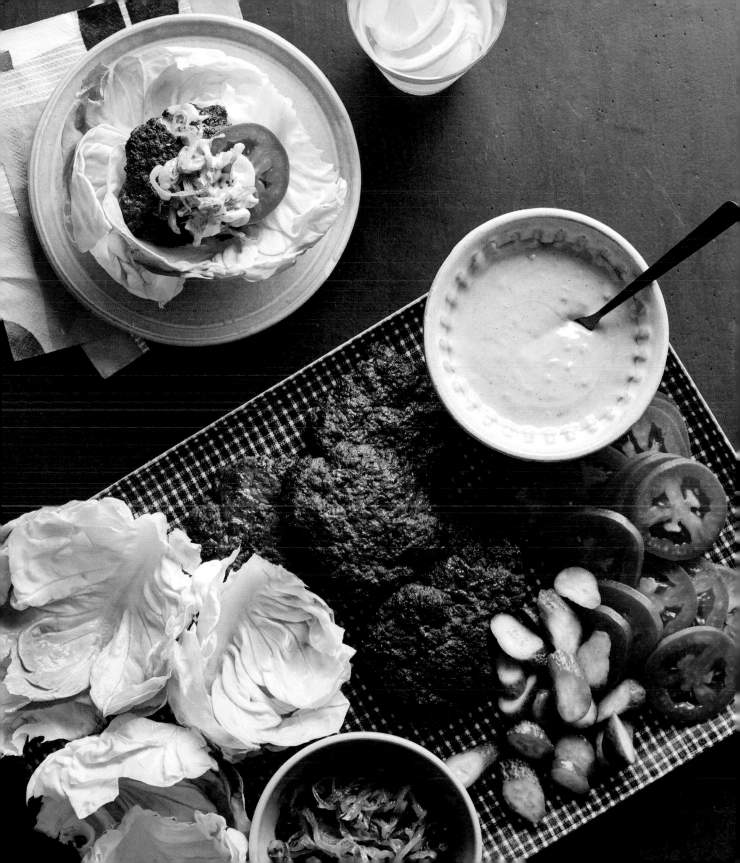

LOW-COUNTRY SHRIMP BOIL

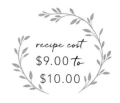

recipe cost
$9.00 to
$10.00

A classic Southern delight, this is a simple shrimp boil made in your pressure cooker! A time saver and a flavor enhancer, enjoy this dish with lemon wedges, olive oil or melted butter, and homemade tartar sauce or hot sauce!

SERVES 4

1½ pounds small red potatoes

½ pound smoked andouille sausage, sliced ½ inch thick diagonally

3 ears corn, husked and cut into thirds

2 bay leaves

1 tablespoon plus 2 teaspoons Old Bay seasoning or Cajun Seasoning (page 328) or store-bought

3 cups water

1 pound medium shrimp, deveined, shells left on

Tartar Sauce (page 212), for serving

Lemon wedges, extra-virgin olive oil, butter, cocktail sauce, and/or hot sauce, for serving

1. In an electric pressure cooker, combine the potatoes, sausage, corn, and bay leaves. In a medium bowl, stir together the 1 tablespoon Old Bay seasoning and water and add to the cooker.

2. Place the lid on the cooker and make sure the vent valve is in the SEALING position. Using the display panel, select the MANUAL/PRESSURE COOK function and HIGH PRESSURE. Use the +/− buttons until the display reads 5 minutes.

3. When the cooker beeps, switch the vent valve from the SEALING to the VENTING position, administering a quick release. Use caution while the steam escapes.

4. Add the shrimp and stir to combine. Sprinkle the 2 teaspoons Old Bay seasoning over the shrimp. Place the lid back on the cooker and let sit for 4 minutes to cook the shrimp in the residual heat.

5. Pour everything into a colander to drain, then transfer to a large serving platter or paper-lined table. Discard the bay leaves.

6. Serve with tartar sauce, lemon wedges, olive oil or butter, cocktail sauce, and/or hot sauce.

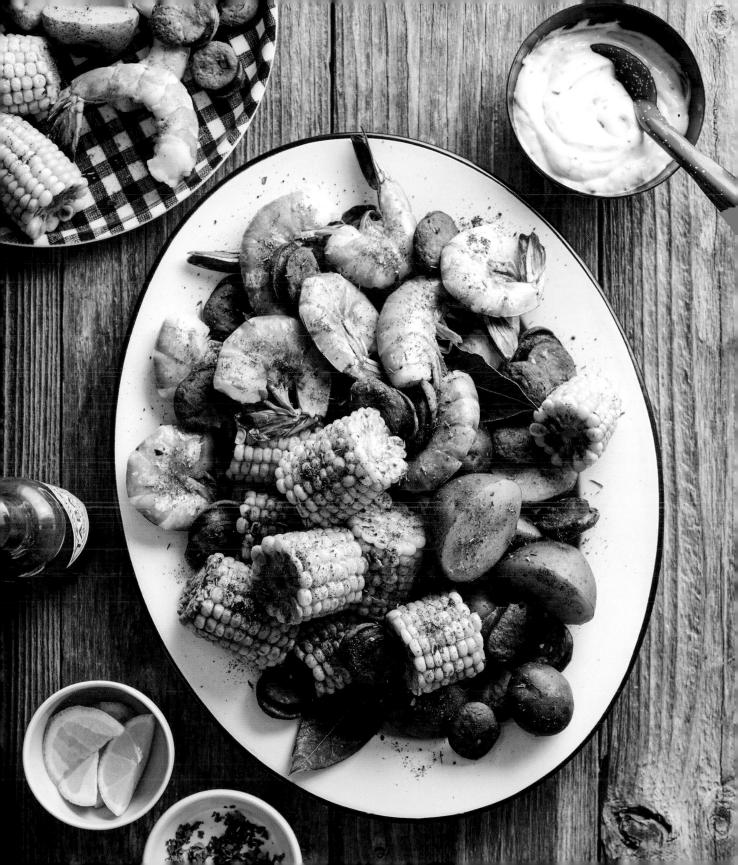

TARTAR SAUCE

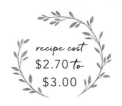

recipe cost $2.70 to $3.00

This is the perfect dairy-free tartar sauce to serve with a shrimp boil or your favorite fish and chips!

In a medium bowl, combine the mayonnaise, vinegar, parsley, dried onion, garlic powder, and salt. Use an immersion blender to puree until smooth. Cover and refrigerate until serving time.

MAKES 1 CUP

1 cup Homemade Mayo (page 330) or store-bought

1 tablespoon apple cider vinegar

¾ teaspoon dried parsley flakes

¾ teaspoon dried minced onion

¾ teaspoon garlic powder

¾ teaspoon fine sea salt

HONEY-GINGER CHICKEN

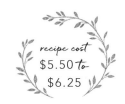

recipe cost
$5.50 *to*
$6.25

This is a great stir-fry for any night of the week! It cooks up quickly in your pressure cooker and is best served over rice with stir-fry vegetables or the Veggie Lo Mein on page 218.

SERVES 4

1 pound boneless, skinless chicken breasts, cut into bite-size pieces

1½ teaspoons extra-virgin olive oil

1 teaspoon toasted sesame oil

½ teaspoon fine sea salt

¼ teaspoon ground black pepper

2 tablespoons naturally sweetened ketchup

2 tablespoons raw honey

1 tablespoon coconut aminos

1 green onion, thinly sliced

1 tablespoon red wine vinegar

½ teaspoon grated fresh ginger

½ teaspoon garlic powder

1. In a large bowl, combine the chicken, olive oil, sesame oil, salt, and black pepper. Stir to coat.

2. Preheat an electric pressure cooker using the SAUTÉ function and adjust the heat to MORE (see Note page 95).

3. When the display panel reads HOT, add the chicken and cook, stirring occasionally, for about 6 minutes. Add the ketchup, honey, coconut aminos, green onion, vinegar, ginger, and garlic powder.

4. Place the lid on the cooker and make sure the vent valve is in the SEALING position. Using the display panel, select the MANUAL/PRESSURE COOK function and HIGH PRESSURE. Use the +/− buttons until the display reads 4 minutes.

5. When the cooker beeps, let it naturally release the pressure until the display reads LO:05. Switch the vent valve from the SEALING to the VENTING position. Use caution while the steam escapes.

6. Transfer the chicken and the sauce from the cooker to a serving plate. Let stand for 5 minutes to allow the sauce to thicken slightly before serving.

NOTE: Store fresh ginger in an airtight container in the freezer—it will keep for up to a year!

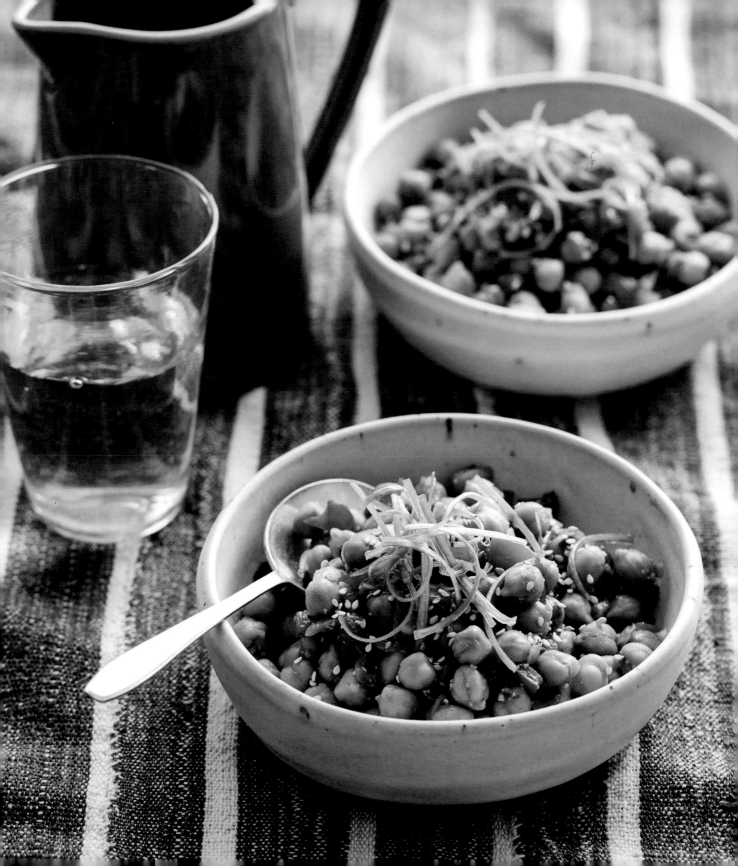

KUNG PAO CHICKPEAS

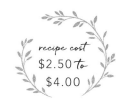

recipe cost
$2.50 to
$4.00

These little chickpeas pack a lot of punch. One of the most difficult things to do when I began eating well was weaning myself off of fast food. Recipes like this made it a lot easier!

SERVES 4

1 cup dried chickpeas

1¾ cups low-sodium chicken broth or Bone Broth (page 331)

1 red bell pepper, seeded and diced

½ yellow onion, diced

⅓ cup coconut aminos

2 tablespoons balsamic vinegar

2 tablespoons raw honey

1 teaspoon garlic powder

1 teaspoon red pepper flakes

1 teaspoon toasted sesame oil

½ teaspoon ground ginger

3 green onions, thinly sliced

1 teaspoon sesame seeds

1. Place the chickpeas in a large bowl and add water to cover by a couple of inches. Let them soak on the countertop, uncovered, for at least 4 hours or overnight. Rinse and drain.

2. In an electric pressure cooker, combine the broth, chickpeas, bell pepper, onion, coconut aminos, vinegar, honey, garlic powder, red pepper flakes, sesame oil, and ginger.

3. Place the lid on the cooker and make sure the vent valve is in the SEALING position. Using the display panel, select the MANUAL/PRESSURE COOK function and HIGH PRESSURE. Use the +/− buttons until the display reads 50 minutes.

4. When the cooker beeps, let it naturally release the pressure until the display reads LO:10. Switch the vent valve from the SEALING to the VENTING position. Use caution while the steam escapes.

5. Using the display panel, select the SAUTÉ function and adjust to NORMAL (see Note page 182). Cook, stirring, until the mixture thickens a bit, about 10 minutes.

6. Top with green onions and sesame seeds and serve.

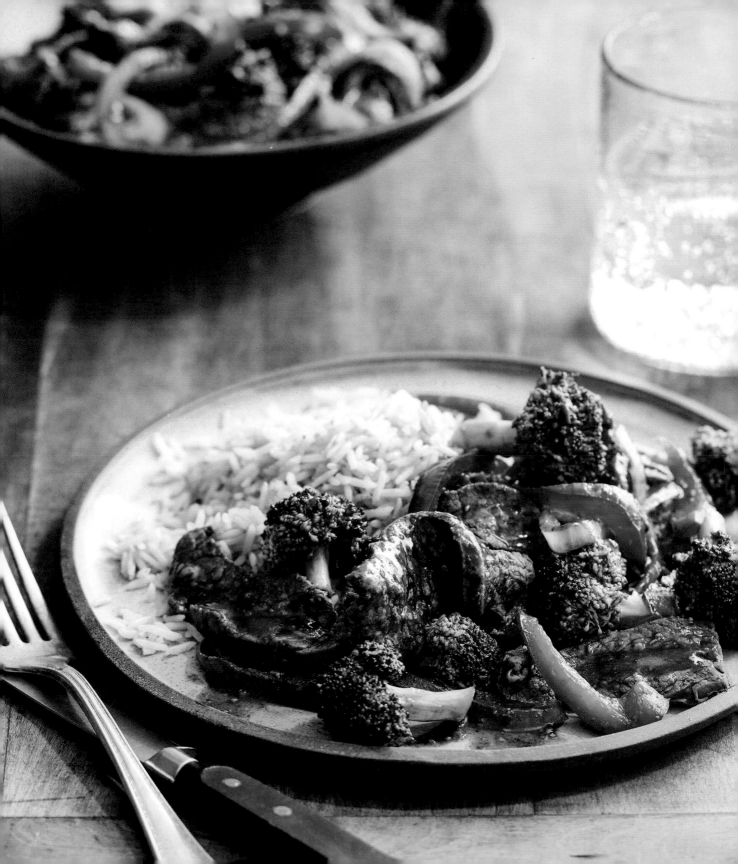

BEIJING BEEF *with* STEAMED BROCCOLI

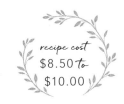

recipe cost
$8.50 *to* $10.00

Brady and I were huge Panda Express fans before we made over our diets. One of his favorite things to order was Beijing Beef, which was typically marinated for days and deep-fried. This is a lighter, less time-consuming take on a family favorite. It's basically like sweet-and-sour chicken, only with beef. A little heat, a lot of flavor! Serve this beef-and-broccoli dish over Veggie Lo Mein (page 218) or cooked brown rice.

SERVES 4

- 1 pound skirt or flank steak, cut into strips
- ½ medium yellow onion, sliced
- ½ red bell pepper, seeded and thinly sliced
- ¼ cup coconut aminos
- 2 tablespoons balsamic vinegar
- 2 tablespoons raw honey
- 1 tablespoon dried minced onion
- 1 teaspoon garlic powder
- 1 teaspoon red pepper flakes (optional)
- 1 teaspoon toasted sesame oil
- ½ teaspoon ground ginger
- 2 teaspoons arrowroot powder
- 2 tablespoons water
- 1 pound broccoli florets
- ½ teaspoon fine sea salt
- ¼ teaspoon ground black pepper

1. In an electric pressure cooker, combine the steak, onion, bell pepper, coconut aminos, vinegar, honey, dried onion, garlic powder, red pepper flakes, sesame oil, and ginger.

2. Place the lid on the cooker and make sure the vent valve is in the SEALING position. Using the display panel, select the MANUAL/PRESSURE COOK function and HIGH PRESSURE. Use the +/− buttons until the display reads 8 minutes.

3. When the cooker beeps, let it naturally release the pressure until the display reads LO:10. Switch the vent valve from the SEALING to the VENTING position. Use caution while the steam escapes.

4. Using the display panel, select the SAUTÉ function and adjust the heat to MORE (see Note page 95).

5. In a small bowl, stir together the arrowroot powder and water to create a slurry. Add the arrowroot mixture to the cooker and stir to combine. Add the broccoli, salt, and black pepper and cook, stirring occasionally, until the broccoli is crisp-tender and the sauce thickens, 6 to 8 minutes.

6. Serve over veggie lo mein or cooked brown rice.

VEGGIE LO MEIN

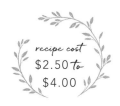

recipe cost
$2.50 *to*
$4.00

This dish is made entirely out of vegetables but it tastes just like the real thing! I promise: One bite, and you'll be hooked! If you do not have an air fryer, you can make this on the stovetop over medium-high heat. Just sauté and let all of the veggies cook down, stirring occasionally, for about 20 minutes. The benefit of the air fryer is that any extra moisture falls through the bottom, enabling the zucchini to crisp up and dehydrate. If cooking on the stovetop, there may be an excess amount of water that you will have to carefully remove.

SERVES 4

- 2 medium zucchini, spiralized (see Note page 51)
- 2 cups shredded green cabbage
- ½ cup seeded and julienned orange bell pepper
- ½ cup julienned carrots (see Note page 51)
- 2 green onions, thinly sliced
- 2 tablespoons extra-virgin olive oil
- 1 tablespoon coconut aminos
- 1 teaspoon toasted sesame oil
- 1 teaspoon fine sea salt
- ½ teaspoon ground black pepper

1. In a large bowl, combine the zucchini, cabbage, bell pepper, carrots, green onions, olive oil, coconut aminos, sesame oil, salt, and black pepper. Stir well to combine.

2. Pour the vegetables into a 5.3-quart air-fryer basket and bake for 15 minutes at 370°F, stirring once halfway through cooking time.

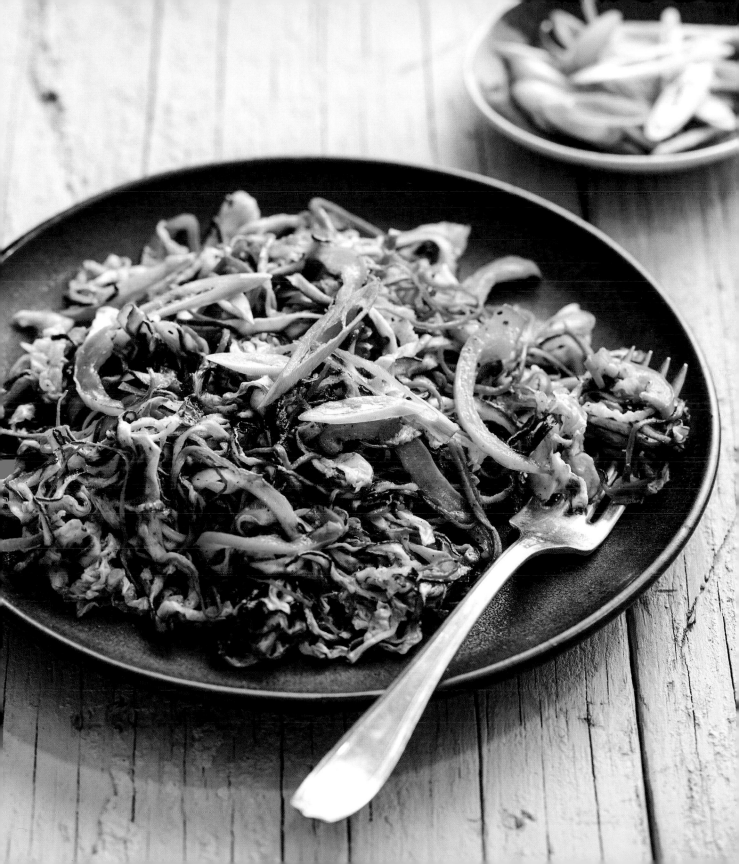

BLACK BEAN TOSTADAS

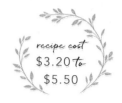

recipe cost
$3.20 to
$5.50

Tostadas were one of my favorites growing up and they are something my children now enjoy. I like them because you can build your own however you like. Don't like tomatoes? Leave them off—or add onions if you like. They're totally customizable, so they're a great dish for the family that has a picky eater or two.

SERVES 4

1 cup dried black beans

2 cups water

3 tablespoons chopped fresh cilantro stems

1 tablespoon dried minced onion

1 teaspoon ground cumin

½ teaspoon fine sea salt

¼ teaspoon cayenne pepper

¼ cup extra-virgin coconut oil

8 corn tortillas

3 cups shredded romaine lettuce

2 Roma tomatoes, cored and diced

1 cup sugar-free salsa

1. Place the beans in a large bowl and add water to cover by a couple of inches. Let them soak on the countertop, uncovered, for at least 8 hours or overnight. Rinse and drain.

2. In an electric pressure cooker, combine the beans, water, cilantro stems, dried onion, cumin, salt, and cayenne.

3. Place the lid on the cooker and make sure the vent valve is in the SEALING position. Using the display panel, select the MANUAL/PRESSURE COOK function and HIGH PRESSURE. Use the +/− buttons until the display reads 15 minutes.

4. While the beans are cooking, heat a 10-inch pan over medium-high heat. Add the coconut oil and let it warm. Working quickly, use tongs to place one corn tortilla in the oil, flip it immediately, then place it on a paper towel–lined plate. Repeat until all the corn tortillas are warmed, stacking each tortilla on top of the one before.

5. When the cooker beeps, let it naturally release the pressure until the display reads LO:25. Switch the vent valve from the SEALING to the VENTING position. Use caution while the steam escapes.

6. Drain the beans, reserving the cooking liquid. Place the beans in a medium bowl and mash with a potato masher, adding small amounts of the cooking liquid until the desired consistency is reached.

7. Spread beans on the tortillas. Top with romaine, tomatoes, and salsa.

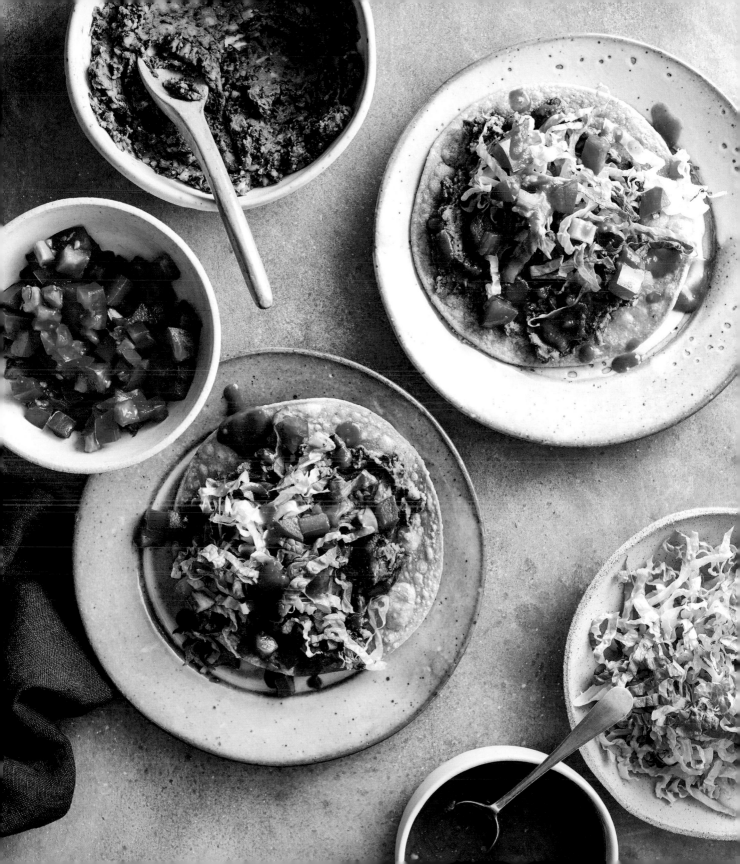

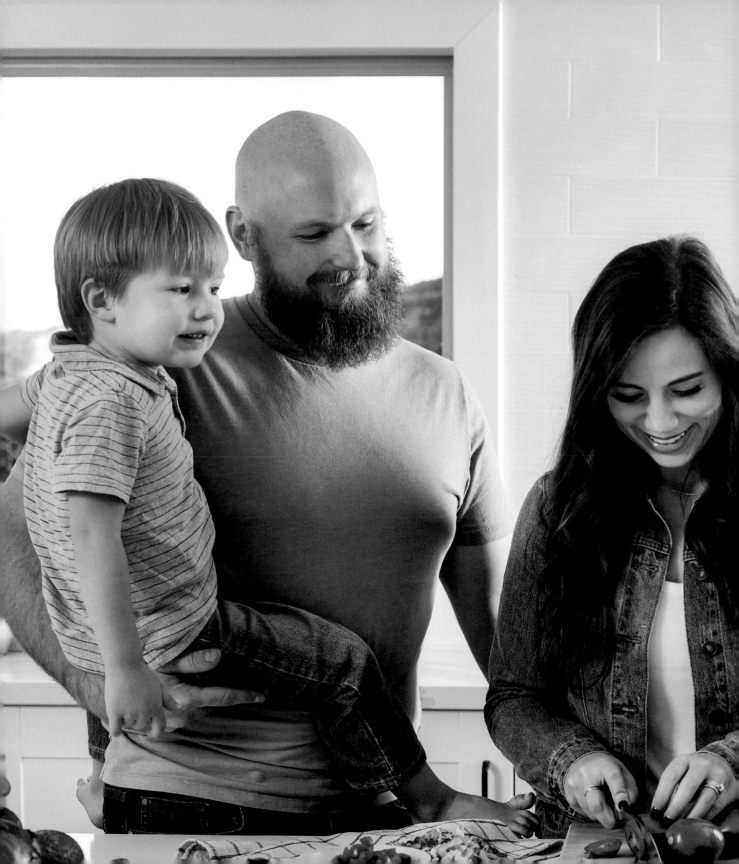

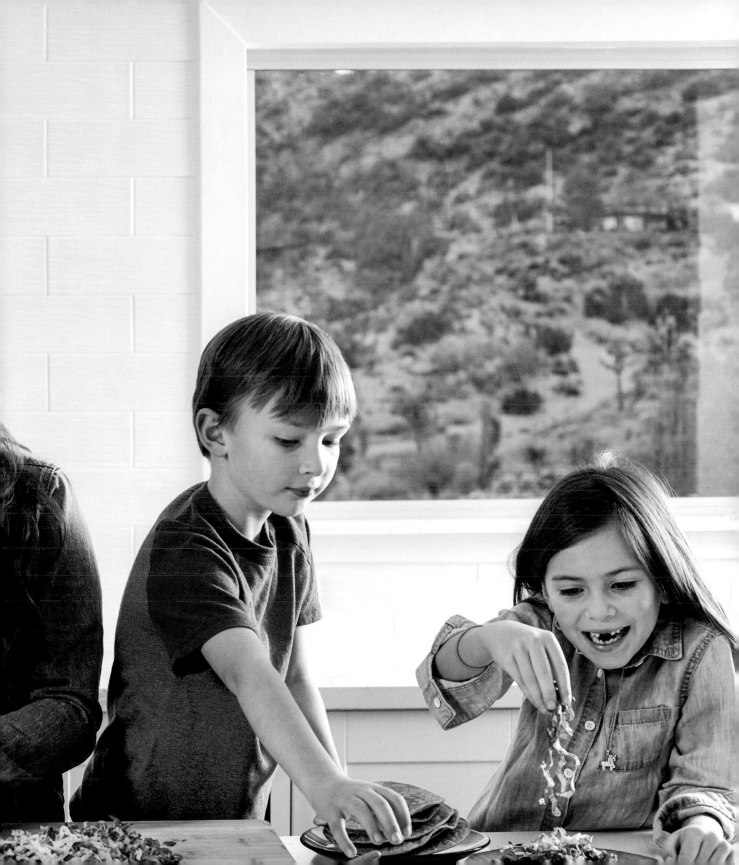

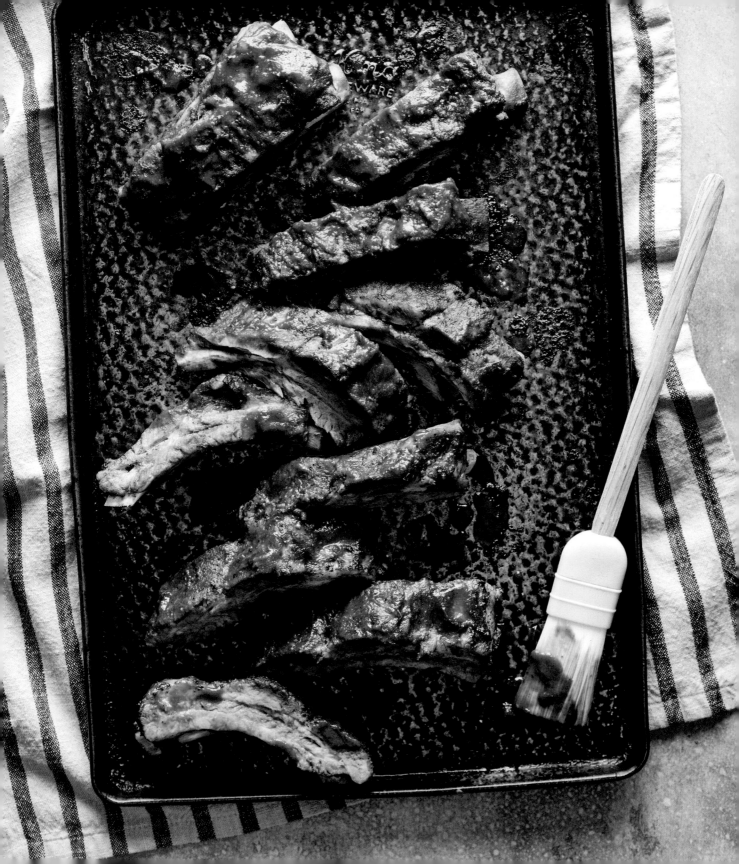

SMOKY BABY BACK RIBS

recipe cost
$5.50 to
$7.00

These ribs are fall off-the-bone tender and delicious. You begin with a dry rub and end with Tangy Barbecue Sauce, which just takes them right over the top! Serve with a vegetable side or green salad.

SERVES 4

1½ teaspoons fine sea salt

1 teaspoon ground black pepper

1 teaspoon onion powder

½ teaspoon garlic powder

¼ teaspoon cayenne pepper

2 to 3 pounds pork baby back ribs

½ cup apple cider vinegar

2 teaspoons liquid smoke

¼ cup Tangy Barbecue Sauce (page 324)

1. In a small bowl, stir together the salt, black pepper, onion powder, garlic powder, and cayenne. Place the ribs on a large plate and thoroughly coat them with the spice mixture, using your fingers to rub the spices into the meat.

2. Pour the vinegar and liquid smoke into an electric pressure cooker and place a trivet inside. Carefully set the rack(s) of ribs on the trivet. If the rack(s) do not fit, cut in half.

3. Place the lid on the cooker and make sure the vent valve is in the SEALING position. Using the display panel, select the MANUAL/PRESSURE COOK function and HIGH PRESSURE. Use the +/− buttons until the display reads 25 minutes.

4. When the cooker beeps, let it naturally release the pressure until the display reads LO:10. Switch the vent valve from the SEALING to the VENTING position. Use caution while the steam escapes.

5. Preheat the broiler on high. Remove the ribs from the cooker and place on a foil-lined baking sheet. Using a silicone pastry brush, brush the ribs with the barbecue sauce. Broil until the sauce browns, 2 to 5 minutes.

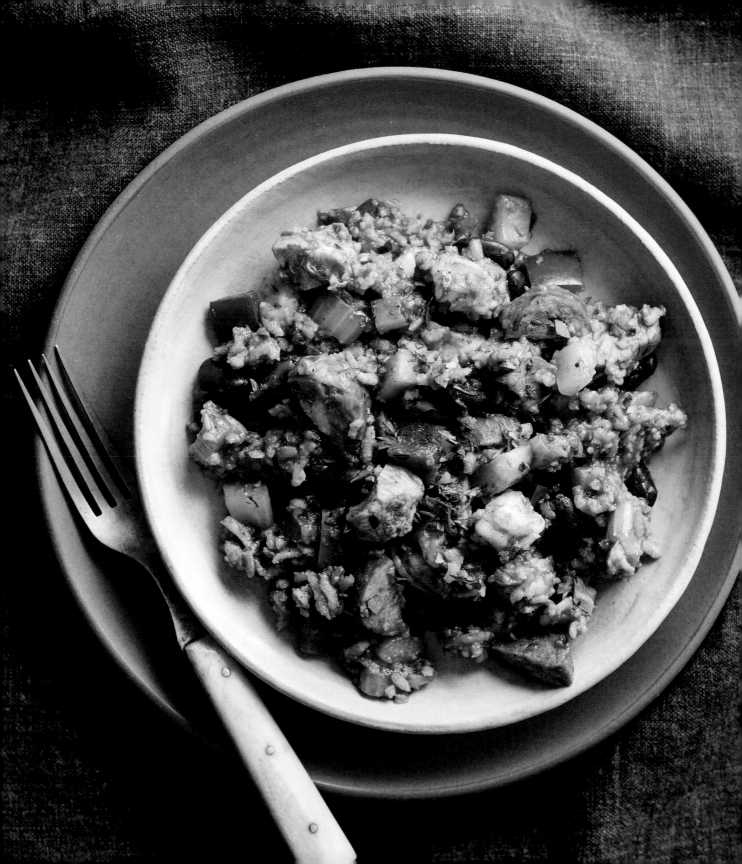

JAMBALAYA

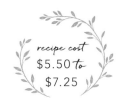

recipe cost
$5.50 to
$7.25

This is a popular Louisiana dish chock full of smoky sausage, chicken, and shrimp! It's a one-pot meal, so there is no need to serve anything else unless you'd like to start with a simple green salad.

SERVES 4 TO 6

2 stalks celery, chopped

½ medium yellow onion, diced

½ cup chopped seeded red bell pepper

8 ounces boneless, skinless chicken breasts, cut into bite-size pieces

5 ounces andouille sausage, diced

1 teaspoon garlic powder

1 teaspoon Cajun Seasoning (page 328) or store-bought

½ teaspoon dried thyme

½ teaspoon fine sea salt

½ teaspoon ground black pepper

2 cups low-sodium chicken broth or water

1 cup uncooked brown rice

1 cup tomato sauce

½ cup canned red kidney beans, rinsed and drained

4 ounces shrimp, peeled and deveined, cut into bite-size pieces

1 tablespoon chopped fresh flat-leaf parsley (optional)

1. Preheat an electric pressure cooker using the SAUTÉ function and adjust the heat to MORE (see Note page 95). When the display panel reads HOT, add the celery, onion, and bell pepper. Cook, stirring frequently, until the onion begins to soften and turn translucent, about 5 minutes.

2. Stir in the chicken, sausage, garlic powder, Cajun seasoning, thyme, salt, and black pepper and cook for 1 minute. Add the broth and scrape up any browned bits stuck to the bottom. Stir in the rice, tomato sauce, and beans.

3. Place the lid on the cooker and make sure the vent valve is in the SEALING position. Using the display panel, select the MANUAL/PRESSURE COOK function and HIGH PRESSURE. Use the +/− buttons until the display reads 28 minutes.

4. When the cooker beeps, switch the vent valve from the SEALING to the VENTING position, administering a quick release. Use caution while the steam escapes.

5. Add the shrimp and stir to combine. Place the lid back on the cooker and allow the shrimp to cook in the residual heat, about 4 minutes. Ladle the jambalaya into bowls.

6. Top with parsley, if desired, and serve.

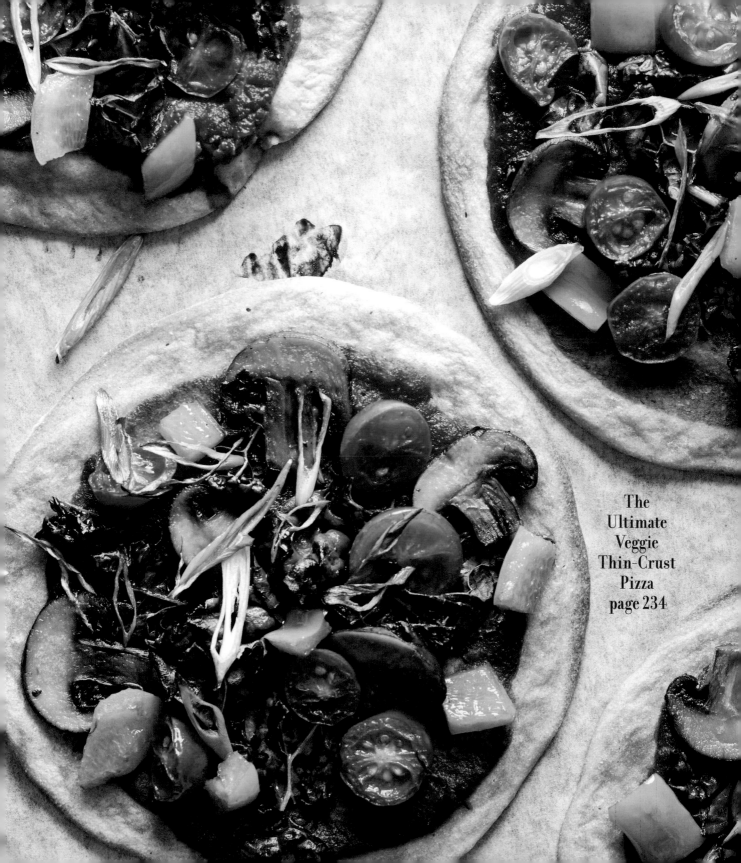

The
Ultimate
Veggie
Thin-Crust
Pizza
page 234

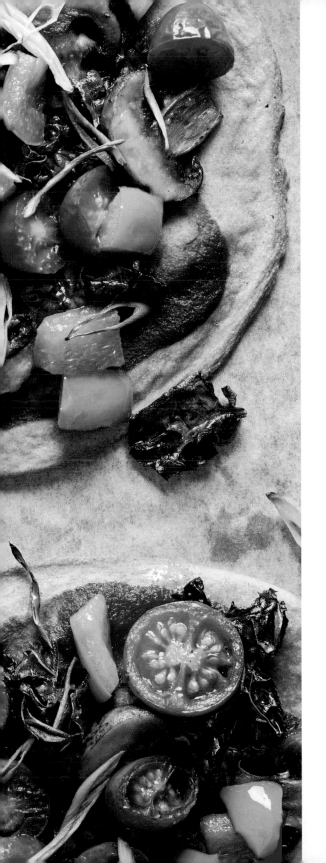

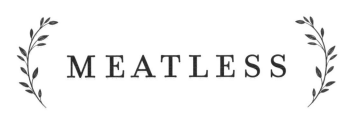

MEATLESS

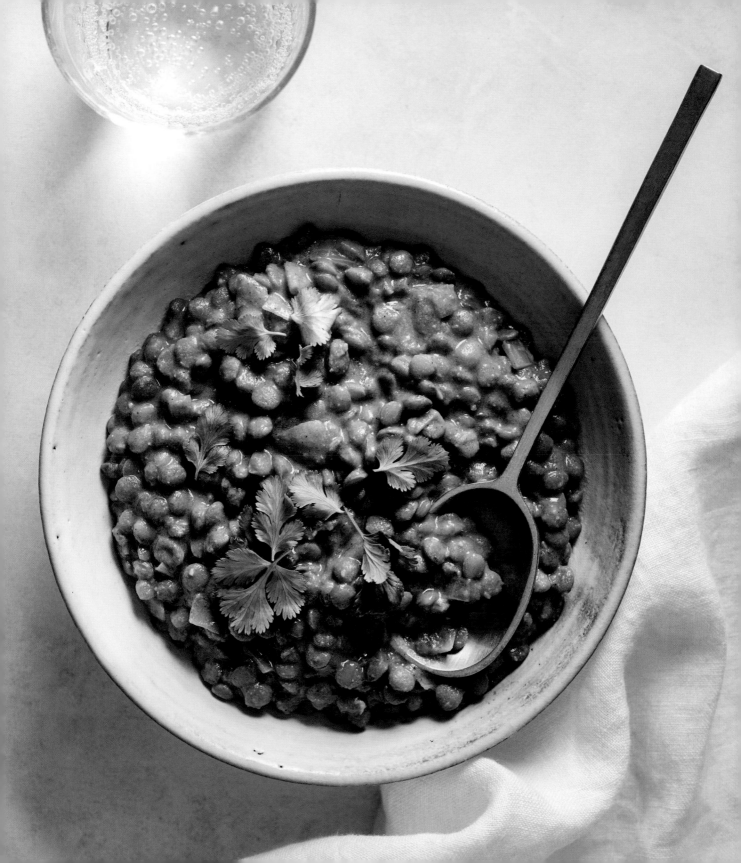

TIKKA MASALA LENTILS

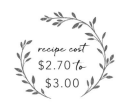

recipe cost
$2.70 to
$3.00

Tikka Masala is traditionally a creamy spiced curry chicken dish that is most often served over rice. In order to cut the cost and make it virtually prep-free, I converted it to a vegan dish with lentils instead—same great taste made with a cheaper plant-protein alternative. I love to serve mine over fresh baby spinach and top with tomato if I have some on hand. It's also fabulous with the Jamaican Rice and Peas on page 242.

1. Preheat an electric pressure cooker using the SAUTÉ function and adjust the heat to MORE (see Note page 95).

2. When the display panel reads HOT, add the onion and cook, stirring frequently, until it softens and becomes translucent, about 5 minutes.

3. Add the curry powder, garlic powder, paprika, turmeric, salt, cayenne, cinnamon, cumin, and black pepper and stir. Add the water, lentils, coconut milk, tomato paste, and lemon juice and stir well.

4. Place the lid on the cooker and make sure the vent is in the SEALING position. Using the display panel, press the CANCEL button to turn off the SAUTÉ function, then select the MANUAL/PRESSURE COOK and LOW PRESSURE. Use the +/− buttons until the display reads 15 minutes.

5. When the cooker beeps, let it naturally release the pressure until the display reads LO:10. Switch the vent valve from the SEALING to the VENTING position. Use caution while the steam escapes.

6. Top with cilantro leaves and serve.

SERVES 4

½ yellow onion, diced

1½ teaspoons curry powder

½ teaspoon garlic powder

½ teaspoon paprika

½ teaspoon turmeric

½ teaspoon fine sea salt

¼ teaspoon cayenne pepper

¼ teaspoon ground cinnamon

¼ teaspoon ground cumin

¼ teaspoon ground black pepper

2 cups water

1 cup brown lentils

½ cup canned full-fat coconut milk

2 tablespoons tomato paste

1 tablespoon fresh lemon juice

2 tablespoons chopped fresh cilantro leaves

POBLANO PEPPER—POTATO STEW

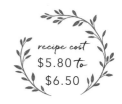

recipe cost
$5.80 *to*
$6.50

If using canned beans in this recipe, you can place everything in the cooker after sautéing the onion and garlic. Cook for ten minutes and serve.

SERVES 4 TO 6

2 poblano peppers

1 medium yellow onion, diced

6 cloves garlic, minced

2 cups low-sodium chicken broth or Bone Broth (page 331)

1 (15-ounce) can diced tomatoes

¾ cup dried black beans

1 tablespoon unfortified nutritional yeast

2 teaspoons paprika

2 teaspoons garlic powder

2 tablespoons dried minced onion

1 teaspoon onion powder

¼ teaspoon ground cumin

¼ teaspoon coriander

1¾ teaspoons fine sea salt

2 cups frozen corn kernels

3 cups quartered red baby potatoes

2 cups Oat Milk (page 288) or other milk

1 tablespoon arrowroot powder

¼ cup chopped fresh cilantro leaves

1 lime, cut into wedges

1. Preheat the broiler on high. Place the peppers on a baking sheet and broil for 10 to 12 minutes, turning them to evenly blacken each side.

2. Using tongs, carefully transfer the peppers to a gallon-size plastic bag and allow to stand until cool enough to be handled, about 5 minutes. (This steams the skin and makes it easier to remove.) Once cool, peel off the outer skin and remove the stems and seeds before dicing; set aside.

3. Preheat an electric pressure cooker using the SAUTÉ function and adjust the heat to MORE (see Note page 95). When the display reads HOT, add the onion and cook, stirring infrequently, until it softens and becomes translucent, about 3 minutes. Stir in the garlic.

4. Add the diced poblano peppers, broth, tomatoes, beans, nutritional yeast, paprika, garlic powder, dried onion, onion powder, cumin, and coriander.

5. Place the lid on the cooker and make sure the vent valve is in the SEALING position. Using the display panel, press the CANCEL button to turn off the SAUTÉ function, then select the MANUAL/PRESSURE COOK function and HIGH PRESSURE. Use the +/− buttons until the display reads 40 minutes.

6. When the cooker beeps, switch the vent valve from the SEALING to the VENTING position, administering a quick release. Use caution while the steam escapes.

7. Remove the lid and stir in the salt, corn, and baby potatoes. Place the lid on the cooker and make sure the vent valve is in the SEALING position. Using the display panel, select the MANUAL/PRESSURE COOK function and HIGH PRESSURE. Use the +/− buttons until the display reads 10 minutes.

8. When the cooker beeps, switch the vent valve from the SEALING to the VENTING position, administering a quick release. Use caution while the steam escapes.

9. Remove the lid and stir in the oat milk and arrowroot powder.

10. Ladle the stew into bowls, garnish with cilantro and a squeeze of lime juice, and serve.

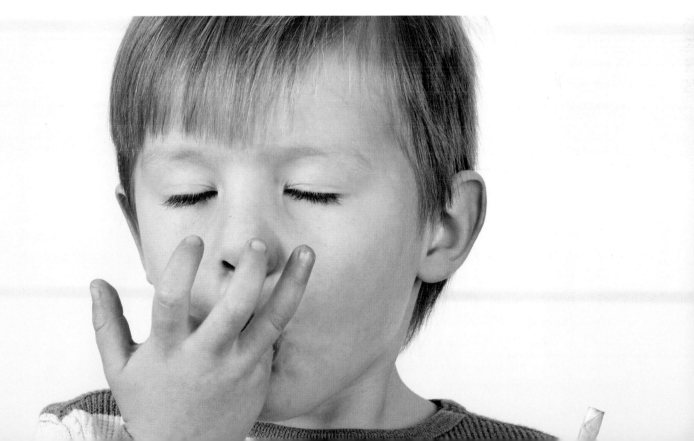

THE ULTIMATE VEGGIE THIN-CRUST PIZZA

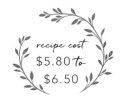

recipe cost
$5.80 to
$6.50

I'm always looking for new and inventive ways to make gluten-free pizza crust. This crust is absolutely fabulous! You don't have to do veggie pizza, though; top the crust however you'd like. Or simply add leftover chicken or chickpeas to the vegetables if you have them on hand. Did you know that quinoa is one of the best sources of plant-based protein? So even though this pizza is dairy-free, you can still get that boost!

MAKES FOUR 8-INCH PIZZAS

1 cup quinoa, rinsed and drained

1 cup water

1 teaspoon fine sea salt, plus more for sprinkling

1 teaspoon garlic powder

½ teaspoon onion powder

1 tablespoon extra-virgin olive oil

1 medium orange bell pepper, seeded and diced

1 medium jalapeño, seeded and diced

4 cups chopped kale (ribs removed) or 4 cups baby spinach

12 cherry tomatoes, cut into thirds

6 cremini mushrooms, thinly sliced

2 green onions, thinly sliced

1 cup tomato sauce

1. Place a pizza stone or baking steel inside the oven and preheat the oven to 425°F.

2. In a high-powered blender, combine the quinoa, water, salt, garlic powder, and onion powder. Blend on high until the batter is smooth, about 60 seconds.

3. On a 12×12-inch piece of parchment paper, spread ¼ cup of batter into a thin 8-inch circle. Carefully transfer the parchment paper and batter to the baking stone and bake for 8 to 10 minutes.

4. While the crust cooks, heat a cast-iron skillet over medium-high heat. Add the olive oil, bell pepper, and jalapeño and cook for 3 minutes. Add the kale, tomatoes, mushrooms, and green onions and stir to combine. Cook until the kale wilts and cooks down, about 2 minutes. Take the pan off the heat.

5. Carefully pull the stone out of the oven. Use a spoon to spread ¼ cup of tomato sauce on the crust. Sprinkle with salt to taste and top with one-quarter of the cooked vegetable mixture. Push the rack back into the oven and bake for an additional 8 to 10 minutes, until the edges of the crust have browned.

6. Use a thin spatula to remove the pizza from the parchment paper and transfer to a cutting board. Slice and serve warm.

7. Repeat with the remaining ingredients to make three additional personal-size pizzas.

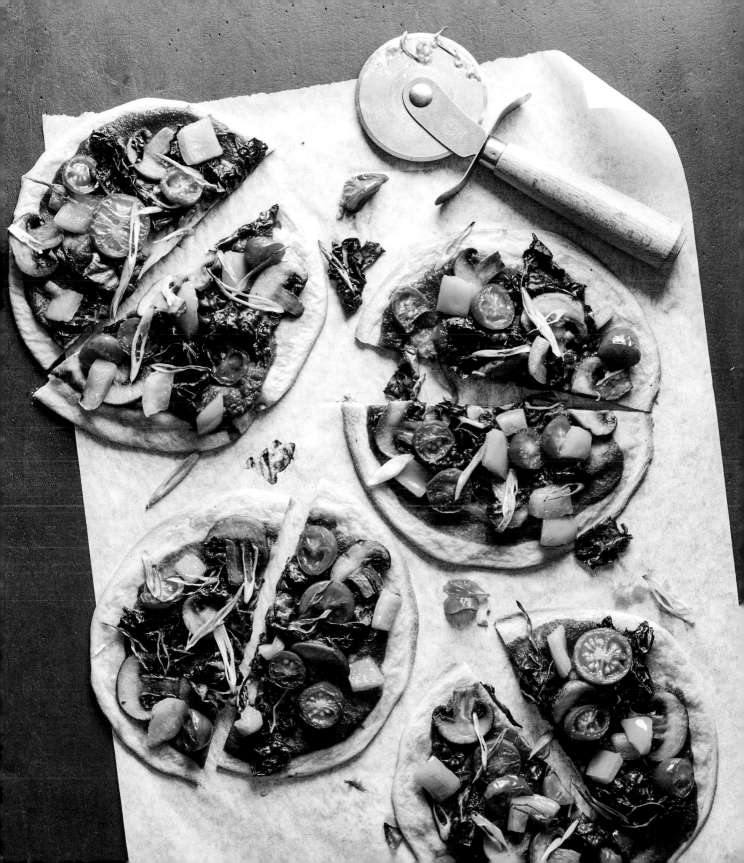

CAULIFLOWER MAC *and* CHEESE

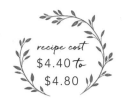

recipe cost
$4.40 *to*
$4.80

This is just as great the day after you make it. If you are cooking for one, save half for lunch tomorrow—or, if you are not a fan of leftovers, simply cut the recipe in half.

SERVES 2

1 cup low-sodium chicken broth or Vegetable Broth (page 332)

½ cup diced carrots (see Note page 51)

¼ cup unfortified nutritional yeast

2 tablespoons raw cashews

1 tablespoon dried minced onion

1¾ teaspoons fine sea salt

1½ teaspoons Taco Seasoning (page 325)

1 teaspoon garlic powder

¼ teaspoon ground black pepper

1 large head cauliflower, cored and trimmed

1. In a high-powered blender, combine the broth, carrots, nutritional yeast, cashews, dried onion, salt, taco seasoning, garlic powder, and black pepper. Blend on high until smooth, about 30 seconds.

2. Place the cauliflower in an electric pressure cooker. Pour the sauce over the top.

3. Place the lid on the cooker and make sure the vent valve is in the SEALING position. Using the display panel, select the MANUAL/PRESSURE COOK function and HIGH PRESSURE. Use the +/− buttons until the display reads 2 minutes.

4. When the cooker beeps, switch the vent valve from the SEALING to the VENTING position, administering a quick release. Use caution while the steam escapes.

5. Remove the lid and using the display panel, select the SAUTÉ function and adjust to NORMAL (see Note page 182). Cook, stirring occasionally, breaking up the cauliflower into pieces and allowing the sauce to thicken, about 3 minutes.

6. Serve hot.

TWO-BEAN *and* LENTIL CHILI

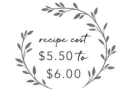

recipe cost
$5.50 *to*
$6.00

Plant-based vegan chili! Don't let that scare you away. This chili is packed full of veggie protein—you won't even miss the meat!

SERVES 4 TO 6

¾ cup dried kidney beans

¾ cup dried pinto beans

½ cup green or brown lentils

1 yellow onion, diced

2 jalapeños, seeded and diced

1 red bell pepper, seeded and diced

1 (15-ounce) can tomato sauce

1 (15-ounce) can diced tomatoes

1½ cups water

1 cup Vegetable Broth (page 332) or store-bought

2 tablespoons dried minced onion

2 tablespoons chili powder

6 cloves garlic, minced

2 tablespoons tomato paste

1½ teaspoons ground cumin

1½ teaspoons fine sea salt

1 teaspoon garlic powder

1 teaspoon onion powder

½ teaspoon liquid smoke

¼ teaspoon chipotle chili powder

¼ teaspoon ground black pepper

1. Place the kidney beans and pinto beans in a large bowl and cover with water by a few inches. Let them soak on the countertop, uncovered, for at least 4 hours or overnight. Rinse and drain. In an electric pressure cooker, combine the drained beans, lentils, onion, jalapeños, bell pepper, tomato sauce, tomatoes, water, broth, dried onion, chili powder, garlic, tomato paste, cumin, salt, garlic powder, onion powder, liquid smoke, chili powder, and black pepper. Stir well to combine.

2. Place the lid on the cooker and make sure the vent valve is in the SEALING position. Using the display panel, select the MANUAL/PRESSURE COOK function and HIGH PRESSURE. Use the +/− buttons until the display reads 50 minutes.

3. When the cooker beeps, let it naturally release the pressure until the display reads LO:10. Switch the vent valve from the SEALING to the VENTING position. Use caution while the steam escapes.

4. Serve hot.

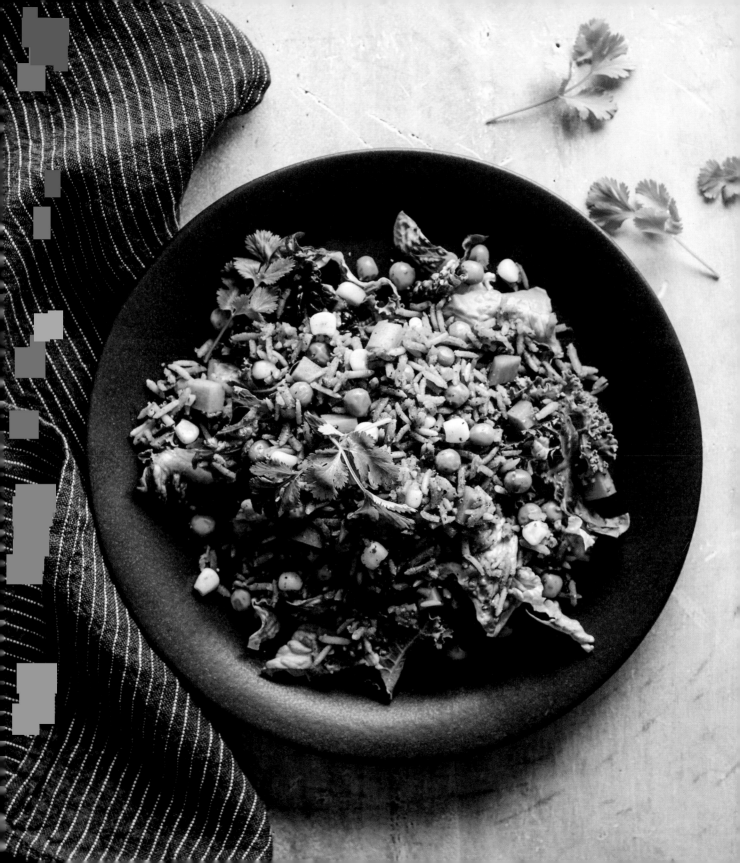

SPICY MEXI-RICE BOWLS

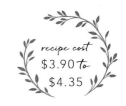

recipe cost
$3.90 *to*
$4.35

This is a quick bowl you can throw together midweek for lunch with your kids. I garnish my children's bowls with organic tortilla chips and maybe crumble up a few on top of my rice for texture as well. If you have fresh cilantro on hand, that is always wonderful sprinkled on top!

SERVES 4

1 cup brown rice

1 cup water

½ cup mild hot sauce or sugar-free salsa

3 tablespoons Taco Seasoning (page 325)

2 cups frozen peas

1 cup cubed frozen carrots

1 cup frozen corn kernels

1 tablespoon extra-virgin olive oil

8 cups mixed greens

1. In an electric pressure cooker, combine the rice, water, hot sauce, and taco seasoning.

2. Place the lid on the cooker and make sure the vent valve is in the SEALING position. Using the display panel, select the MANUAL/PRESSURE COOK function and HIGH PRESSURE. Use the +/− buttons until the display reads 28 minutes.

3. When the cooker beeps, switch the vent valve from the SEALING to the VENTING position, administering a quick release. Use caution while the steam escapes.

4. Remove the lid and using the display panel, select the SAUTÉ function and adjust to NORMAL (see Note page 182). Add the peas, carrots, corn, and olive oil. Cook, stirring continuously, 3 to 5 minutes.

5. To serve, divide the mixed greens into four bowls and top with the rice.

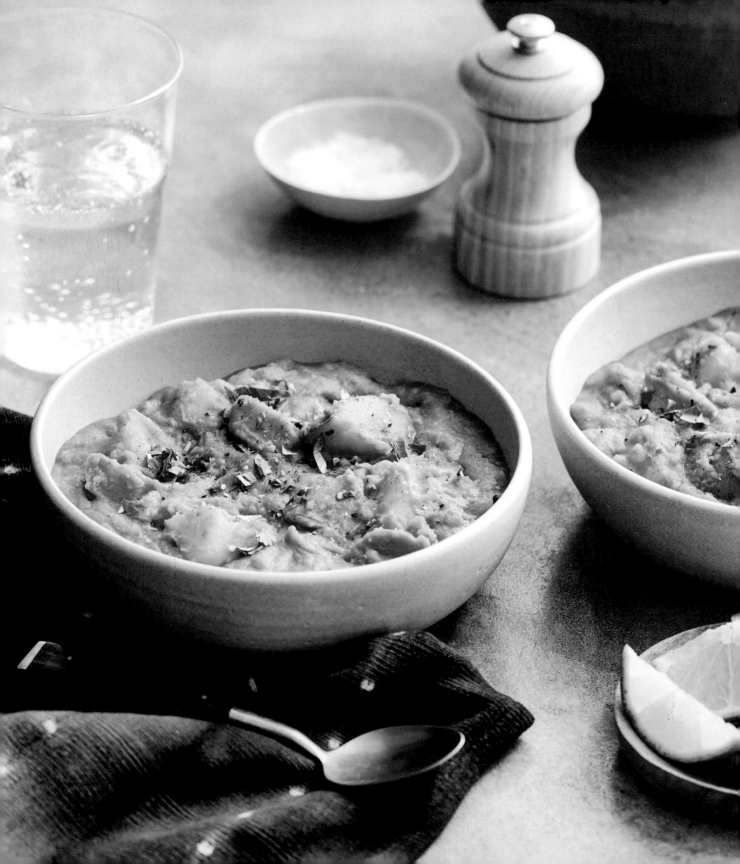

THAI RED CURRY *with* POTATOES *and* LENTILS

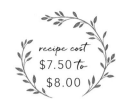

recipe cost
$7.50 *to*
$8.00

This is one of my favorite plant-based dishes in this book. I love to serve it over the Jamaican Rice and Peas on page 242. If you're trying to cut carbs, omit the potatoes.

SERVES 6

1 pound sweet potatoes or red potatoes, diced

1 large carrot, diced (see Note page 51)

½ medium yellow onion, diced

1 tablespoon grated fresh ginger

3 cloves garlic, minced

1½ cups water

1 cup red lentils

1 (14-ounce) can diced tomatoes

1 (14-ounce) can full-fat coconut milk

5 tablespoons red curry paste

½ teaspoon fine sea salt

1 lime, cut into wedges

1. Preheat an electric pressure cooker using the SAUTÉ function and adjust the heat to MORE (see Note page 95). When the display panel reads HOT, add the potatoes, carrot, and onion. Cook, stirring frequently, until the onion softens and is translucent, about 3 minutes. Stir in the ginger and garlic.

2. Add the water and scrape up any browned bits stuck to the bottom of the cooker. Stir in the lentils, tomatoes, coconut milk, curry paste, and salt.

3. Place the lid on the cooker and make sure the vent valve is in the SEALING position. Using the display panel, press the CANCEL button to turn off the SAUTÉ function, then select the MANUAL/PRESSURE COOK function and HIGH PRESSURE. Use the +/− buttons until the display reads 12 minutes.

4. When the cooker beeps, switch the vent valve from the SEALING to the VENTING position, administering a quick release. Use caution while the steam escapes.

5. Serve with a squeeze of lime juice.

JAMAICAN RICE *and* PEAS

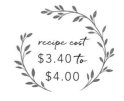

recipe cost
$3.40 *to*
$4.00

Rice and peas is a traditional Caribbean dish. The peas referred to here are not green garden peas, but beans—called "peas" in the Caribbean. Creamy and delicious, this pairs really well with the Thai Red Curry (page 241) because of the coconut milk base.

SERVES 4

1 cup brown rice

1 cup cooked red kidney beans

1 (14-ounce) can full-fat coconut milk

½ large yellow onion, diced

2 green onions, thinly sliced

3 cloves garlic, minced

1 tablespoon extra-virgin olive oil

1 teaspoon dried thyme

¾ teaspoon fine sea salt

¼ teaspoon ground black pepper

⅛ teaspoon ground allspice

1. In an electric pressure cooker, combine the rice, beans, coconut milk, onion, green onions, garlic, olive oil, thyme, salt, black pepper, and allspice and stir.

2. Place the lid on the cooker and make sure the vent valve is in the SEALING position. Using the display panel, select the MANUAL/PRESSURE COOK function and HIGH PRESSURE. Use the +/− buttons until the display reads 28 minutes.

3. When the cooker beeps, switch the vent valve from the SEALING to the VENTING position, administering a quick release. Use caution while the steam escapes.

4. Serve hot.

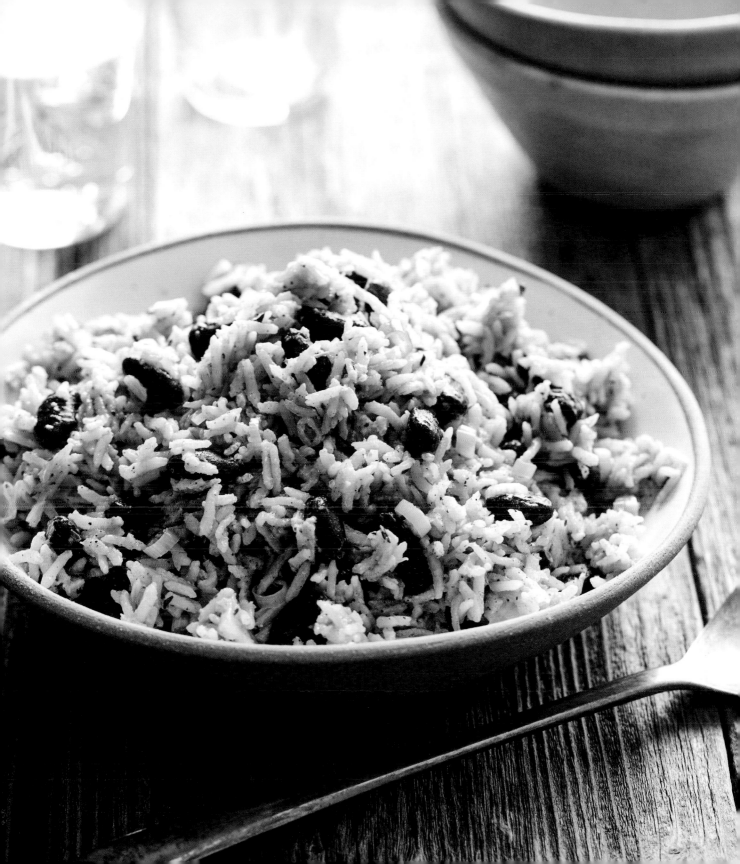

CABBAGE STEAKS

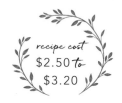

recipe cost
$2.50 to
$3.20

This is obviously not a big, juicy, beefy steak. Called cabbage "steaks" for their shape, the thickness of the cut does lend a certain meatiness to a bite! Seasoned well with garlic and lemon, this is a great vegetable main. Serve with Garlic-Chive Mashed Potatoes (page 184) and a healthy serving of Green Beans Amandine (page 187).

SERVES 4

1 medium to large head green cabbage, cut into 1½-inch-thick "steaks"

3 tablespoons extra-virgin olive oil

2 teaspoons fine sea salt

1 teaspoon garlic powder

1 teaspoon fresh lemon juice

½ teaspoon ground black pepper

1. Preheat the oven to 400°F.

2. Arrange the cabbage steaks on a large baking sheet. Drizzle with half of the olive oil, gently flip, and drizzle the other side with the remaining olive oil. Sprinkle the steaks evenly with the salt, garlic powder, lemon juice, and black pepper.

3. Roast for 20 to 24 minutes, gently flipping halfway through the cooking time, until the edges begin to brown and the cabbage is tender.

4. Serve hot.

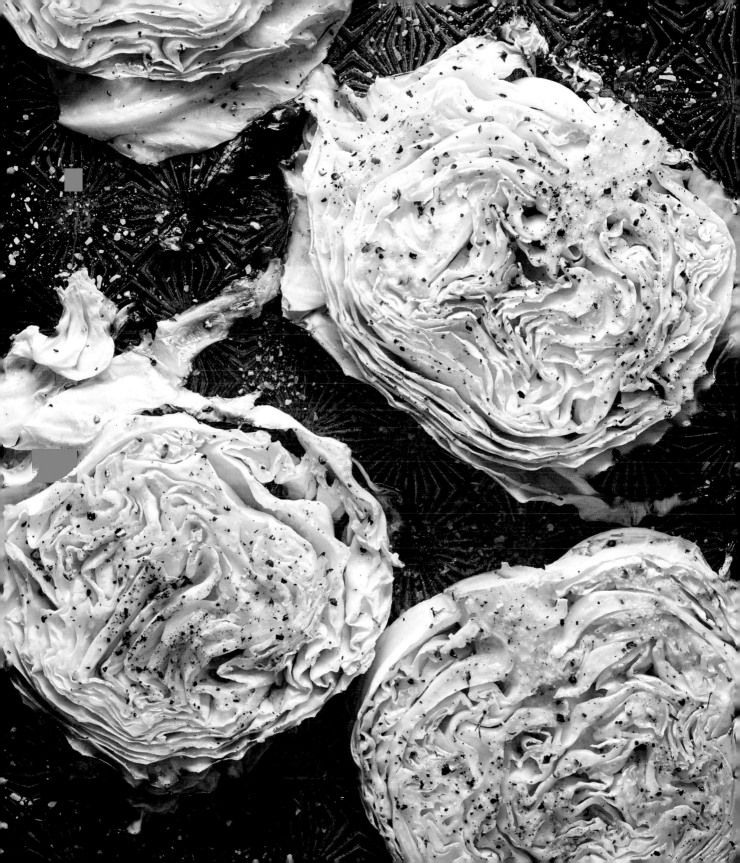

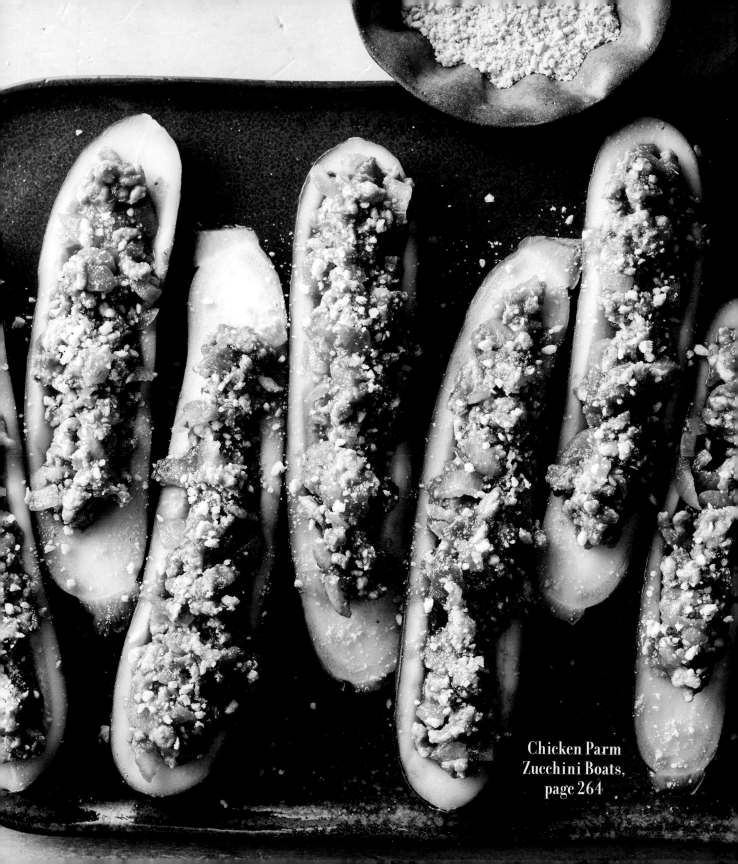

Chicken Parm
Zucchini Boats,
page 264

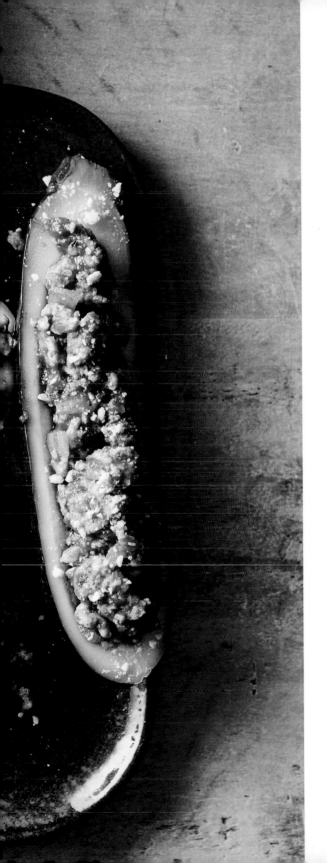

 # LAND AND SEA

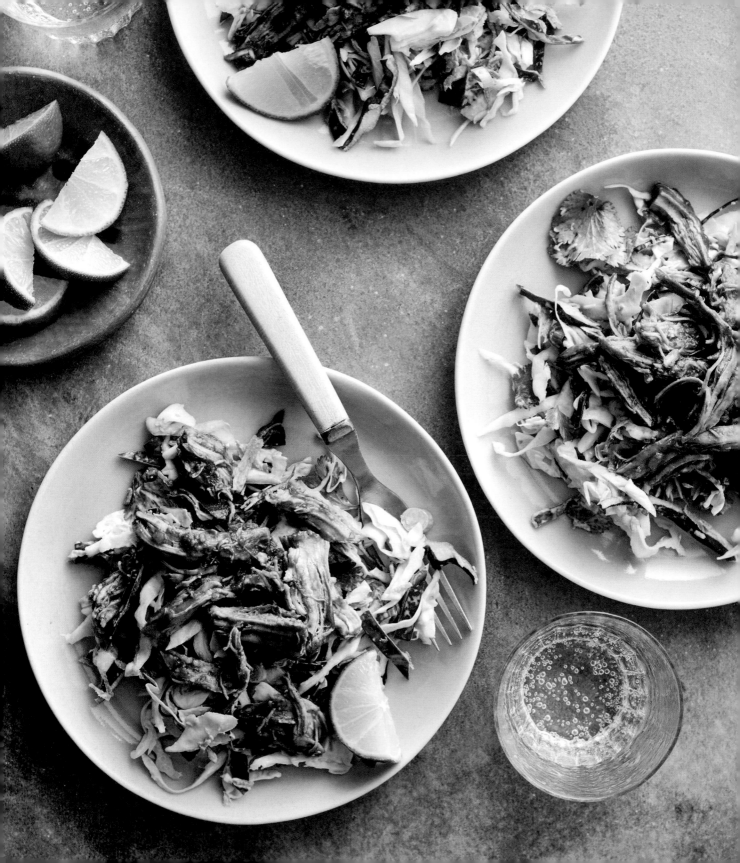

BARBECUE CHICKEN *with* CILANTRO–LIME COLESLAW

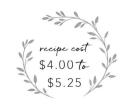

My family is crazy for everything barbecue. I, however, take exception to most store-bought barbecue sauces. Not only are they usually high in processed sugars—like high-fructose corn syrup—but in order to stay shelf-stable, they're usually chock-full of preservatives, too!

   This barbecue chicken is special because you make your barbecue sauce from scratch. And there's no need to dirty any extra dishes—simply toss everything into your pressure cooker and close the lid for a tangy chicken dish that's ready in less than thirty minutes. As an added bonus, this whole meal only costs $8 to make for a family of four—that's only $2 per person!

SERVES 4

1 pound boneless, skinless chicken breasts, cut into 1-inch pieces (see Note)

1 cup tomato sauce

2½ tablespoons raw honey

1 tablespoon tomato paste

4 teaspoons apple cider vinegar

1½ teaspoons low-sodium Worcestershire sauce

1 teaspoon liquid smoke

1 teaspoon fine sea salt

1 teaspoon dried minced onion

½ teaspoon chili powder

Cilantro-Lime Coleslaw (page 250)

1. Place the chicken in the bottom of an electric pressure cooker. Add the tomato sauce, honey, tomato paste, vinegar, Worcestershire, liquid smoke, salt, dried onion, and chili powder. Do not stir.

2. Place the lid on the cooker and make sure the vent valve is in the SEALING position. Using the display panel, select the MANUAL/PRESSURE COOK function and HIGH PRESSURE. Use the +/− buttons until the display reads 15 minutes.

3. When the cooker beeps, let it naturally release the pressure until the display reads LO:05. Switch the vent valve from the SEALING to the VENTING position. Use caution while the steam escapes.

4. Shred the chicken into the sauce and let stand for 5 minutes. (If the sauce has not thickened after standing, select the SAUTÉ function and adjust to NORMAL [see Note page 182] and stir continuously to allow some of the moisture to evaporate.)

5. Serve the chicken over the coleslaw.

NOTE: You can use frozen chicken in this recipe; no additional cook time is required.

CILANTRO-LIME COLESLAW

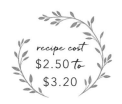
recipe cost
$2.50 *to*
$3.20

This simple, tangy slaw recipe is a perfect side to pair with spicy chicken or fish. Light and refreshing, it's also a breeze to whip up. If you'd like to save yourself some chopping time, simply use a 9-ounce bag of coleslaw mix in place of the carrots and cabbage.

In a medium bowl, stir together all the ingredients. Chill until serving time.

SERVES 4

2 cups shredded green cabbage

1½ cups shredded purple cabbage

½ cup shredded carrots

¼ cup fresh cilantro leaves

2 green onions, thinly sliced

3 tablespoons Homemade Mayo (page 330) or store-bought

3 tablespoons fresh lime juice

LEMON-GARLIC DRUMSTICKS

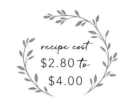

recipe cost
$2.80 to
$4.00

It doesn't get much easier than these tasty drumsticks. Make sure to stick them in the oven after cooking to crisp up the outside!

SERVES 4

4 chicken drumsticks (1 to 1¼ pounds)

2 tablespoons extra-virgin olive oil

1 teaspoon garlic powder

½ teaspoon fine sea salt

¼ teaspoon ground black pepper

¼ cup water

2 tablespoons coconut aminos

1 tablespoon rice vinegar

3 cloves garlic, minced

1 tablespoon freshly grated lemon zest

Juice of 1 lemon

1. In a small bowl, combine the chicken, 1 tablespoon of the olive oil, garlic powder, salt, and black pepper.

2. Preheat an electric pressure cooker using the SAUTÉ function and adjust the heat to MORE (see Note page 95). When the display panel reads HOT, add the remaining 1 tablespoon olive oil and chicken. Cook the chicken for 3 minutes per side. Add the water, coconut aminos, vinegar, garlic, lemon zest, and lemon juice.

3. Place the lid on the pressure cooker and make sure the vent valve is in the SEALING position. Using the display panel, select the MANUAL/PRESSURE COOK function and HIGH PRESSURE. Use the +/− buttons until the display reads 8 minutes.

4. When the cooker beeps, let it naturally release the pressure until the display reads LO:05. Switch the vent valve from the SEALING to the VENTING position. Use caution while the steam escapes.

5. Remove the chicken from the cooker and let rest for 5 minutes before serving. If desired, preheat the broiler and transfer the chicken to a rimmed baking sheet. Broil the chicken until the skin is crisp, about 5 minutes.

SESAME-CHILI TURKEY MEATBALLS

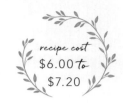

If you are new to Paleo or a more whole-foods way of eating, this recipe may seem intimidating at first. It may contain a few ingredients you've never heard of. Let me demystify it for you. Coconut aminos are just a healthier alternative to low-sodium soy sauce. Rice vinegar is a vinegar made out of fermented rice and is traditionally used in a lot of Asian cooking. If you do not have it on hand, you can substitute cider vinegar or white wine vinegar. Fish sauce—I use Red Boat brand—may not be in your pantry, either. A fabulous sauce used to flavor Thai and Vietnamese dishes, it's made out of fermented anchovies and salt. It's one of those things that you purchase once and lasts several years. It's a little bit of an investment up front, but well worth it. If you do not wish to make the investment, that's okay! You can omit that ingredient and still have a wonderful dish.

1. **MAKE THE MEATBALLS:** In a medium bowl, combine the ground turkey, coconut aminos, vinegar, garlic powder, fish sauce, salt, and black pepper. Mix using your hands. (You can also use a spoon, but I find hands work best.) Divide into twelve equal portions and roll into balls.

2. Place the meatballs in a 5.3-quart air-fryer basket and lightly spray with cooking oil spray. Bake at 360°F for 10 minutes, carefully turning with tongs halfway through the cooking time.

3. **MAKE THE CHILI OIL:** While the meatballs cook, in a small bowl, combine the avocado oil, coconut aminos, vinegar, black pepper, red pepper flakes, sesame oil, fish sauce, and garlic powder and stir well.

4. **TO SERVE:** Transfer the meatballs to a serving platter and drizzle with the chili oil. Sprinkle with sesame seeds and green onion.

MAKES 12 MEATBALLS (SERVES 4)

FOR THE MEATBALLS
1 pound ground turkey
1½ teaspoons coconut aminos
1 teaspoon rice vinegar
½ teaspoon garlic powder
½ teaspoon fish sauce
½ teaspoon fine sea salt
¼ teaspoon ground black pepper
Cooking oil spray

FOR THE CHILI OIL
2 tablespoons avocado oil
1 tablespoon coconut aminos
1 tablespoon rice vinegar
½ teaspoon ground black pepper
½ teaspoon red pepper flakes
½ teaspoon sesame oil
½ teaspoon fish sauce
¼ teaspoon garlic powder

FOR SERVING
½ teaspoon sesame seeds
1 green onion, thinly sliced

NOTE: These can also be made on the stovetop. Preheat a pan over medium-high heat. Add 1 tablespoon avocado oil and cook until browned all over and cooked through, about 12 minutes.

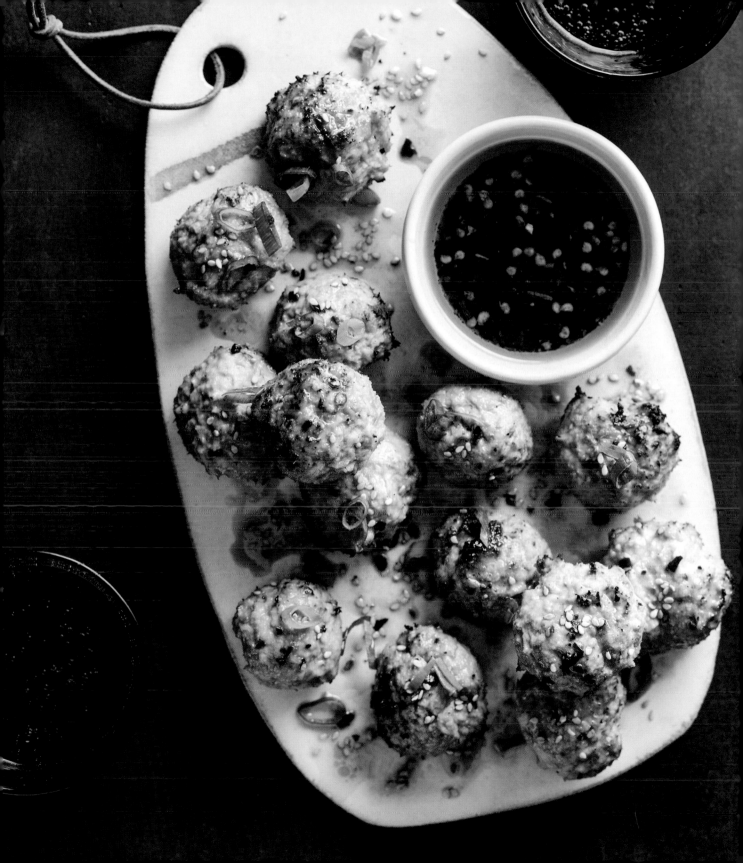

TURKEY CABBAGE CUPS

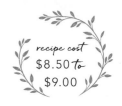

recipe cost
$8.50 *to*
$9.00

If you like lettuce-wrap tacos, you will love these cabbage cups! With lean ground turkey as the base and a combination of coconut aminos (a soy-free soy sauce replacement), ginger, and green onions, these are full of flavor and healthy phytonutrients.

    If you have extra vegetables laying around in the fridge that need to be used up, this is great dish to toss them into. Bell peppers, onions, carrots, or broccoli add a nice bright pop of color!

SERVES 4

- 2 tablespoons extra-virgin olive oil
- 1½ pounds lean ground turkey
- 2 tablespoons coconut aminos
- 3 cloves garlic, minced
- ½ teaspoon toasted sesame oil
- ½ teaspoon grated fresh ginger
- ½ teaspoon fine sea salt
- ¼ teaspoon red pepper flakes
- ¼ teaspoon ground black pepper
- 8 large green or purple cabbage leaves
- 4 green onions, thinly sliced

1. Preheat an electric pressure cooker using the SAUTÉ function and adjust the heat to MORE (see Note page 95). When the display panel reads HOT, add the olive oil, ground turkey, coconut aminos, garlic, sesame oil, ginger, salt, red pepper flakes, and black pepper. Cook, stirring occasionally, until browned, 5 to 7 minutes.

2. Serve the turkey in cabbage leaves topped with a sprinkle of green onion.

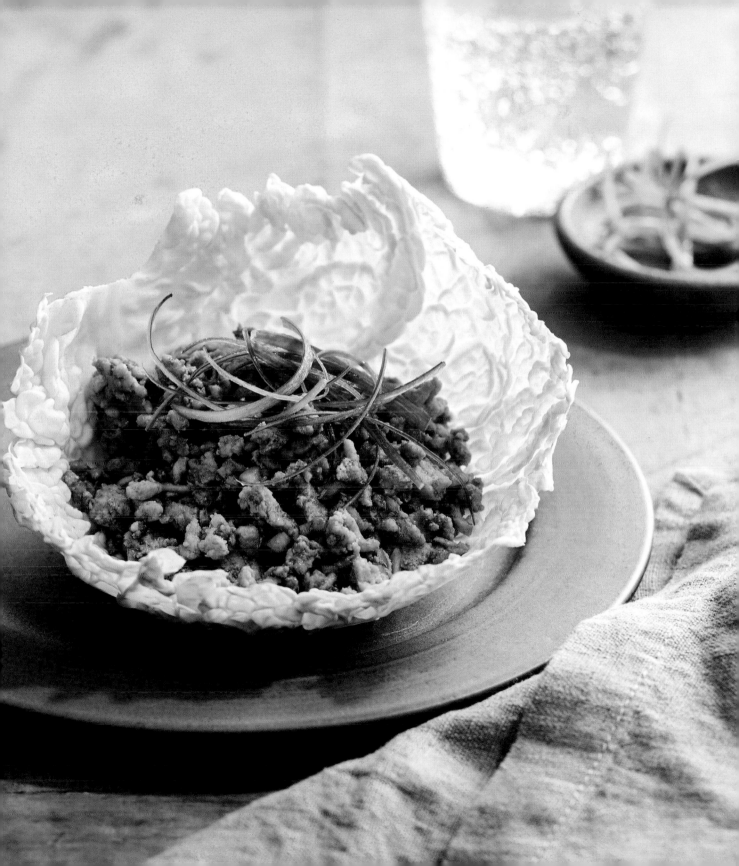

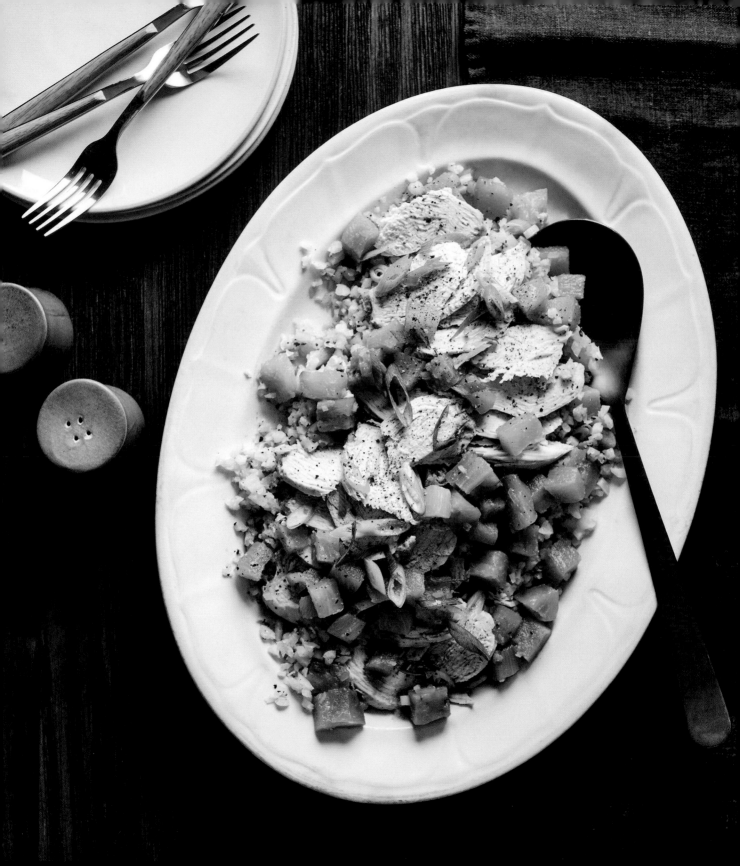

SUMMER PINEAPPLE CHICKEN *over* CAULIFLOWER RICE

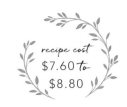

recipe cost
$7.60 *to*
$8.80

Take a bite out of summer with this Whole30-approved classic dump meal! The sweet-and-savory chicken dish is light and refreshing. Top it with a little sprinkle of green onion or chives if you have some on hand.

1. MAKE THE CHICKEN: In an electric pressure cooker, combine the chicken breasts, pineapple, coconut aminos, water, garlic powder, dried onion, salt, ginger, and black pepper.

2. Place the lid on the cooker and make sure the vent valve is in the SEALING position. Using the display panel, select the MANUAL/PRESSURE COOK function and HIGH PRESSURE. Use the +/− buttons until the display reads 15 minutes.

3. MAKE THE RICE: While the chicken cooks, heat a large pan on the stove over medium heat. Add the olive oil, riced cauliflower, lemon juice, salt, and black pepper. Cook, uncovered, until the rice has softened and the liquid has evaporated, 10 minutes.

4. When the cooker beeps, let it naturally release the pressure until the display reads LO:05. Switch the vent valve from the SEALING to the VENTING position. Use caution while the steam escapes.

5. Remove the chicken from the cooker and cut into strips. Serve the chicken and pineapple over the cauliflower rice, drizzled with juices from the cooker and topped with green onion.

SERVES 4

FOR THE PINEAPPLE CHICKEN

1 pound boneless, skinless chicken breasts

2 cups diced fresh pineapple

¼ cup coconut aminos

2 tablespoons water

1 teaspoon garlic powder

1 teaspoon dried minced onion

½ teaspoon fine sea salt

¼ teaspoon grated fresh ginger

¼ teaspoon ground black pepper

FOR THE CAULIFLOWER RICE

1 tablespoon extra-virgin olive oil

4 cups riced cauliflower

1 tablespoon fresh lemon juice

¼ teaspoon fine sea salt

¼ teaspoon ground black pepper

1 green onion, thinly sliced

SALSA VERDE CHICKEN NACHOS *and* MEXICAN LASAGNA

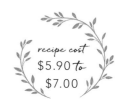

recipe cost
$5.90 *to*
$7.00

A huge time-saver in our home is two-for-one meals. You only spend the amount of time it takes to prepare one meal, but get two! We usually consume one right away and put one in the fridge or freezer for later in the week when I don't feel like cooking.

SERVES 4

FOR THE SALSA VERDE CHICKEN

1 pound boneless, skinless chicken breasts, cubed

1 cup sugar-free salsa verde or jalapeño salsa

½ teaspoon cumin

½ teaspoon fine sea salt

FOR THE NACHOS

3 ounces corn tortilla chips

2 cups shredded romaine lettuce

½ cup canned black beans, rinsed and drained

¼ cup fresh cilantro leaves

FOR THE MEXICAN LASAGNA

½ cup water

¼ cup raw cashews

1½ teaspoons unfortified nutritional yeast

2 teaspoons Taco Seasoning (page 325)

½ teaspoon fine sea salt

10 corn tortillas, quartered

1 small Roma tomato, diced

½ cup frozen yellow corn

½ cup canned black beans, rinsed and drained

¼ cup fresh cilantro leaves

1. **MAKE THE CHICKEN:** Place the chicken in the bottom of an electric pressure cooker. Add the salsa verde, cumin, and salt. Do not stir.

2. Place the lid on the cooker and make sure the vent valve is in the SEALING position. Using the display panel, select the MANUAL/PRESSURE COOK function and HIGH PRESSURE. Use the +/− buttons until the display reads 15 minutes.

3. **MAKE THE NACHOS:** While the chicken cooks, arrange the tortilla chips on a large baking sheet. Top with the romaine lettuce and black beans; set aside.

4. When the cooker beeps, let it naturally release the pressure until the display reads LO:05. Switch the vent valve from the SEALING to the VENTING position. Use caution while the steam escapes. Shred the chicken into the sauce and let stand for 5 minutes. (If the sauce has not thickened after standing, select the SAUTÉ function and adjust to NORMAL [see Note page 182] and stir continuously to allow some of the moisture to evaporate.)

5. Divide the meat mixture into two equal portions. Use one half of it to top the nachos, which can be sprinkled with

cilantro and served immediately. Use the remaining meat to assemble the lasagna.

6. **MAKE THE LASAGNA:** In a high-powdered blender (see Note), combine the water, cashews, nutritional yeast, taco seasoning, and salt. Blend on high until the sauce warms and begins to thicken, 3 to 5 minutes. Lightly coat the bottom of an 8×8-inch baking dish with a little bit of the cashew sauce.

7. Layer the bottom of the dish with 10 of the tortilla quarters and about one-quarter each of the chicken, remaining cashew sauce, tomato, corn, and beans. Repeat three times with remaining ingredients.

8. Cover the lasagna with foil and store in the refrigerator for up to 5 days.

9. To serve, bake at 350°F for 30 minutes, removing the foil 10 minutes before the end of the baking time. Sprinkle with the cilantro before serving.

NOTE: If you have one, use a small blender like a Magic Bullet, or use a small blender cup. If you only have a wide-base blender or a large food processor, double the recipe so that nothing gets trapped beneath the blades.

TIDBIT: This chicken is also a great addition to taco night, salad bowls, or over rice and beans!

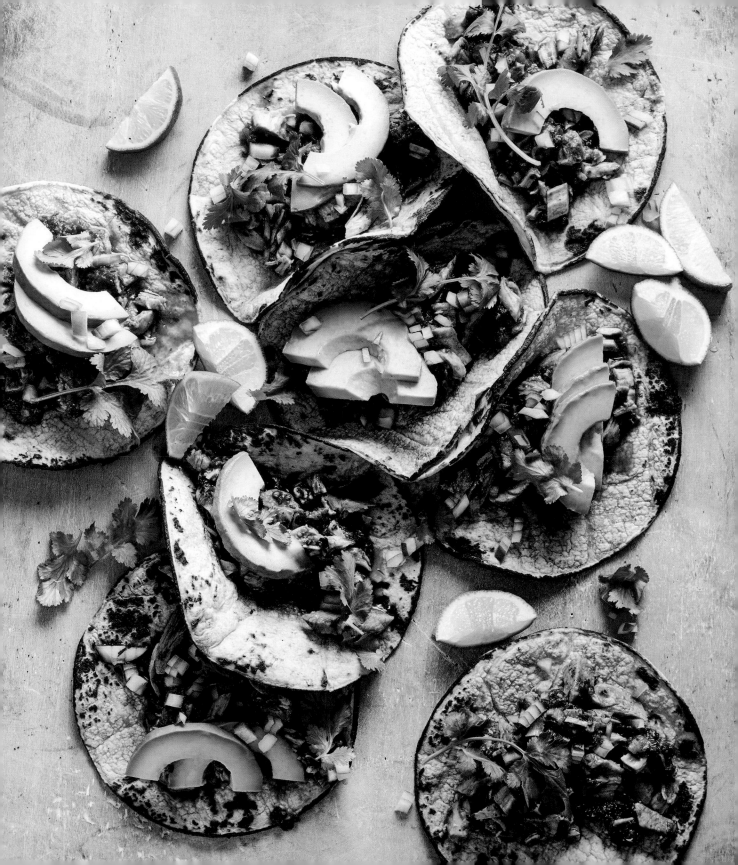

CHICKEN TINGA TACOS

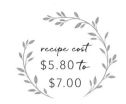

recipe cost
$5.80 to
$7.00

Tinga de pollo is a traditional Mexican shredded chicken dish filled with wonderful bold and smoky chipotle flavor. The chicken is stewed right in the tasty sauce—the longer it sits in the sauce, the better, meaning this dish is great to make ahead and reheat!

1. **MAKE THE CHICKEN:** Preheat an electric pressure cooker using the SAUTÉ function and adjust the heat to MORE (see Note page 95). When the display panel reads HOT, add the olive oil, chicken, and onion. Cook, stirring occasionally, for 3 minutes. Add the garlic, chipotle peppers, oregano, cumin, and salt. Cook, stirring frequently, for 1 minute.

2. Add the tomatoes and chicken broth. Place the lid on pressure cooker and make sure the vent valve is in the SEALING position. Using the display panel, select the MANUAL/PRESSURE COOK function and HIGH PRESSURE. Use the +/− buttons until the display reads 3 minutes.

3. When the cooker beeps, let it naturally release the pressure until the display reads LO:05. Switch the vent valve from the SEALING to the VENTING position. Use caution while the steam escapes.

4. Shred the chicken into the sauce.

5. **TO SERVE:** Divide the chicken among the tortillas. Top with avocado, cilantro, red onion, and a squeeze of lime juice.

SERVES 4

FOR THE CHICKEN

1 tablespoon extra-virgin olive oil

1 pound boneless, skinless chicken breasts, cut into bite-size pieces

½ yellow onion, diced

3 cloves garlic, minced

2 canned chipotle peppers in adobo sauce, finely chopped

2 teaspoons dried oregano

1 teaspoon ground cumin

1 teaspoon fine sea salt

¾ cup fire-roasted diced tomatoes

¼ cup low-sodium chicken broth

FOR SERVING

8 to 10 corn tortillas, warmed

1 large ripe avocado, pitted, peeled, and sliced

¼ cup fresh cilantro leaves

¼ cup diced red onion

1 large lime, cut into wedges

EASY WEEKNIGHT CHICKEN
and POTATOES

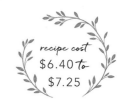

recipe cost
$6.40 *to*
$7.25

This is a weeknight, after-football-practice type of dinner. Serve with a side salad or the Bacon and Broccoli on page 179.

1. Preheat an electric pressure cooker using the SAUTÉ function and adjust the heat to MORE (see Note page 95).

2. **MAKE THE CHICKEN:** In a medium bowl, combine the chicken breasts, olive oil, garlic powder, salt, and black pepper. Stir well to coat.

3. When the display panel reads HOT, add the chicken and cook for 3 minutes on each side.

4. **MAKE THE POTATOES:** While the chicken is cooking, in a large bowl, combine the potatoes, olive oil, parsley, salt, and garlic powder. Toss well to coat.

5. Add the broth to the cooker and place the potatoes on top. Place the lid on pressure cooker and make sure the vent valve is in the SEALING position. Using the display panel, select the MANUAL/PRESSURE COOK function and HIGH PRESSURE. Use the +/− buttons until the display reads 5 minutes.

6. When the cooker beeps, let it naturally release the pressure until the display reads LO:05. Switch the vent valve from the SEALING to the VENTING position. Use caution while the steam escapes. Transfer the potatoes from the cooker to a bowl.

7. Remove the chicken and cut into portions, if necessary. Serve with the potatoes.

SERVES 4

FOR THE CHICKEN
1 pound boneless, skinless chicken breasts
1 tablespoon extra-virgin olive oil
1 teaspoon garlic powder
1 teaspoon fine sea salt
½ teaspoon ground black pepper

FOR THE POTATOES
1½ pounds baby creamer potatoes
1 tablespoon extra-virgin olive oil
1 teaspoon dried parsley flakes
1 teaspoon fine sea salt
½ teaspoon garlic powder
⅓ cup low-sodium chicken broth or Bone Broth (page 331)

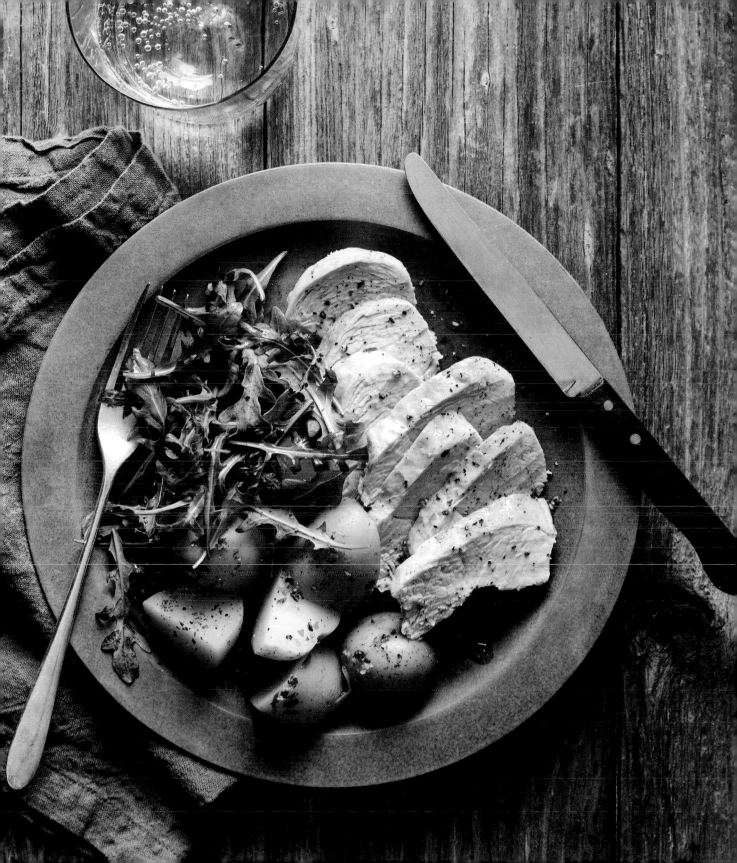

CHICKEN PARM ZUCCHINI BOATS

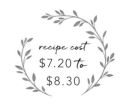

recipe cost
$7.20 *to*
$8.30

This lightened up version of chicken parm is easy to make and stuffed with yummy chicken, herbs—and actually no cheese at all! You can make the boats dairy-free with the Cashew Parmesan, or use regular freshy grated Parmesan if you are not dairy-free.

SERVES 4

1 cup water

4 medium zucchini

1 tablespoon extra-virgin olive oil

1 medium yellow onion, diced

1 pound lean ground chicken

½ teaspoon fine sea salt

½ teaspoon garlic powder

¼ teaspoon ground black pepper

¼ teaspoon dried basil

¼ teaspoon dried thyme

¼ teaspoon dried oregano

1 cup sugar-free marinara sauce

1 recipe Cashew Parmesan (page 266) or ½ cup grated fresh Parmesan

1. Pour the water into an electric pressure cooker and place a trivet in the cooker. Arrange the whole zucchini on the trivet, angling as needed to fit.

2. Place the lid on the cooker and make sure the vent valve is in the SEALING position. Using the display panel, select the MANUAL/PRESSURE COOK function and HIGH PRESSURE. Use the +/− buttons until the display reads 4 minutes.

3. While the zucchini cooks, heat a large skillet over medium-high heat. Once the pan has preheated, add the olive oil. Add the onion and cook, stirring occasionally, until softened, about 5 minutes. Add the chicken, salt, garlic powder, black pepper, basil, thyme, and oregano. Break up the chicken and cook for another 5 minutes.

4. Stir in the marinara sauce and reduce the heat to low.

5. When the cooker beeps, switch the vent valve from the SEALING to the VENTING position, administering a quick release. Use caution while the steam escapes.

6. Carefully transfer the zucchini from the cooker to a cutting board. Once cool, cut in half lengthwise and scoop out the seeds, leaving a ¼-inch shell.

7. Scoop a few tablespoons of the chicken mixture into each boat and sprinkle with the Cashew Parmesan.

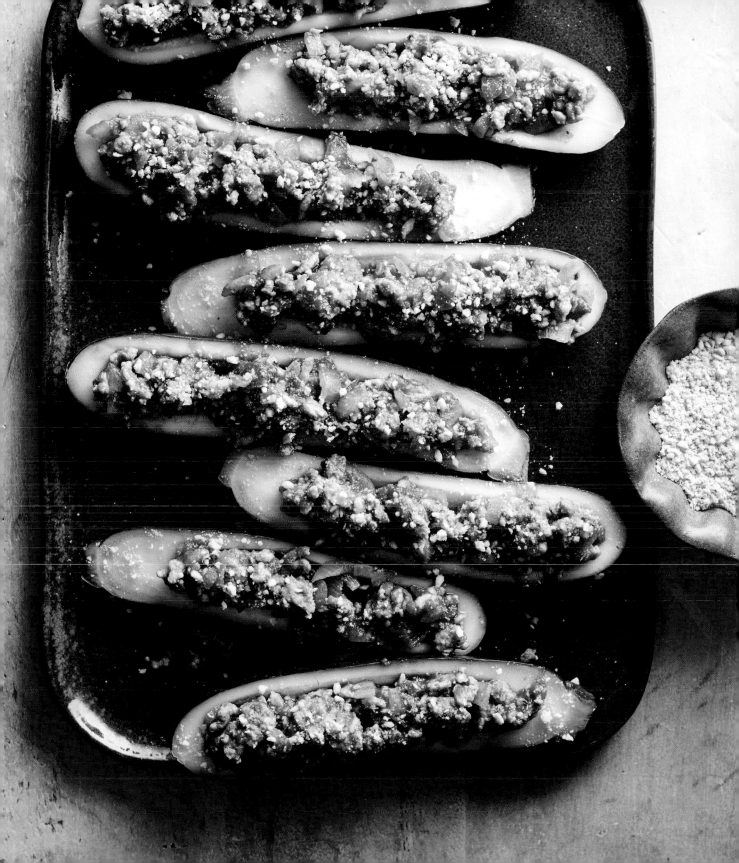

CASHEW PARMESAN

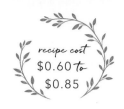

recipe cost
$0.60 to
$0.85

This is a great substitute for Parmesan cheese! You can of course substitute fresh shredded Parmesan in any recipe if you are not dairy-free.

MAKES ½ CUP

½ cup raw cashews

1 tablespoon unfortified nutritional yeast

¼ teaspoon fine sea salt

⅛ teaspoon garlic powder

In a food processor, combine the cashews, nutritional yeast, salt, and garlic powder. Pulse until the cashews are finely ground and resemble grated Parmesan cheese.

Store in an airtight container in the refrigerator for up to 2 weeks.

CILANTRO-LIME CHICKEN

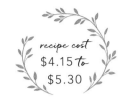

recipe cost
$4.15 *to*
$5.30

Depending on the thickness of the chicken breast, cook for 3 to 5 minutes on each side. Serve on top of a salad, as tacos, or with Casamiento (page 173).

SERVES 4

1 pound boneless, skinless chicken breasts

3 cloves garlic, minced

½ cup chopped fresh cilantro leaves

2 tablespoons fresh lime juice

2 tablespoons extra-virgin olive oil

½ teaspoon fine sea salt

¼ teaspoon black pepper

¼ cup water or low-sodium chicken broth

1. In a medium bowl, combine the chicken breasts, garlic, cilantro, lime juice, 1 tablespoon of the olive oil, salt, and black pepper. Cover and marinate in the refrigerator for 4 to 12 hours.

2. Preheat an electric pressure cooker using the SAUTÉ function and adjust the heat to MORE (see Note page 95). When the display panel reads HOT, add the remaining 1 tablespoon olive oil to the cooker. Arrange the chicken on the bottom in a single layer. Cook for 3 to 5 minutes on each side. Add the water.

3. Place the lid on the cooker and make sure the vent valve is in the SEALING position. Using the display panel, select the MANUAL/PRESSURE COOK function and HIGH PRESSURE. Use the +/− buttons until the display reads 6 minutes.

4. When the cooker beeps, let it naturally release the pressure until the display reads LO:05. Switch the vent valve from the SEALING to the VENTING position. Use caution while the steam escapes.

5. Remove the chicken from the cooker and serve.

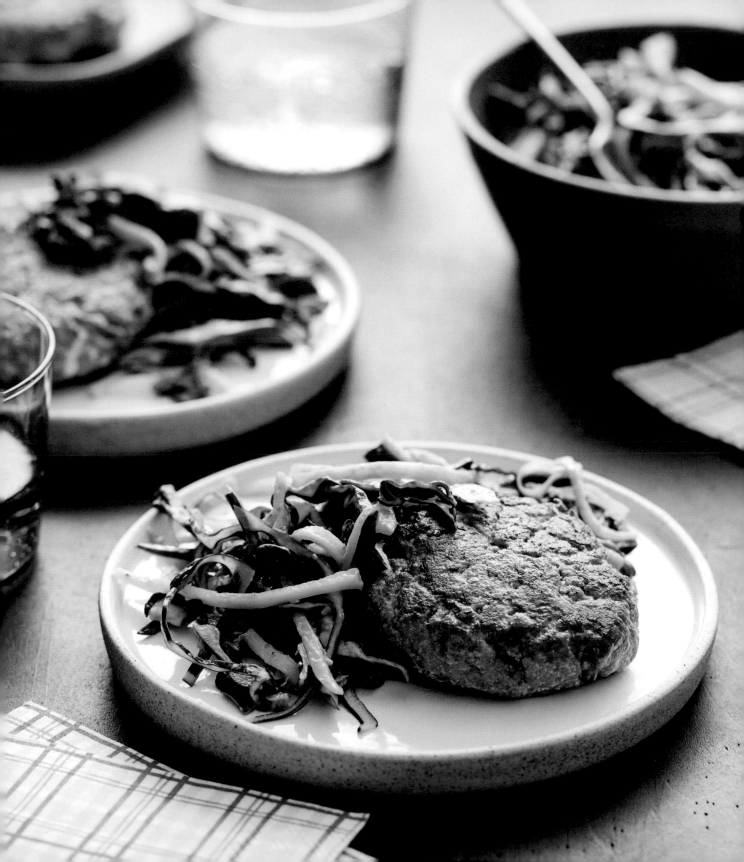

SALMON BURGERS *with* BROCCOLI SLAW

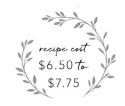

recipe cost $6.50 *to* $7.75

My children are the weirdest. If I put salmon fillets in front of them, they won't eat them, but if I put salmon burgers in front of them, they gobble them right up! I prefer to buy wild-caught Alaskan salmon (in the freezer section at Costco, or fresh if they have it) instead of the farmed fish. Not only is wild-caught salmon higher in nutrients like omega-3s, but farmed fish isn't always well-cared for and, from an ethics standpoint, it's worth it to me to invest in causes I believe in.

Not everyone feels as strongly, though, and that's okay. The quality of your fish will affect the price of the dish—it has a large range because I priced it with both farmed and wild-caught fillets.

1. MAKE THE BURGERS: Pulse the salmon in a food processor until it resembles coarse-ground meat, about 3 seconds. Transfer to a bowl and add the mustard, lemon juice, chives, salt, black pepper, and cayenne. Using your hands, gently combine (don't overwork or your burgers will be tough).

2. Divide the mixture into four equal portions and form into patties.

3. Preheat a 12-inch pan over medium-high heat. Once the pan has preheated, add the olive oil.

4. Add the patties and cook until golden brown and cooked through, 3 to 4 minutes on each side.

5. MAKE THE SLAW: In a large bowl, combine the cabbage and broccoli slaw.

6. In a wide-mouth jar, combine the avocado, water, chives, lemon juice, vinegar, salt, garlic powder, dried onion. Using an immersion blender, puree until smooth. Pour the dressing over the slaw mixture and toss to coat.

7. Serve the salmon burgers with the slaw.

SERVES 4

FOR THE SALMON BURGERS

14 ounces salmon fillets, skinned

1 tablespoon Dijon mustard

1½ teaspoons fresh lemon juice

1½ teaspoons chopped fresh chives

¾ teaspoon fine sea salt

½ teaspoon ground black pepper

¼ teaspoon cayenne pepper

1 tablespoon extra-virgin olive oil

FOR THE BROCCOLI SLAW

3 cups thinly sliced purple cabbage

2 cups broccoli slaw

1 ripe medium avocado, pitted and peeled

¼ cup water

1½ teaspoons chopped fresh chives

1 teaspoon fresh lemon juice

1 teaspoon apple cider vinegar

½ teaspoon fine sea salt

¼ teaspoon garlic powder

¼ teaspoon dried minced onion

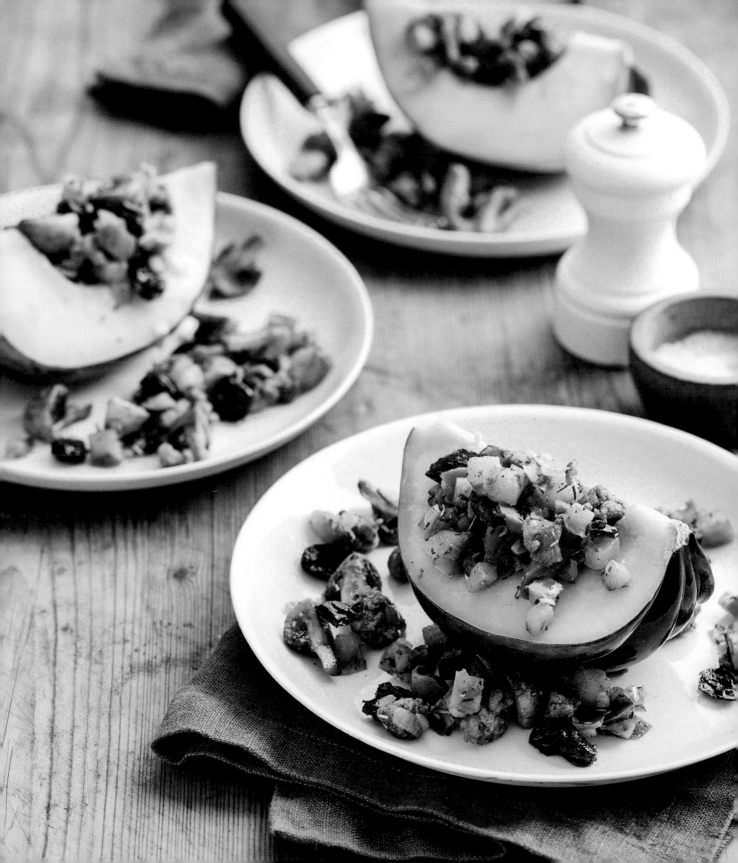

ACORN SQUASH *with* SAUSAGE *and* CRANBERRIES

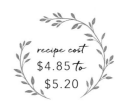

recipe cost $4.85 *to* $5.20

Make sure to save the seeds of your squash! Do not throw those little gems in the trash. Use the recipe on page 272 to toast acorn squash seeds. They are like pumpkin seeds, but better! It's extremely difficult to find naturally sweetened cranberries, so I use cranberries sweetened with cane sugar. Just make sure your cranberries aren't sweetened with any artificial sweeteners. You can also use pomegranate seeds instead of cranberries. If serving this dish as your whole meal, it will serve two. If serving it with something else, like a side salad, it will serve four.

SERVES 2 TO 4

1 cup water

1 (1½- to 2-pound) acorn squash, halved and seeded

2 tablespoons extra-virgin olive oil

6 ounces white mushrooms, chopped

4 ounces ground pork sausage

1 Gala apple, cored and diced

½ yellow onion, diced

1½ teaspoons minced garlic

1 teaspoon fine sea salt

½ teaspoon dried rosemary

½ teaspoon dried thyme

¼ teaspoon dried sage

¼ teaspoon ground black pepper

⅓ cup dried cranberries

1. Pour the water into an electric pressure cooker and place a trivet inside. Set the squash halves on the trivet. Place the lid on the cooker and make sure the vent valve is in the SEALING position. Using the display panel, select the MANUAL/PRESSURE COOK function and HIGH PRESSURE. Use the +/− buttons until the display reads 10 minutes.

2. When the cooker beeps, switch the vent valve from the SEALING to the VENTING position, administering a quick release. Use caution while the steam escapes.

3. Carefully remove the squash halves from the cooker. Remove the trivet. Remove the liner and pour out the water. Place the liner back in the cooker.

4. Preheat the cooker using the SAUTÉ function and adjust the heat to MORE (see Note page 95). When the display reads HOT, add the olive oil, mushrooms, sausage, apple, onion, garlic, salt, rosemary, thyme, sage, and black pepper. Cook, stirring occasionally, until the pork is browned, about 8 minutes. Stir in the cranberries.

5. Cut each squash half in half again. Fill each quarter with one-fourth of the sausage mixture. Serve immediately.

TOASTED ACORN SQUASH SEEDS

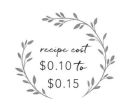

recipe cost
$0.10 *to*
$0.15

Every squash is different and will yield a different amount of seeds. Depending on how many cups of seeds your squash yields, you will need to adjust this recipe accordingly.

Preheat the oven to 300°F.

In a medium bowl, toss together the squash seeds, olive oil, and salt. Transfer the seeds to a baking sheet. Bake for 15 to 20 minutes, or until lightly toasted and crunchy.

MAKES ½ CUP

½ cup fresh acorn squash seeds, strings and guts rinsed off

1½ teaspoons extra-virgin olive oil

¼ to ½ teaspoon fine sea salt

BRUNSWICK STEW

recipe cost
$5.90 to
$7.00

This is a classic Southern stew that's usually served over mashed potatoes. The barbecue sauce and a little hot sauce give the stew its bold flavor and make it a super-popular dish to serve at a barbecue!

SERVES 4

1 pound beef brisket, fat trimmed and cut into ½-inch pieces

1 cup frozen corn

1 cup lima beans

½ cup Tangy Barbecue Sauce (page 324)

½ cup diced tomatoes

½ cup tomato sauce

2 tablespoons mild hot sauce

1 tablespoon reduced-sodium Worcestershire sauce

½ yellow onion, diced

1½ teaspoons garlic powder

1½ teaspoons onion powder

1 teaspoon fine sea salt

½ teaspoon ground black pepper

2 cups water

1 recipe garlic Garlic-Chive Mashed Potatoes (page 184)

1. In an electric pressure cooker, combine the brisket, corn, beans, barbecue sauce, tomatoes, tomato sauce, hot sauce, Worcestershire sauce, onion, garlic powder, onion powder, salt, black pepper, and water.

2. Place the lid on the cooker and make sure the vent valve is in the SEALING position. Using the display panel, select the MANUAL/PRESSURE COOK function and HIGH PRESSURE. Use the +/− buttons until the display reads 45 minutes.

3. When the cooker beeps, let it naturally release the pressure until the display reads LO:10. Switch the vent valve from the SEALING to the VENTING position. Use caution while the steam escapes.

4. To serve, ladle the stew over the mashed potatoes.

BARBACOA LETTUCE WRAP TACOS

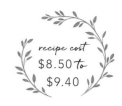

recipe cost
$8.50 to $9.40

Saucy and savory, peppery shredded beef barbacoa is a fabulous addition to taco night! There are so many ways to serve it, too: on top of fresh mixed greens, in a lettuce leaf or cabbage cup, or in a corn tortilla! If you have any leftover cilantro, green onion, or chives, add a generous sprinkling to the top of each wrap for a fresh bite of flavor!

SERVES 4

1 pound beef stew meat, cut into 1-inch pieces

½ cup low-sodium beef broth or Bone Broth (page 331)

1 tablespoon extra-virgin olive oil

1 tablespoon apple cider vinegar

1½ teaspoons chipotle chili powder

1½ teaspoons tomato paste

¾ teaspoon fine sea salt

½ teaspoon cumin

½ teaspoon garlic powder

½ teaspoon dried oregano

½ teaspoon ground black pepper

1 large head butterleaf lettuce or green cabbage, leaves separated

1 medium Roma tomato, diced

½ small red onion, cored and thinly sliced

1. In an electric pressure cooker, combine the meat, broth, olive oil, vinegar, chili powder, tomato paste, salt, cumin, garlic powder, oregano, and black pepper.

2. Place the lid on the cooker and make sure the vent valve is in the SEALING position. Using the display panel, select the BEEF/STEW function and HIGH PRESSURE. Use the +/− buttons until the display reads 35 minutes.

3. When the cooker beeps, let it naturally release the pressure until the display reads LO:15. Switch the vent valve from the SEALING to the VENTING position. Use caution while the steam escapes.

4. Remove the lid and using the display panel, select the SAUTÉ function and adjust the heat to MORE (see Note page 95). Shred the beef into the sauce and cook until it thickens and the liquid reduces by half, about 5 minutes.

5. Fill each lettuce leaf with 2 to 4 tablespoons of meat. Garnish with tomato and onion.

NOTE: Freeze any excess tomato paste in 1-tablespoon quantities: Lay a piece of parchment paper over a baking sheet and scoop the tomato paste onto the sheet in equal portions. Lay flat inside the freezer and freeze for a minimum of 2 hours or until you can combine the tomato paste in an airtight container without it clumping together. Store in the freezer for up to 6 months.

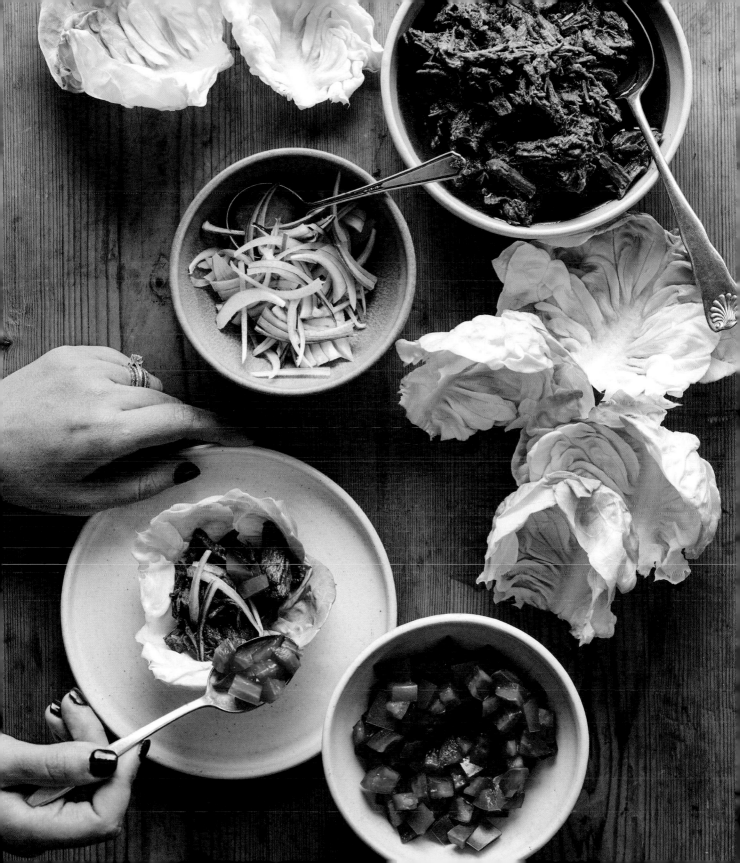

EASY STEAK BITES *with* PEPPERS

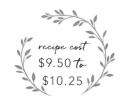

recipe cost
$9.50 *to*
$10.25

With just the right hint of spice, this steak-and-pepper recipe is a perfect way to end the night! Packed full of nutrients, this veggie-heavy dinner will leave you feeling satisfied.

SERVES 4

- 1 pound sirloin steak strips
- 1 medium red bell pepper, seeded and diced
- 1 small yellow onion, thinly sliced
- 1 medium to large zucchini, spiralized (see Note page 51)
- ½ small jalapeño, seeded and thinly sliced
- 2 tablespoons extra-virgin olive oil
- 6 cloves garlic, minced
- 1 tablespoon dried parsley flakes
- 2 teaspoons Taco Seasoning (page 325)
- 1¼ teaspoons fine sea salt
- ½ teaspoon ground black pepper
- ¼ cup fresh cilantro or flat-leaf parsley
- 1 lime, cut into wedges

1. In a large bowl, combine the steak strips, bell pepper, onion, zucchini, jalapeño, olive oil, garlic, parsley, taco seasoning, salt, and black pepper. Toss to combine.

2. Transfer the steak to a 5.3-quart air-fryer basket and bake at 370°F for 12 to 15 minutes, stirring halfway through the cooking time.

3. Divide among four plates. Garnish with cilantro and a squeeze of lime.

NOTE: If you do not have an air fryer, this dish can be made on the stovetop in a large pan. Sauté everything over medium-high heat until the vegetables are soft and the meat is cooked to your liking.

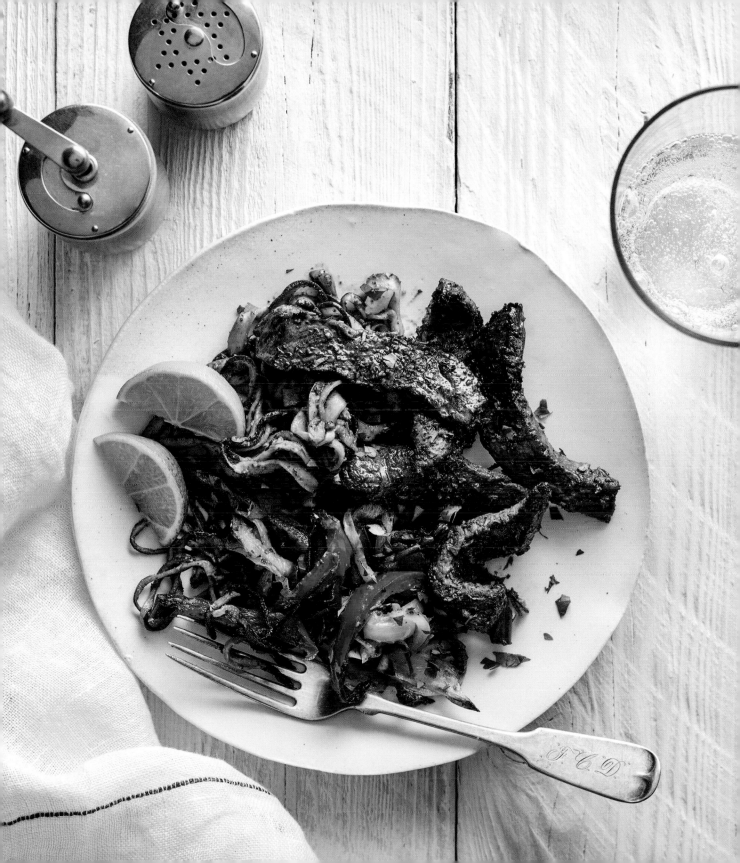

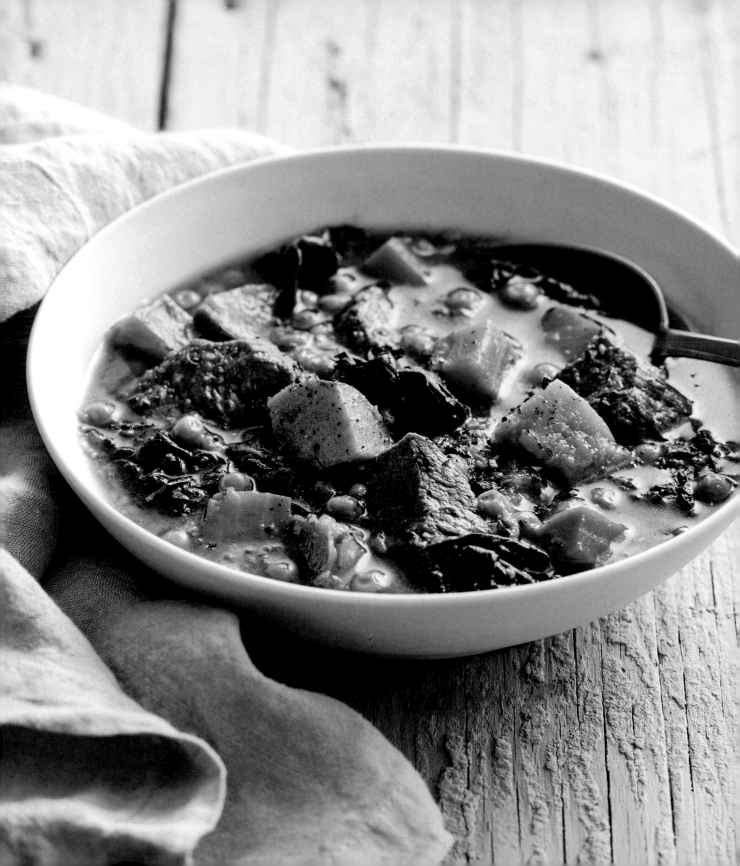

MAMA'S BARE-BONES BEEF STEW

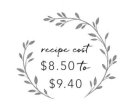

recipe cost
$8.50 to $9.40

I have a stew recipe in each of my books because this was 100 percent a dinner staple for our family while I was working to get well and shed some weight. There are so many different variations to make it feel like it's new and fresh, but at its core it's the same base with delicious ingredients that have been keeping my whole family happy for years. It's an excellent Sunday-night dinner that requires very little time in the kitchen.

SERVES 4

- 1 pound beef stew meat, cut into 1-inch pieces
- 2 large carrots, peeled and diced (see Note page 51)
- 2 medium sweet potatoes, peeled and cut into 1½-inch cubes
- 1 large yellow onion, diced
- ½ bunch kale (ribs removed), shredded
- 2 cups low-sodium beef broth or Bone Broth (page 331)
- 1 cup water
- 2 tablespoons dried minced onion
- 1 tablespoon dried parsley flakes
- 2 teaspoons arrowroot powder or cornstarch
- 1½ teaspoons fine sea salt
- ½ teaspoon garlic powder
- ½ teaspoon ground black pepper
- 1 cup frozen peas, thawed

1. In an electric pressure cooker, combine the meat, carrots, sweet potatoes, onion, kale, broth, water, dried onion, parsley, arrowroot powder, salt, garlic powder, and black pepper.

2. Place the lid on the cooker and make sure the vent valve is in the SEALING position. Using the display panel, select the MANUAL/PRESSURE COOK function and HIGH PRESSURE. Use the +/− buttons until the display reads 35 minutes.

3. When the cooker beeps, let it naturally release the pressure until the display reads LO:10. Switch the vent valve from the SEALING to the VENTING position. Use caution while the steam escapes. Remove the lid, stir in the peas, and serve.

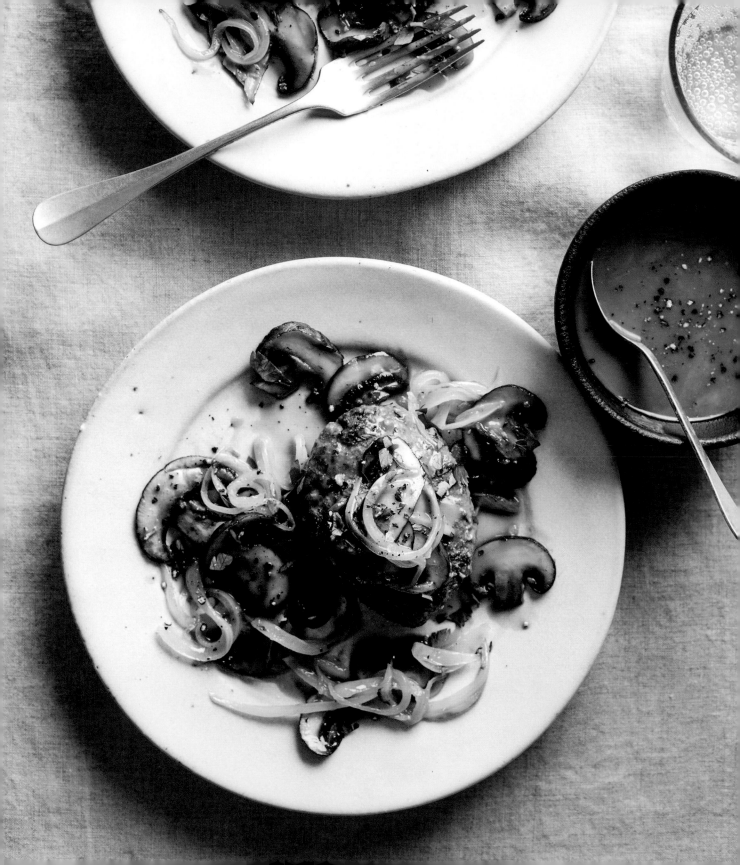

SALISBURY STEAK *with* MUSHROOM GRAVY

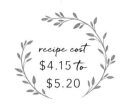

recipe cost $4.15 *to* $5.20

Classic TV-dinner heaven, this handmade steak is smothered in a mushroom and onion gravy and is ready in under 30 minutes!

SERVES 4

1 pound lean ground beef

1 tablespoon extra-virgin olive oil

1 teaspoon fine sea salt

½ teaspoon ground black pepper

½ teaspoon onion powder

½ teaspoon garlic powder

½ teaspoon Cajun Seasoning (page 328) or store-bought

½ teaspoon dried basil

½ yellow onion, thinly sliced

1 cup sliced mushrooms

¾ cup low-sodium beef broth or Bone Broth (page 331)

1 tablespoon yellow mustard

1 teaspoon apple cider vinegar

1 tablespoon arrowroot powder or cornstarch

1 cup Oat Milk (page 288) or other milk

1 tablespoon chopped fresh flat-leaf parsley (optional)

1. Divide the ground beef into four equal portions. Shape each portion into a patty. Arrange the patties in the bottom of an electric pressure cooker in a single layer. (It's okay if they touch.)

2. Sprinkle the steaks evenly with the olive oil, salt, black pepper, onion powder, garlic powder, Cajun seasoning, and basil. Scatter the onion and mushrooms on top.

3. In a bowl, combine the broth, mustard, and vinegar. Stir to combine. Pour the mixture over the mushrooms and onions. Place the lid on the cooker and make sure the vent valve is in the SEALING position. Using the display panel, select the MANUAL/PRESSURE COOK function and HIGH PRESSURE. Use the +/− buttons until the display reads 6 minutes.

4. When the cooker beeps, switch the vent valve from the SEALING to the VENTING position, administering a quick release. Use caution while the steam escapes.

5. Remove the steaks, onions, and mushrooms.

6. Using the display panel, select the SAUTÉ function and adjust to NORMAL (see Note page 182). Stir in the arrowroot powder and oat milk and let simmer, stirring frequently, until the gravy thickens, about 2 minutes.

7. Serve the steaks topped with mushrooms, onions, and gravy. Sprinkle with parsley, if desired.

CABBAGE *and* QUINOA BOWL

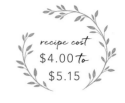

recipe cost
$4.00 *to*
$5.15

It's so important to rinse your quinoa in a fine-mesh strainer. Quinoa has a natural coating, called saponin, which can make it taste bitter or soapy. Most quinoa is prerinsed now, but make sure to read the label and rinse your quinoa well if it isn't. I purchase my prerinsed quinoa in a large bag at Costco.

SERVES 4

½ pound lean ground beef

½ medium yellow onion, diced

3 cloves garlic, minced

1 teaspoon fine sea salt

¼ teaspoon ground black pepper

1 tablespoon dried oregano

1 cup low-sodium beef broth or water

¾ cup quinoa, rinsed and drained

½ cup tomato sauce

½ large head of cabbage, cored and chopped (6 to 8 cups)

1. Preheat an electric pressure cooker using the SAUTÉ function and adjust the heat to MORE (see Note page 95). When the display panel reads HOT, add the ground beef, onion, garlic, salt, black pepper, and oregano. Cook, stirring occasionally, until the beef is lightly browned, about 3 minutes.

2. Add the broth, quinoa, tomato sauce, and cabbage and stir well.

3. Place the lid on the cooker and make sure the vent valve is in the SEALING position. Using the display panel, select the MANUAL/PRESSURE COOK function and HIGH PRESSURE. Use the +/− buttons until the display reads 2 minutes.

4. When the cooker beeps, let it naturally release the pressure until the display reads LO:10. Switch the vent valve from the SEALING to the VENTING position. Use caution while the steam escapes.

5. Serve hot.

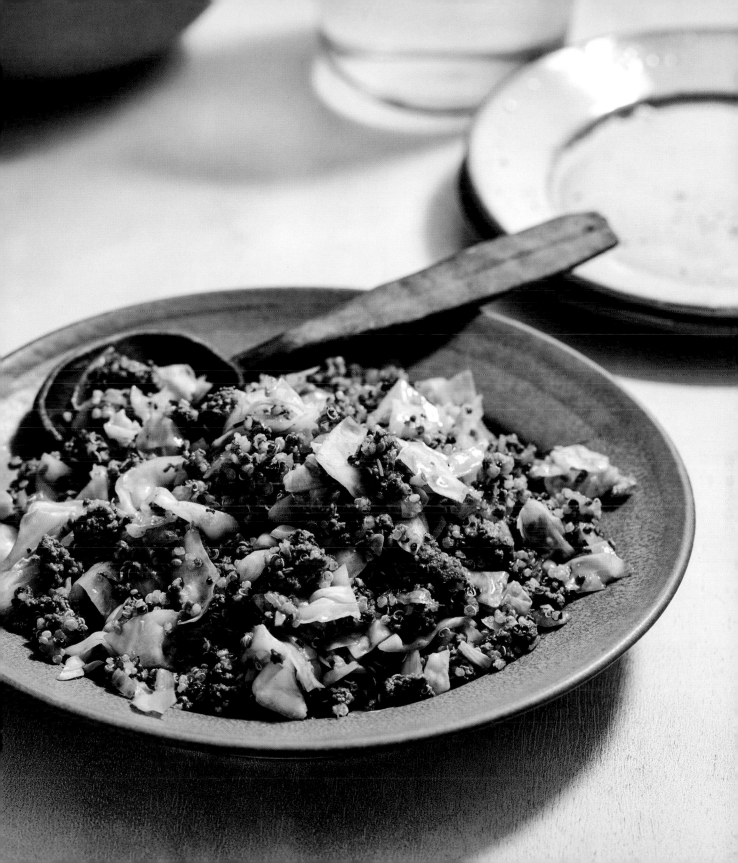

BLACK BEAN BURRITO BOWLS

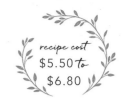

recipe cost
$5.50 to
$6.80

Sometimes you just need a no-fuss dinner, fast. This meal comes together in under thirty minutes from start to finish. It is packed full of vegetables and tasty sauces that satisfy even the strongest craving for Taco Bell. It's also super-versatile, so serve it in a bowl or as a burrito stuffing.

SERVES 4

½ pound lean ground beef

¼ cup Taco Seasoning (page 325)

½ yellow onion, diced

½ small jalapeño, seeded and thinly sliced

½ red bell pepper, seeded and diced

2 cups cooked black beans

2 cups sliced green cabbage

1 cup frozen corn kernels

½ cup low-sodium chicken broth or water

1 large head romaine, cored and sliced

½ large avocado, pitted, peeled, and sliced

No-Queso Queso (page 121)

1 Roma tomato, cored and diced

2 tablespoons fresh cilantro

1. Preheat an electric pressure cooker using the SAUTÉ function and adjust the heat to MORE (see Note page 95).

2. When the display panel reads HOT, add the ground beef, taco seasoning, onion, jalapeño, and bell pepper. Cook, stirring occasionally, until the beef is lightly browned. Add the beans, cabbage, corn, and broth.

3. Place the lid on pressure cooker and make sure the vent valve is in the SEALING position. Using the display panel, select the MANUAL/PRESSURE COOK function and HIGH PRESSURE. Use the +/− buttons until the display reads 2 minutes.

4. When the cooker beeps, switch the vent valve from the SEALING to the VENTING position, administering a quick release. Use caution while the steam escapes.

5. Serve over romaine and avocado. Top with No-Queso Queso, tomato, and cilantro.

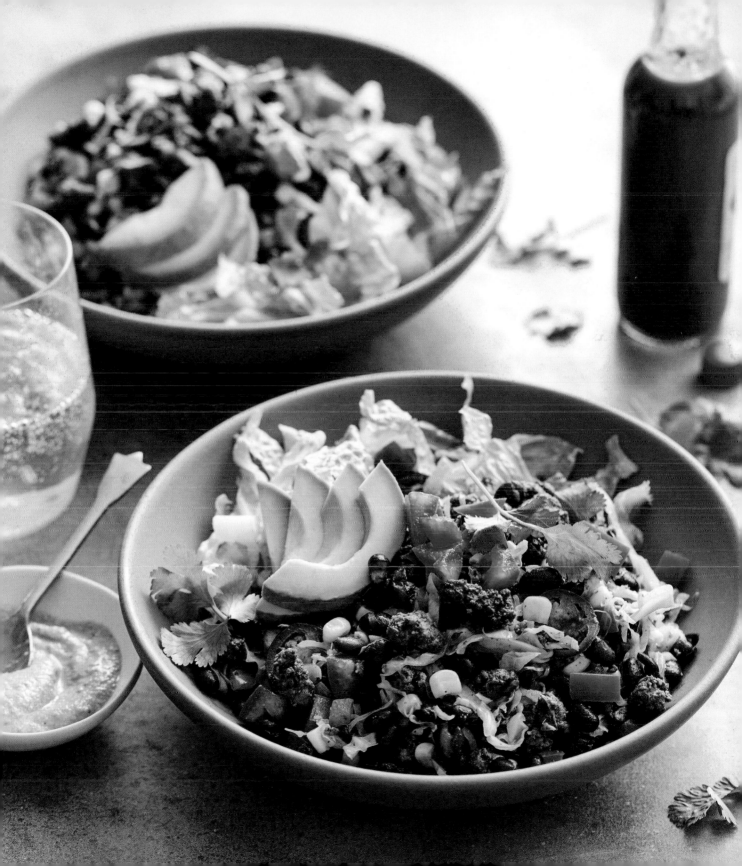

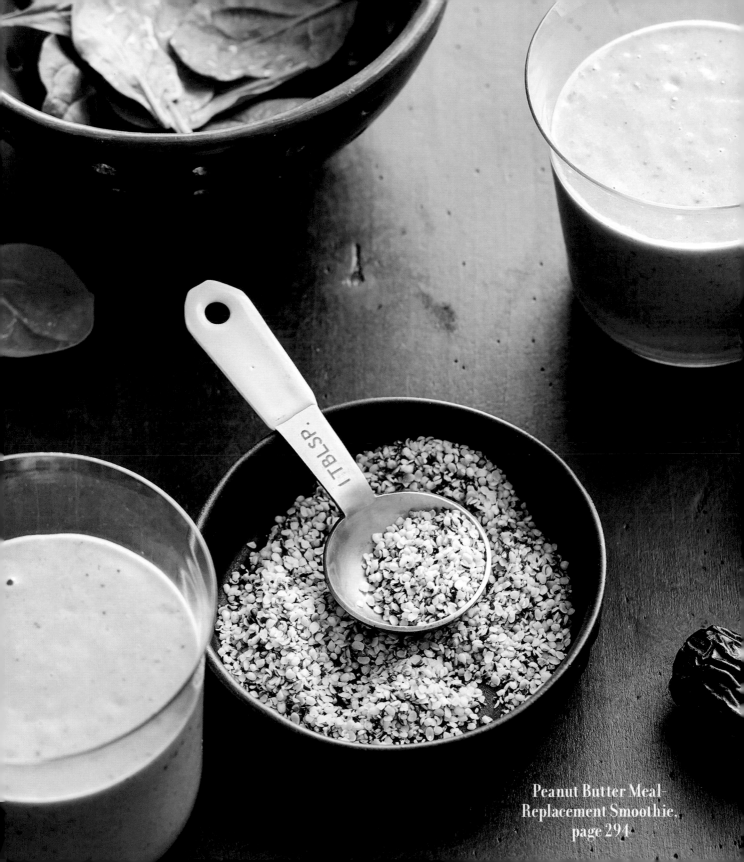

Peanut Butter Meal-
Replacement Smoothie,
page 294

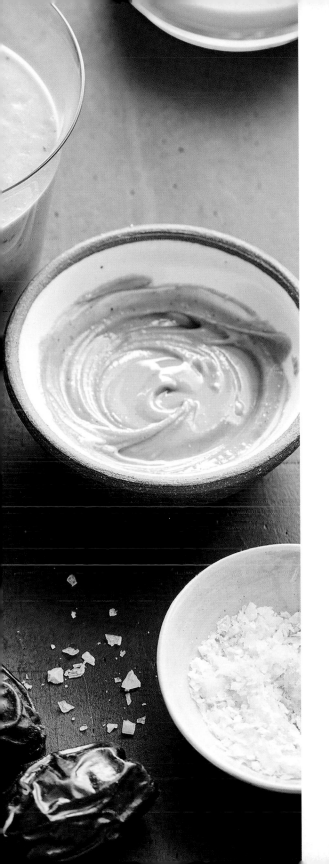

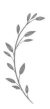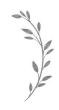

DRINKS

HOMEMADE NONDAIRY MILK

Purchasing nondairy alternative milks at the store adds up quickly. Not only is it costly, but most store-bought plant-based milk is full of gums, preservatives, and fillers in order to keep them shelf-stable.

I held off and refused to make my own milk for a long time because it seemed intimidating and time-consuming. At the prodding of the Instant Loss Facebook community, I decided to put on my big girl pants and give it a try. I felt awfully embarrassed that I made such a big deal about it after my first attempt because it's honestly one of the easiest things I whip up in my kitchen. It's truly as simple as blend, strain, and refrigerate!

If you can make a smoothie, you can make your own plant-based milk. Oat milk is by far the most cost-effective alternative milk—just pennies per cup!

MAKES 4 CUPS

THINGS YOU'LL NEED
Blender (I use a Vitamix)
Fine-mesh nut milk bag (super-cheap on Amazon)
Glass container/pitcher (got mine in the $1 spot at Target)

MILK	PLANT BASE	WATER	BLEND / STRAIN	STORE	COST
Oat Milk	1 cup gluten-free old-fashioned rolled oats (see Note)	4 cups	20 seconds; gently squeeze	Up to 1 week	$0.06 to $0.10
Hemp Milk	1 cup hemp seeds or hearts	4 cups	30 to 60 seconds; gently squeeze	Up to 1 week	$1.80 to $2.60
Coconut Milk	1 cup unsweetened shredded coconut	4 cups	30 to 60 seconds; gently squeeze	Up to 1 week	$0.80 to $1.00
Almond Milk	1 cup whole raw almonds	4 cups	60 seconds; wring as hard as you can	3 to 5 days	$1.20 to $2.45
Cashew Milk	1 cup whole raw cashew	4 cups	30 to 60 seconds; gently squeeze	3 to 5 days	$1.40 to $2.45

1. Simply combine the plant base and water in a blender and blend on high for the time indicated in the chart. Strain the milk through a nut milk bag, squeeze as indicated, and store in a glass container in the refrigerator. Make sure to consume it within the time indicated.

2. To make a lightly sweetened variation, add two pitted Medjool dates to the blender. For vanilla milk, stir in a splash of vanilla extract and 1 tablespoon pure maple syrup.

3. This recipe can be cut in half or quartered if you know you will not consume 4 cups of milk within 5 days.

NOTE: It's important not to overblend oat milk because the water can get too warm and heat the oats, making them gummy or slimy. If you find that your oat milk is yielding slimy results, try soaking the oats with digestive enzymes before you blend; the amylase enzyme helps break down starches. (This is a tip I learned from Downshiftology). Soak 1 cup oats in 2 cups water with two emptied capsules (powder only, outside capsule removed) of digestive enzymes for 15 minutes. Strain and rinse the oats and proceed with the recipe.

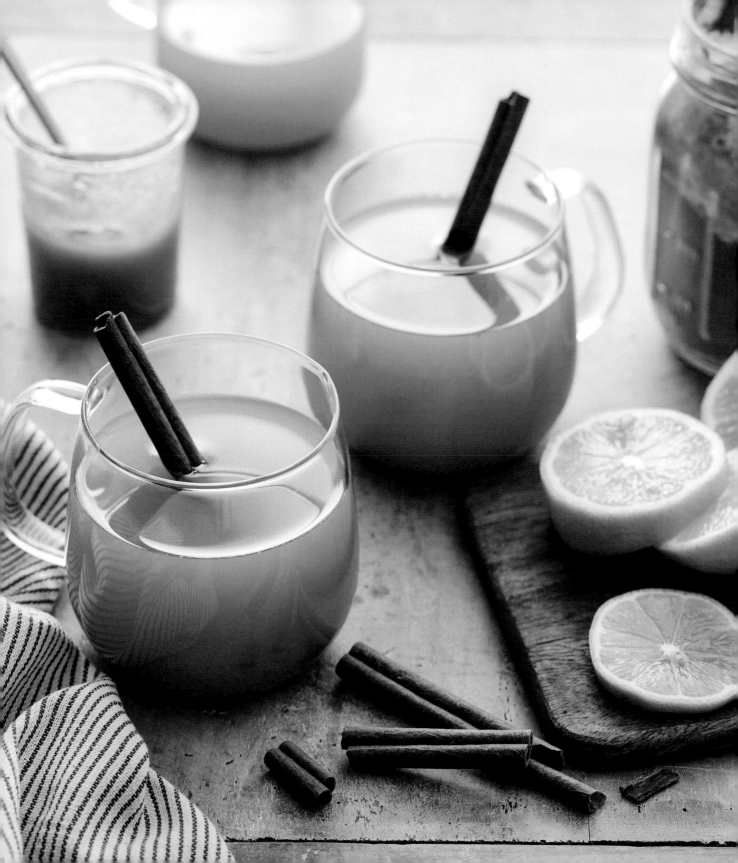

LEMON-TURMERIC TEA

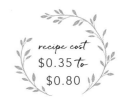

recipe cost
$0.35 *to*
$0.80

This tea is fabulous hot or cold. Turmeric is so beneficial for reducing inflammation in the body and improving digestion! I include black pepper here because a compound in it, piperine, enhances absorption of curcumin (a beneficial compound in turmeric) in the body by up to 2,000 percent, so combining spices truly magnifies their effects.

MAKES 4 CUPS

4 cups water
2 tablespoons raw honey
½ cinnamon stick
1 teaspoon ground turmeric
⅛ teaspoon ground black pepper
Juice of 1 lemon
1 bay leaf

1. In an electric pressure cooker, combine the water, honey, cinnamon stick, turmeric, black pepper, lemon juice, and bay leaf and stir well.

2. Place the lid on the cooker and make sure the vent valve is in the SEALING position. Using the display panel, select the MANUAL/PRESSURE COOK function and LOW PRESSURE. Use the +/− buttons until the display reads 5 minutes.

3. When the cooker beeps, let it naturally release the pressure until the display reads LO:10. Switch the vent valve from the SEALING to the VENTING position. Use caution while the steam escapes.

4. Discard the cinnamon stick and bay leaf. Ladle into cups and serve.

DINOSAUR JUICE

recipe cost
$0.75 to
$0.90

As a mother of young children, I know it isn't always easy getting the good stuff into those bellies. But add a fun name and all of a sudden it gets a whole lot easier!

In a blender, combine the oat milk, spinach, kale, strawberries, banana, and date. Blend on high until smooth, about 30 seconds.

SERVES 1 TO 2

1 cup Oat Milk (page 288) or water

1 cup baby spinach

½ cup chopped kale (ribs removed)

½ cup frozen strawberries

½ frozen banana, peeled

1 Medjool date, pitted

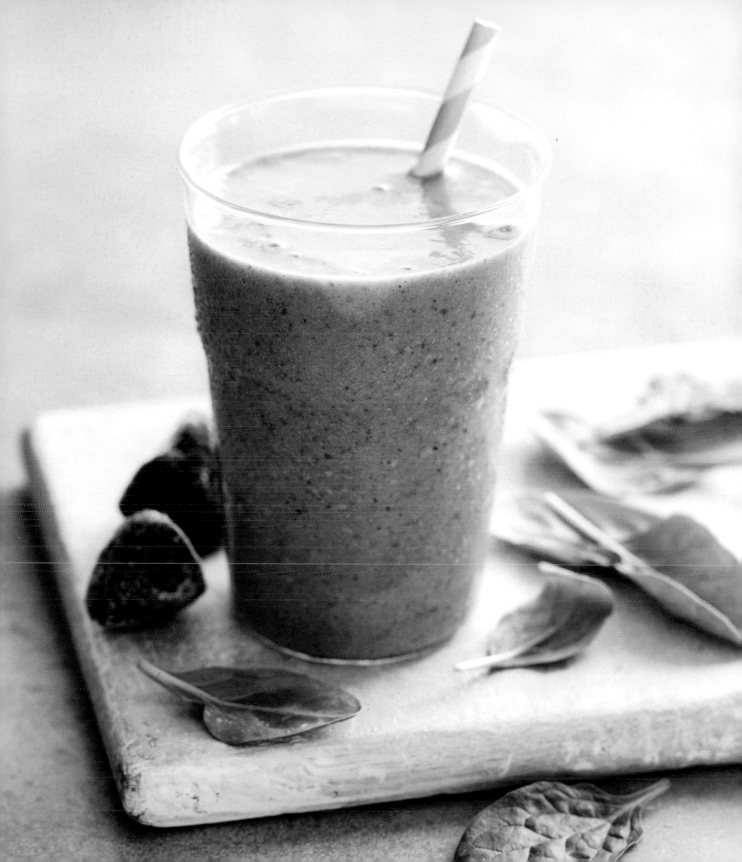

PEANUT BUTTER MEAL-REPLACEMENT SMOOTHIE

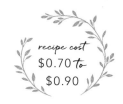

recipe cost
$0.70 to
$0.90

This protein-packed smoothie is the perfect meal replacement for busy days on the go. Packed full of fiber and rich in vitamins and heart-healthy fats, this smoothie will keep you feeling powered up!

In a blender, combine the oat milk, spinach, peaches, banana, peanut butter, hemp hearts, collagen peptides (if using), date, and salt. Blend on high until smooth, about 30 seconds.

SERVES 1

1 cup Oat Milk (page 288) or water

1 cup baby spinach

½ cup frozen peaches

½ frozen banana, peeled

1 tablespoon organic peanut butter

1 tablespoon hemp hearts

1 tablespoon collagen peptides (optional)

1 Medjool date, pitted

⅛ teaspoon fine sea salt

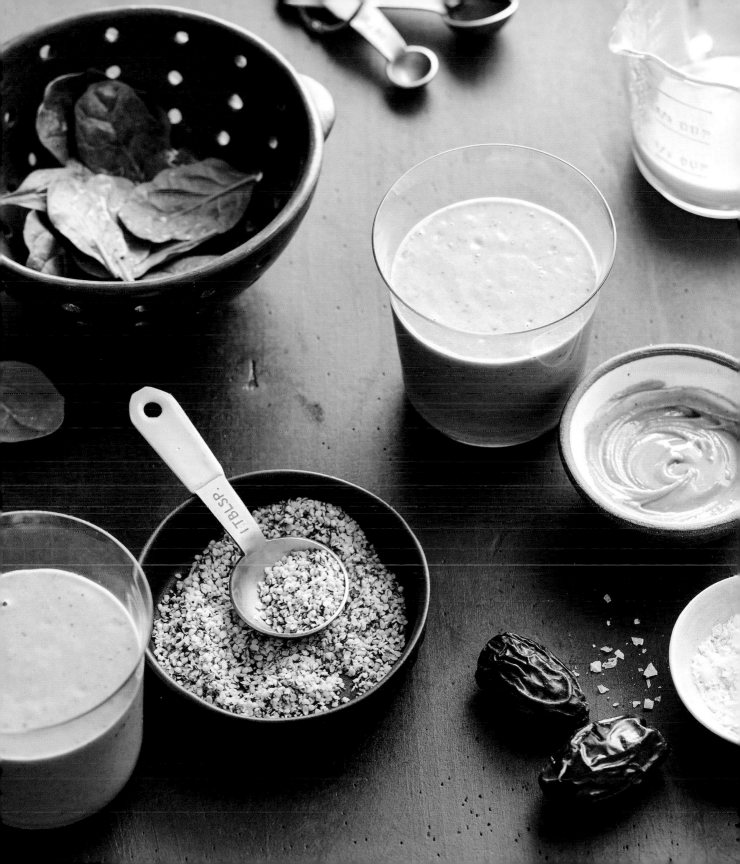

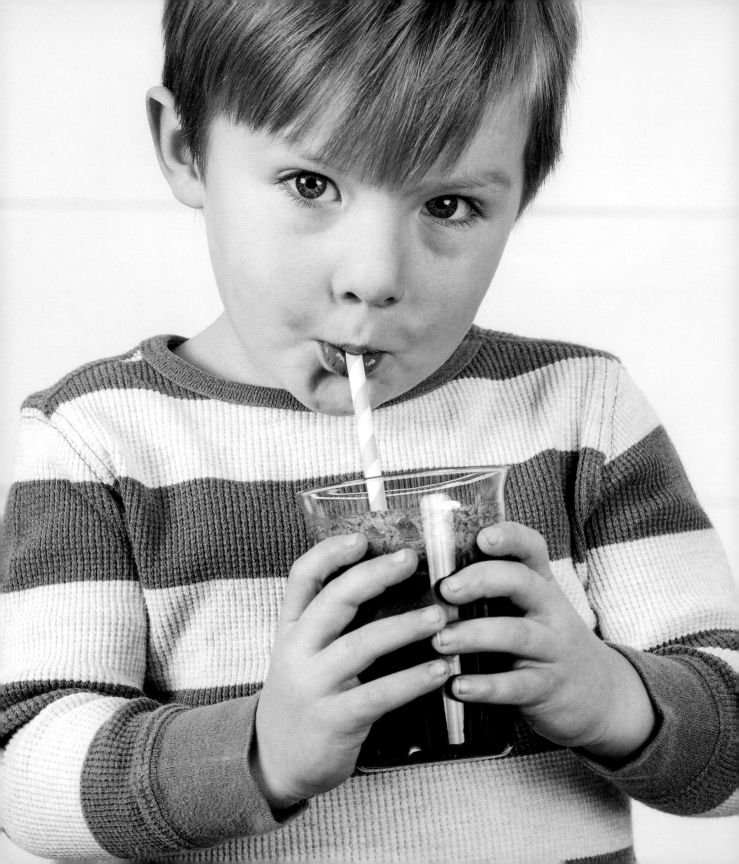

TART APPLE–BLUEBERRY JUICE

recipe cost
$0.40 *to*
$0.65

We stopped buying store-bought juice because I noticed their ability to make my mild-mannered children go from calm to crazy in ten minutes. That doesn't mean they can't still enjoy their favorite drinks, though! Making them at home not only gives me control over the ingredients, but also the ability to add a little extra veggie without them noticing.

SERVES 1

1 cup baby spinach
1 cup water
⅓ cup frozen blueberries
½ green apple, cored and sliced
1 tablespoon fresh lemon juice

In a blender, combine the spinach, water, blueberries, apple, and lemon juice. Blend on high until smooth, about 30 seconds.

SNOWY DAY HOT COCOA

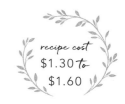

recipe cost
$1.30 *to*
$1.60

The kids will love this creamy homemade hot chocolate! Rich and easy to make, its intense chocolate flavor pairs well with your favorite dairy-free whipped cream. So Delicious brand is very tasty, or see the Note on page 316 to make your own. This is a treat for the kid in all of us!

SERVES 4

4 cups Oat Milk (page 288) or other milk

⅓ cup dairy-free chocolate chips

3 tablespoons cacao powder

4½ teaspoons 100 percent pure maple syrup

Dairy-free whipped cream (optional)

1. In an electric pressure cooker, combine the oat milk, chocolate chips, cacao powder, and maple syrup and stir well.

2. Place the lid on the cooker and make sure the vent valve is in the SEALING position. Using the display panel, select the MANUAL/PRESSURE COOK function and HIGH PRESSURE. Use the +/− buttons until the display reads 1 minute.

3. When the cooker beeps, let it naturally release the pressure until the display reads LO:05. Use caution while the steam escapes.

4. Remove the lid. Use an immersion blender or whisk to blend the cocoa. Serve warm, with whipped cream if you like.

SUMMERTIME SWEET TEA

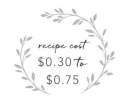

recipe cost
$0.30 *to*
$0.75

The tea bags in this recipe can be reused once—three used tea bags plus three new ones will yield the same result. Sub in two chai tea bags for a lightly spiced flavor and add a splash of milk!

MAKES 6 CUPS

6 green, white, or black tea bags, paper tabs removed

6 cups water

¼ cup raw honey

1. In an electric pressure cooker, combine the tea bags, water, and honey and stir well.

2. Place the lid on the cooker and make sure the vent valve is in the SEALING position. Using the display panel, select the MANUAL/PRESSURE COOK function and HIGH PRESSURE. Use the +/− buttons until the display reads 5 minutes.

3. When the cooker beeps, let it naturally release the pressure until the display reads LO:15. Switch the vent valve from the SEALING to the VENTING position. Use caution while the steam escapes.

4. Allow the tea to cool before serving over ice.

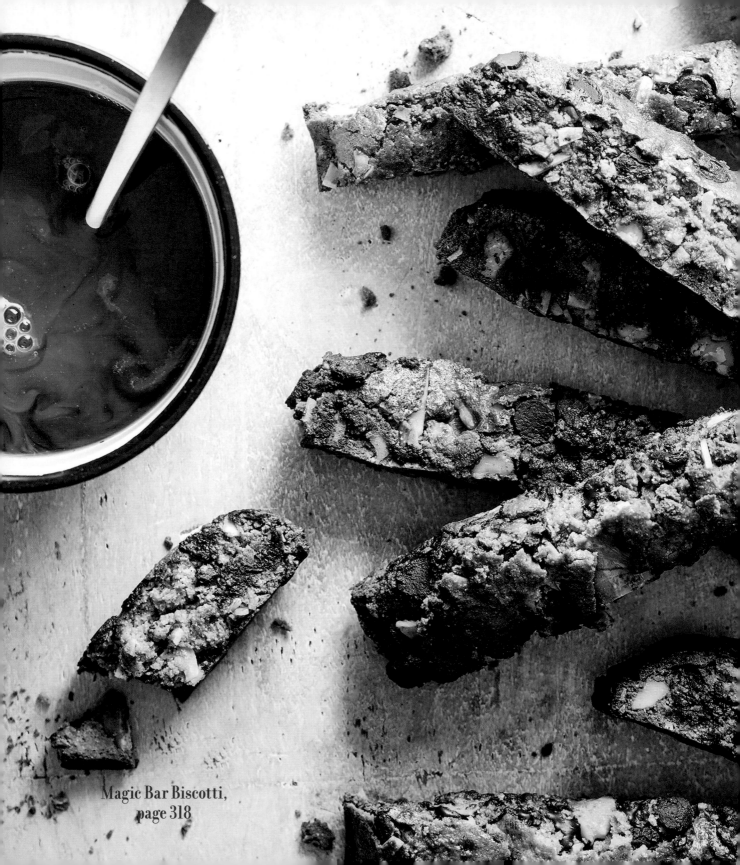

Magic Bar Biscotti,
page 318

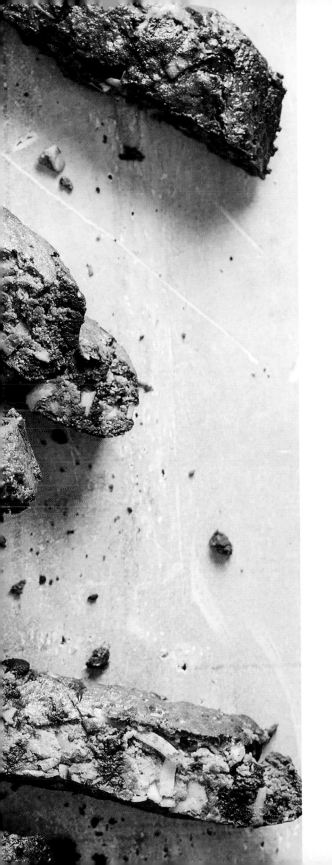

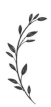 # DESSERTS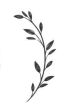

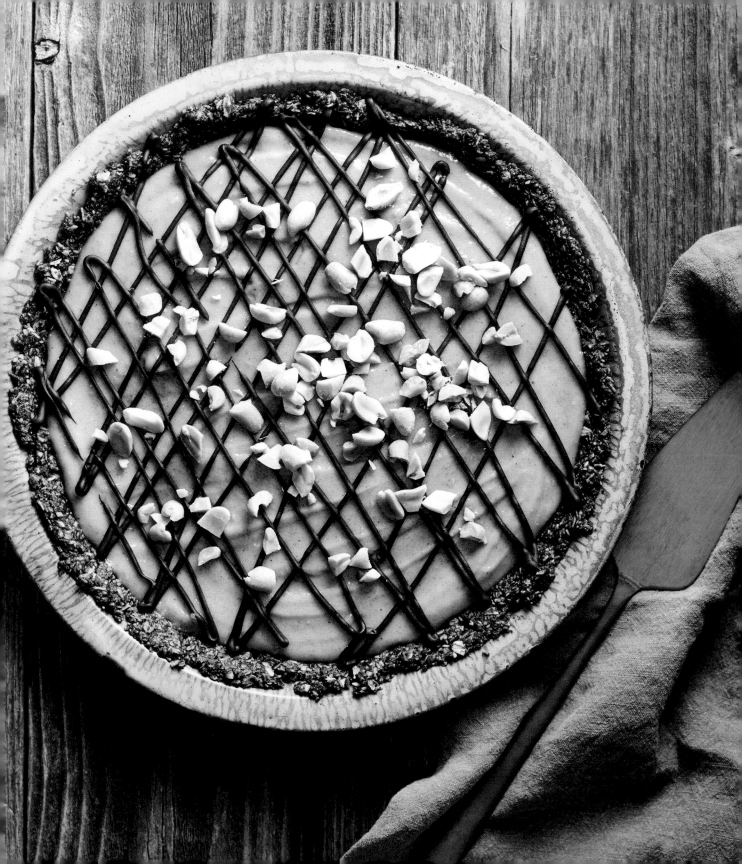

FROZEN CHOCOLATE—PEANUT BUTTER PIE

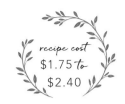

recipe cost $1.75 *to* $2.40

Who doesn't love a fabulous no-bake dessert? This pretty little pie is mini-sized but maxi on flavor and a treat any time of the year. I took to making smaller desserts a few years back as they suit our family of five better and helped me control my portions. I typically find that desserts taste so rich now that I only need a few bites to be satisfied.

SERVES 6 TO 8

Cooking oil spray

1 cup gluten-free old-fashioned rolled oats

¼ cup 100 percent pure maple syrup

2 tablespoons cacao powder

¼ cup plus 2 tablespoons organic peanut butter

¼ teaspoon fine sea salt

¼ cup raw cashews

¼ cup water

2 tablespoons dairy-free chocolate chips

1 tablespoon chopped peanuts (optional)

1. Spray a 6-cup baking dish or a 7-inch round dish with cooking oil spray.

2. In a food processor, combine the rolled oats, 2 tablespoons of the maple syrup, cacao powder, 2 tablespoons of the peanut butter, and salt. Pulse ten times, or until the mixture is sticky and crumbly.

3. Press the dough firmly into the bottom of the prepared dish and partially up the sides.

4. In a food processor, combine the cashews, water, remaining ¼ cup peanut butter, and remaining 2 tablespoons maple syrup. Process on high until a smooth batter forms, about 30 seconds. Pour into the crust.

5. Microwave the chocolate chips in a microwave-safe dish until softened, about 15 seconds.

6. Transfer the melted chocolate to a sandwich bag, pushing it down into one corner. Cut a ⅛-inch hole in the corner. Pipe the chocolate over the pie in a crisscross design.

7. Sprinkle the top with peanuts, if desired. Freeze, uncovered, for at least 45 minutes before serving.

8. Store in the freezer.

BREAD PUDDING *with* CARAMEL SAUCE

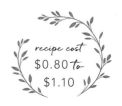

recipe cost
$0.80 *to*
$1.10

This is an easy bread pudding recipe made with the Oat Bread on page 65 and other simple ingredients. It's a total comfort food and a family favorite. Top it with dairy-free caramel sauce and sprinkle it with a little nutmeg, if you're into that kind of thing. You can also add raisins, but we prefer it without.

SERVES 6

4 cups cubed (1-inch) Oat Bread (page 65)

1¼ cups Oat Milk (page 288) or other milk

¼ cup coconut sugar

1 tablespoon raw honey

1 large egg

1 teaspoon pure vanilla extract

½ teaspoon ground cinnamon, plus more for sprinkling

⅛ teaspoon fine sea salt

1 cup water

1 recipe Caramel Sauce (page 306)

Dairy-free whipped cream (see page 316; optional)

Sliced bananas (optional)

1. Arrange the bread cubes in a 7-inch round baking pan.

2. In a medium bowl, whisk together the oat milk, coconut sugar, honey, egg, vanilla, cinnamon, and salt. Pour the mixture over the bread. Cover with foil and chill for 30 minutes.

3. Set the dish on a trivet and pour the water into the cooker. Carefully lower the trivet into the cooker.

4. Place the lid on the cooker and make sure the vent valve is in the SEALING position. Using the display panel, select the MANUAL/PRESSURE COOK function and HIGH PRESSURE. Use the +/− buttons until the display reads 30 minutes.

5. When the cooker beeps, let it naturally release the pressure until the display reads LO:10. Switch the vent valve from the SEALING to the VENTING position. Use caution while the steam escapes.

6. Remove the dish from the cooker. Remove the foil. Sprinkle with cinnamon and drizzle with the caramel sauce. Top with whipped cream and bananas, if you like. Serve immediately.

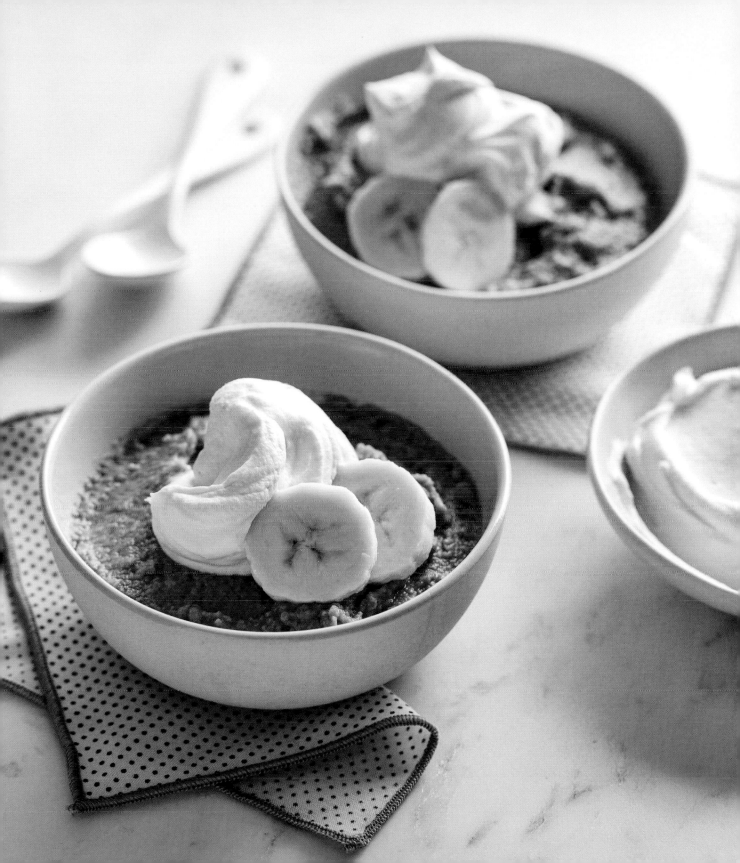

CARAMEL SAUCE

recipe cost $0.75 to $1

This dreamy dairy-free sauce comes together in seconds from just three simple ingredients. It's a great, inexpensive alternative to store-bought sauces that are packed with stabilizers and corn syrups. Use it to top ice cream, pancakes, cakes, or muffins. If you cannot consume sesame seeds, then almond butter or sunflower seed butter will work just as well in place of tahini.

MAKES ABOUT ¼ CUP

2 tablespoons avocado oil

2 tablespoons 100 percent pure maple syrup

1 tablespoon Homemade Tahini (page 329) or store-bought

1. In a small bowl, combine the avocado oil, maple syrup, and tahini and stir until smooth.

2. Store in an airtight container in the refrigerator for up to 1 week.

CREAMY BANANA PUDDING

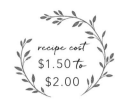

recipe cost
$1.50 to $2.00

My boys love this creamy pudding, which is so healthy you could eat it for breakfast—and in actuality my children do! You can dress it up with gluten-free shortbread cookies (the Jam Thumbprint Cookies in *Instant Loss: Eat Real, Lose Weight*, sans jam, work great!) and dairy-free whipped cream (see Note page 316) for an over-the-top dessert.

SERVES 4

Cooking oil spray

1 medium ripe banana, peeled

4 large egg yolks

2 tablespoons arrowroot powder

1 teaspoon pure vanilla extract

2 Medjool dates, pitted

⅛ teaspoon fine sea salt

1 cup Oat Milk (page 288) or other milk

1 cup water

1. Spray a 6-inch round baking dish with cooking oil spray.

2. In a blender, combine the banana, egg yolks, arrowroot powder, vanilla, dates, salt, and oat milk. Blend on high until smooth, about 60 seconds. Transfer to the prepared dish.

3. Pour the water into an electric pressure cooker and place a trivet inside. Set the dish on the trivet.

4. Place the lid on the cooker and make sure the vent is in the SEALING position. Using the display panel, select the MANUAL/PRESSURE COOK function and LOW PRESSURE. Use the +/− buttons until the display reads 6 minutes.

5. When the cooker beeps, switch the vent valve from the SEALING position to the VENTING position, administering a quick release. Use caution while the steam escapes.

6. Stir and serve warm or cold.

7. Store, covered, in the refrigerator for up to 3 days.

RASPBERRY CRUMBLE

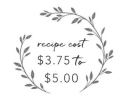

recipe cost $3.75 *to* $5.00

This dreamy little crumble is best served with a dairy-free ice cream or whipped cream. So Delicious is my favorite store-bought brand for both—or you can make your own! I have recipes for ice cream in my *Instant Loss Cookbook,* and see the Note on page 316 to make dairy-free whipped cream.

1. Spray a 6- or 7-inch round baking dish with cooking oil spray.

2. **MAKE THE CRUMBLE:** In a food processor, combine the almond flour, rolled oats, maple syrup, coconut flour, olive oil, and tahini and pulse about ten times.

3. Press half of the crumble mixture into the bottom and partially up the sides of the prepared dish.

4. **MAKE THE FILLING:** In a small bowl, combine the raspberries, maple syrup, vanilla, and salt and stir well. Pour the filling into the crust and top with the remaining crumble. Cover the pan with foil and set on a trivet. Pour the water into an electric pressure cooker and carefully lower the trivet and dish into the cooker.

5. Place the lid on the cooker and make sure the vent valve is in the SEALING position. Using the display panel, select the MANUAL/PRESSURE COOK function and HIGH PRESSURE. Use the +/− buttons until the display reads 30 minutes.

6. When the cooker beeps, let it naturally release the pressure until the display reads LO:10. Switch the vent valve from the SEALING to the VENTING position. Use caution while the steam escapes.

7. Remove the dish from the cooker and discard the foil. Serve warm.

SERVES 6

Cooking oil spray

FOR THE CRUMBLE
¾ cup superfine almond flour

½ cup gluten-free old-fashioned rolled oats

3 tablespoons 100 percent pure maple syrup

2 tablespoons coconut flour

2 tablespoons extra-virgin olive oil

2 tablespoons Homemade Tahini (page 329) or store-bought

FOR THE FILLING
1 (6-ounce) container fresh raspberries

2 tablespoons 100 percent pure maple syrup

½ teaspoon pure vanilla extract

¼ teaspoon fine sea salt

1 cup water

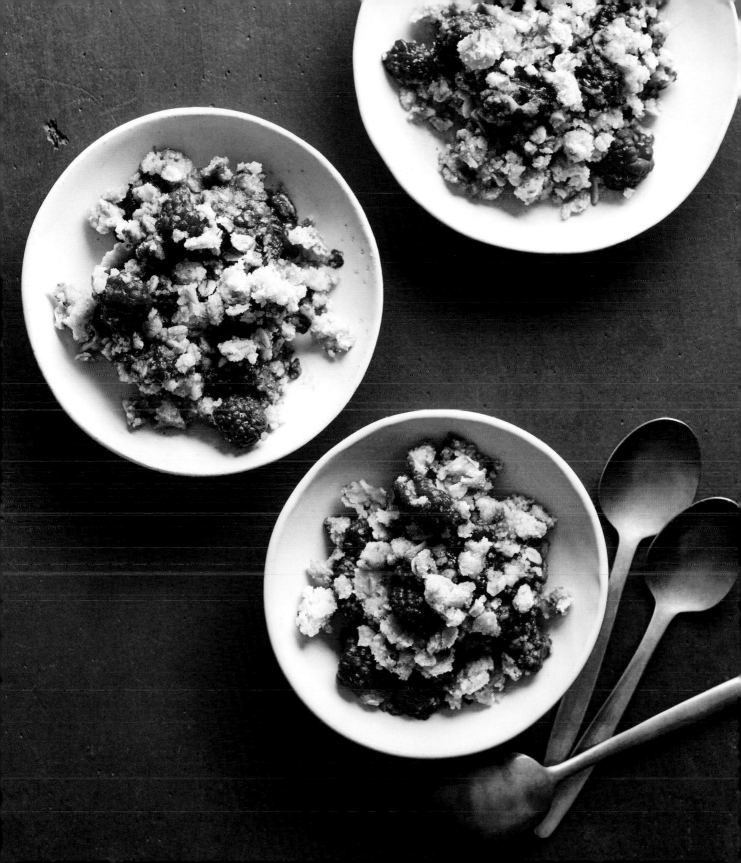

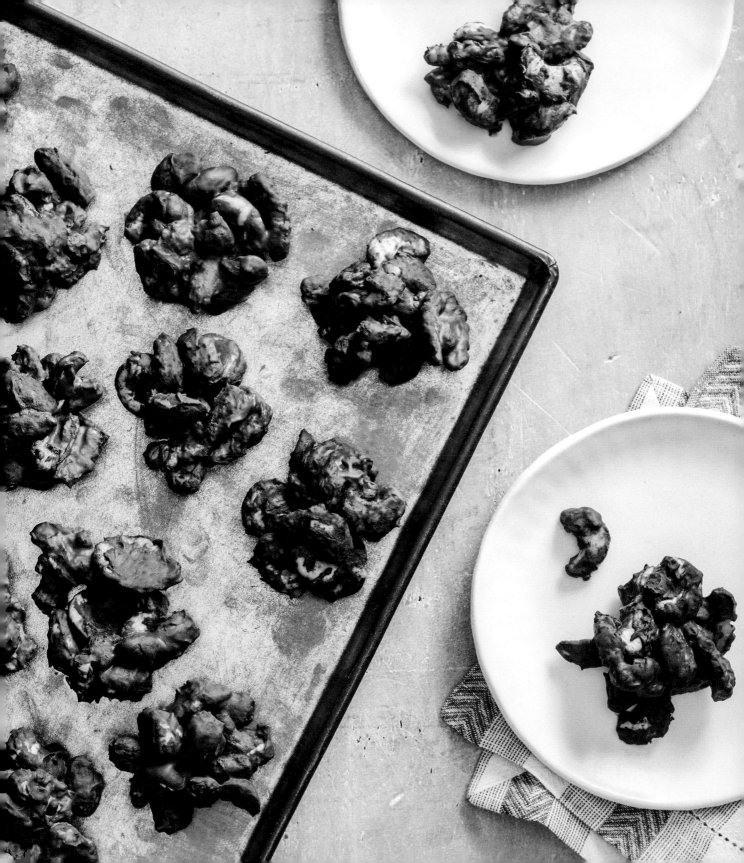

CHOCOLATE-MOCHA NUT CLUSTERS

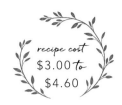

recipe cost
$3.00 *to*
$4.60

Make these right now! Dear heavens, y'all! This is my favorite after-dinner snack as of late. Don't let the instant coffee weird you out, it really heightens the chocolatey flavor. If you are a sweet lover, this will hit the spot when you need some chocolatey goodness. Make 'em, toss 'em in an airtight container in the freezer, and then pull one out whenever you need a little extra something-something.

MAKES 18 CLUSTERS

1 tablespoon extra-virgin olive oil

½ cup raw cashews

½ cup raw almonds

½ cup raw walnuts

½ teaspoon fine sea salt

½ cup dairy-free chocolate chips

2 tablespoons full-fat coconut milk

1 teaspoon instant coffee

1. Line a baking sheet with parchment paper.

2. Preheat an electric pressure cooker using the SAUTÉ function and adjust the heat to NORMAL (see Note page 182).

3. When the display panel reads HOT, add the olive oil, cashews, almonds, walnuts, and salt. Cook, stirring continuously, until the nuts begin to toast, 1 to 2 minutes. Using the display panel, press the CANCEL button to turn off the SAUTÉ function.

4. Add the chocolate chips, coconut milk, and instant coffee. Cook, stirring continuously, until the chocolate melts and the nuts are coated, 30 to 60 seconds.

5. Working quickly, use a tablespoon measuring spoon to scoop the nuts into little clusters on the lined baking sheet. (There should be about 18 clusters.)

6. Chill in the freezer for 2 hours, then store in an airtight container in the freezer.

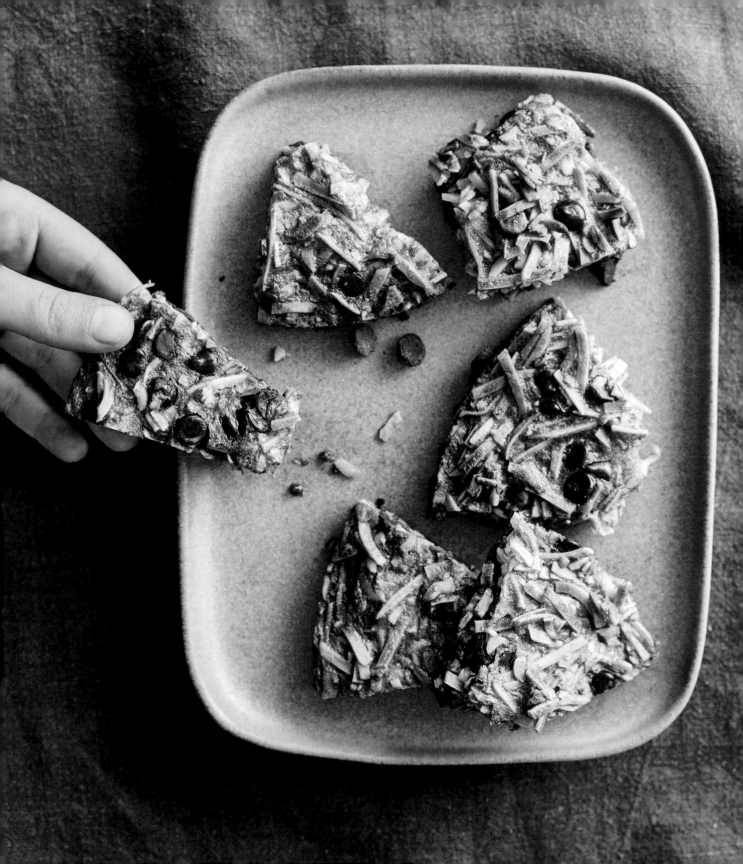

MACAROON COOKIE BARS

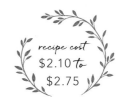

recipe cost
$2.10 *to*
$2.75

Simple and sweet, these cookie bars are a light dessert that will satiate any sweet tooth! I use Enjoy Life brand dairy-free chocolate chips. They are free of the most common food allergens.

SERVES 6

Cooking oil spray

⅓ cup coconut sugar

2 large eggs

¼ teaspoon pure vanilla extract

⅛ teaspoon fine sea salt

1 cup packed unsweetened shredded coconut

¼ cup dairy-free mini chocolate chips

1. Spray a 6-inch round baking dish with cooking oil spray.

2. In a large bowl, whisk together the coconut sugar, eggs, vanilla, and salt. Stir in the shredded coconut and chocolate chips. Pour the batter into the prepared dish.

3. Place in a 5.3-quart air-fryer basket and bake at 370°F for 4 minutes. Reduce heat to 300°F and bake for an additional 8 to 10 minutes.

4. Carefully remove the pan from the air fryer and let the bars cool for 15 minutes on a wire rack before slicing and serving.

NOTE: If you do not have an air fryer, you can bake these in a conventional oven at 350°F for 15 minutes.

FUDGY PEANUT BUTTER BROWNIES

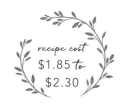

recipe cost
$1.85 *to*
$2.30

My kids go crazy over these brownies! We love them with a little dairy-free whipped cream (see Note page 316), but they're perfect on their own as well. Portion control tip: If you're only baking for one or two, portion the brownies out, wrap them in plastic wrap, and store in an airtight container in the freezer for up to six months. Pull one out when you get a hankering, and the rest are out of sight, out of mind.

SERVES 6 TO 8

Cooking oil spray

½ cup organic peanut butter or raw almond butter

¼ cup Oat Milk (page 288) or other milk

3 tablespoons cacao powder

2 tablespoons raw honey

1 large egg

1 teaspoon pure vanilla extract

¼ teaspoon baking soda

⅛ teaspoon fine sea salt

3 tablespoons dairy-free chocolate chips

1 cup water

1. Spray a 6-inch round baking dish with cooking oil spray.

2. In a large bowl, whisk together the peanut butter, oat milk, cacao powder, honey, egg, vanilla, baking soda, and salt. Add the chocolate chips and stir well.

3. Pour the batter into the prepared dish and cover with foil. Pour the water into an electric pressure cooker and set the dish on a trivet. Carefully lower the trivet and dish into the cooker.

4. Place the lid on the cooker and make sure the vent valve is in the SEALING position. Using the display panel, select the MANUAL/PRESSURE COOK function and HIGH PRESSURE. Use the +/− buttons until the display reads 30 minutes.

5. When the cooker beeps, switch the vent valve from the SEALING to the VENTING position, administering a quick release. Use caution while the steam escapes.

6. Let cool for 10 minutes on a wire rack before cutting.

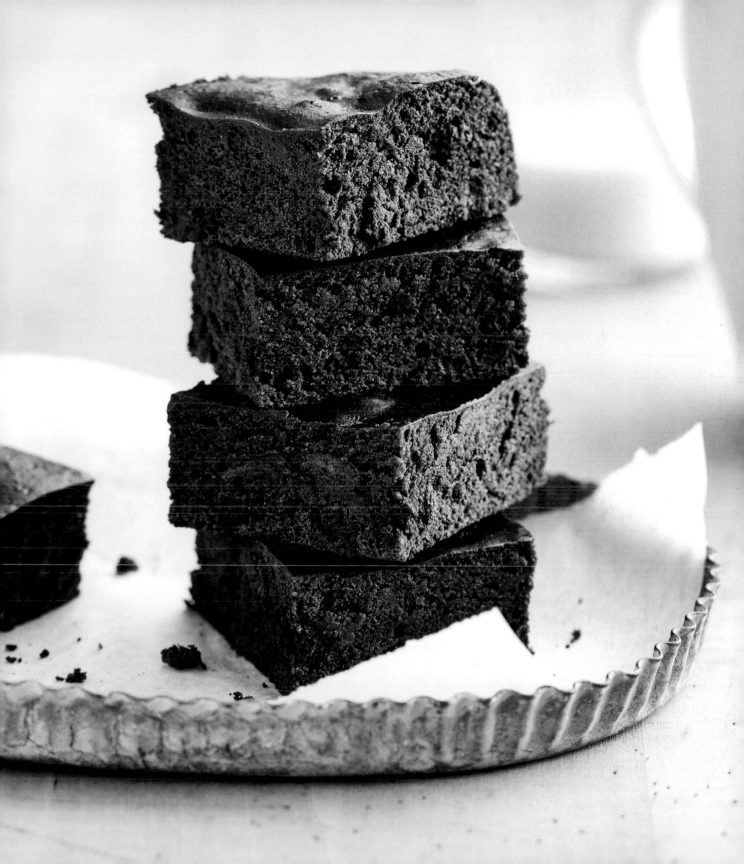

PEACH DUMP CAKE

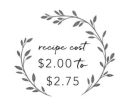

recipe cost
$2.00 *to*
$2.75

Who doesn't love a good dump cake? This dessert is usually made with boxed cake mix, but cake mixes that are refined sugar– and preservative-free are difficult to find, not to mention extremely expensive. Make your own cake mix out of a few ingredients you probably have in your pantry and enjoy this yummy treat with dairy-free whipped cream or dairy-free ice cream!

SERVES 4 TO 6

- 1 (15-ounce) can sliced peaches in natural juice, drained
- 2 tablespoons juice from canned peaches
- ¾ cup oat flour
- ¼ cup coconut sugar
- 1½ teaspoons baking powder
- 1 teaspoon pure vanilla extract
- ½ teaspoon ground cinnamon
- ⅛ teaspoon fine sea salt
- 2 tablespoons unsalted butter or ghee, cut into ¼-inch cubes
- 1 cup water
- 1 cup dairy-free whipped cream (optional; see Note)

1. Arrange the peaches into the bottom of a 6-inch round baking dish. Drizzle the peach juice over the top.

2. In a large bowl, combine the oat flour, coconut sugar, baking powder, vanilla, cinnamon, and salt. Sprinkle the mixture over the peaches and dot the butter evenly over the top. Cover the dish with foil and set on a trivet.

3. Pour the water into an electric pressure cooker and carefully lower the trivet and dish into the cooker.

4. Place the lid on the cooker and make sure the vent valve is in the SEALING position. Using the display panel, select the MANUAL/PRESSURE COOK function and HIGH PRESSURE. Use the +/− buttons until the display reads 25 minutes.

5. When the cooker beeps, switch the vent valve from the SEALING to the VENTING position, administering a quick release. Use caution while the steam escapes.

6. Serve immediately with whipped cream, if desired.

NOTE: To make dairy-free whipped cream, chill one can of coconut cream (not coconut milk) in the refrigerator for at least 12 hours. Add the chilled cream, ¼ cup powdered sugar, and 1 teaspoon pure vanilla extract to a medium bowl. With a hand mixer or stand mixer, beat on high until fluffy (it will be thicker than dairy whipped cream). Serve immediately, or refrigerate for up to 1 week.

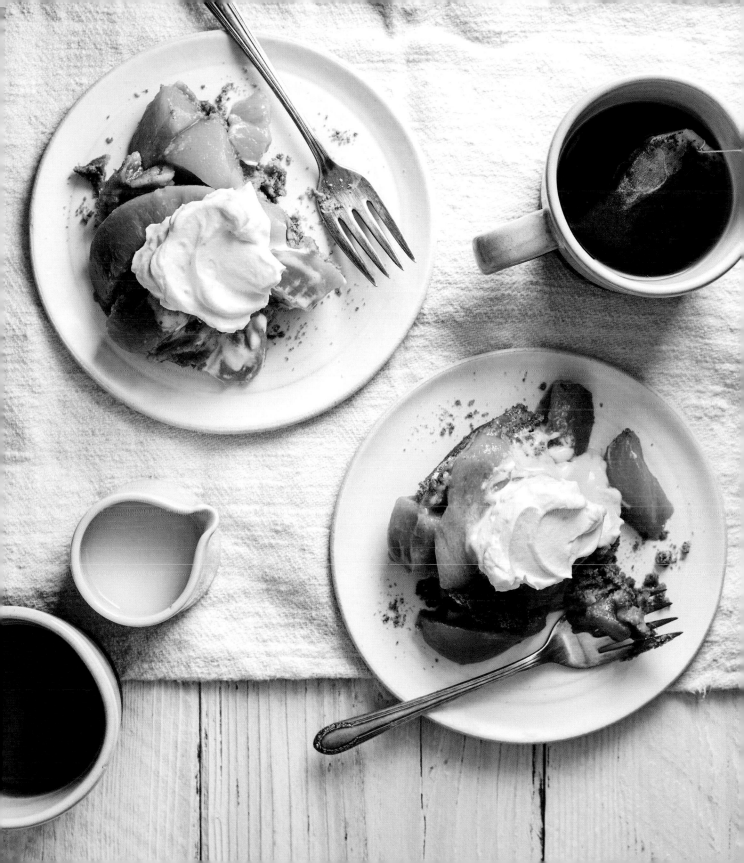

MAGIC BAR BISCOTTI

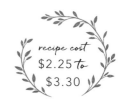

recipe cost
$2.25 *to*
$3.30

This recipe comes together like magic! *Biscotti* means "twice-baked" in Italian. Simply shape the dough and bake it twice to create this amazing grain-free classic. Perfect with tea or your morning coffee, this is one of my favorite recipes in this book!

MAKES 12 BISCOTTI

¾ cup chickpea flour

3 tablespoons coconut sugar

3 tablespoons raw honey

2 tablespoons coconut flour

2 tablespoons extra-virgin olive oil or unsalted butter

1 large egg

¼ teaspoon fine sea salt

¼ cup dairy-free chocolate chips

¼ cup unsweetened shredded coconut

¼ cup chopped raw walnuts

1. In a large bowl, combine the chickpea flour, coconut sugar, honey, coconut flour, olive oil, egg, and salt and mix well. Stir in the chocolate chips, shredded coconut, and walnuts.

2. Form the dough into a ball and place between two pieces of parchment paper cut to the size of a 5.3-quart air-fryer basket. Press the dough through the parchment into a circle 1 inch thick and 3 inches wide. Remove the top piece of parchment paper and place the parchment with the dough inside the air-fryer basket and bake at 300°F for 15 minutes.

3. Remove the dough and carefully cut into ¼-inch slices. Arrange slices cut-side up on the paper in a single layer.

4. Place the biscotti back inside the basket and bake at 280°F for an additional 12 to 15 minutes.

5. Remove the biscotti from the basket. Cool on a wire rack (the cookies will get crunchy as they cool completely).

6. Store in an airtight container at room temperature for up to 1 week.

NOTE: If you do not have an air fryer, you can bake these in a conventional oven. Bake the dough circle on a parchment-lined baking sheet at 325°F oven for 15 minutes. Slice, then bake cookies for an additional 15 to 20 minutes.

MOLTEN LAVA CAKES *for* SHARING

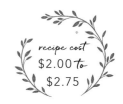

recipe cost
$2.00 *to*
$2.75

These cakes come with a chocolate surprise in the center! Gooey and delicious, these cakes love to be served with dairy-free ice cream or whipped cream (see Note page 316) and are perfect for sharing with the ones you love!

MAKES 2 CAKES (SERVES 4)

4 tablespoons unsalted ghee or butter, plus more for greasing

1 tablespoon cacao powder

⅓ cup dairy-free chocolate chips

⅓ cup coconut sugar

2 large eggs

4½ teaspoons arrowroot powder

1 tablespoon coconut flour

1 teaspoon instant coffee (optional)

⅛ teaspoon fine sea salt

1 cup water

1. Grease 2 (8-ounce) oven-safe ramekins with some ghee. Lightly dust the inside of the ramekins with a little bit of the cacao powder.

2. In a high-powered blender, combine the 4 tablespoons ghee, chocolate chips, coconut sugar, eggs, arrowroot powder, flour, instant coffee (if using), and salt. Blend on high until the mixture forms a smooth batter, about 30 seconds.

3. Fill the ramekins three-quarters full, dividing the batter evenly between the two, and cover each with foil. Set the ramekins on a trivet. Pour the water into an electric pressure cooker and carefully lower the trivet and ramekins into the cooker.

4. Place the lid on the cooker and make sure the vent valve is in the SEALING position. Using the display panel, select the MANUAL/PRESSURE COOK function and HIGH PRESSURE. Use the +/− buttons until the display reads 14 minutes.

5. When the cooker beeps, switch the vent valve from the SEALING to the VENTING position, administering a quick release. Use caution while the steam escapes.

6. Carefully remove the ramekins, discard the foil, and let cool on a wire rack for 10 minutes.

7. Run a butter knife around the inside of each ramekin, then carefully turn the cakes over onto serving plates. Dust each cake with the remaining cacao powder and share with three friends.

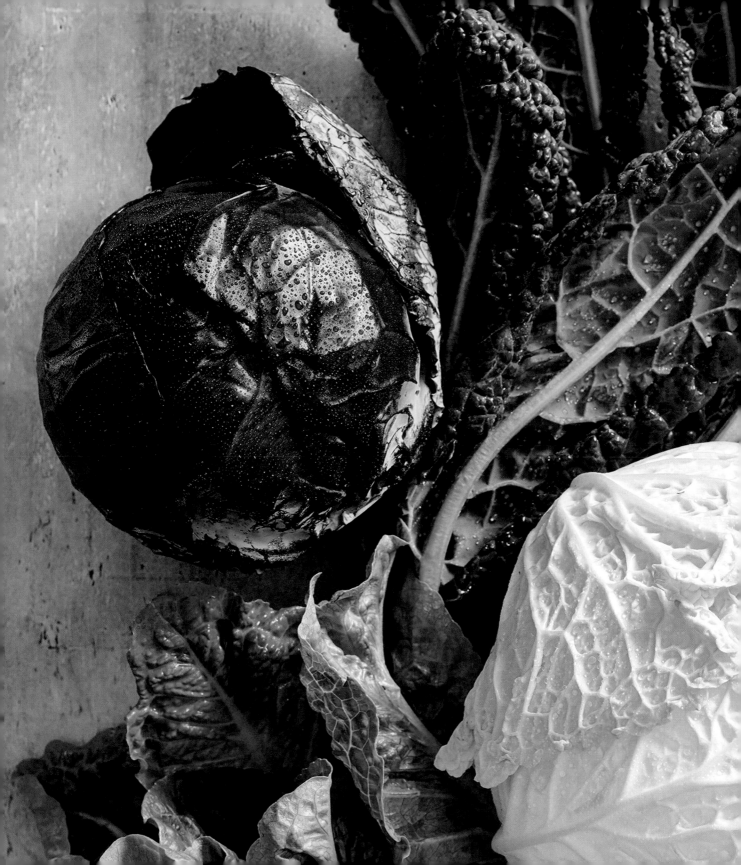

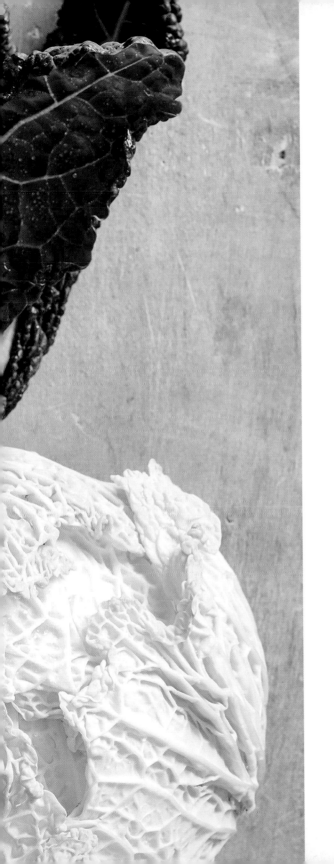

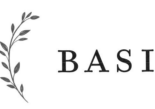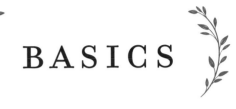

BASICS

CHOCOLATE FROSTING

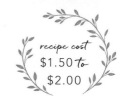

recipe cost
$1.50 to
$2.00

This simple and satisfying frosting is dairy-free and made with only two ingredients! It's great for frosting cakes and muffins, or as a dessert-y addition to pancakes.

MAKES 1 CUP

¾ cup dairy-free chocolate chips
¼ cup plus 2 tablespoons
    coconut cream

In a small microwave-safe bowl, stir together the chocolate chips and coconut cream. Microwave for 15 to 30 seconds and stir. Store in the refrigerator for up to 1 week.

SUPER-SIMPLE GRANOLA

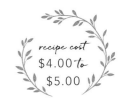

recipe cost
$4.00 *to*
$5.00

Have you priced granola at the grocery store lately? It's crazy expensive! I gave that stuff up a long time ago and now make mine at home. Y'all, it is so dang easy! We like to sprinkle it over oatmeal for a nice little crunch, dairy-free ice cream as a tasty treat, or dairy-free yogurt with some berries. With this pantry staple, the sky really is the limit!

MAKES 5 CUPS

3 cups gluten-free old-fashioned rolled oats

1 cup slivered raw almonds

¾ cup shredded unsweetened coconut flakes

¼ cup 100 percent pure maple syrup

¼ cup creamy organic peanut butter, raw almond butter, or Homemade Tahini (page 329)

¼ cup extra-virgin olive oil

¾ teaspoon fine sea salt

1. Preheat the oven to 350°F. Line a baking sheet with parchment paper.

2. In a large bowl, combine the oats, almonds, coconut flakes, maple syrup, peanut butter, olive oil, and salt. Stir well to ensure all of the ingredients are evenly coated.

3. Spread the mixture on the prepared baking sheet and bake for 18 to 20 minutes, or until crisp and golden.

4. Remove the baking sheet from the oven and allow the granola to cool completely.

5. Store in an airtight container in the pantry for up to 1 month.

TANGY BARBECUE SAUCE

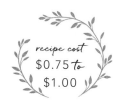

recipe cost
$0.75 *to*
$1.00

Our family absolutely loves barbecue sauce, but unfortunately most of the sauces sold in stores have artificial colors and highly refined sugars. No problem though, because barbecue sauce is easy to make at home and comes together in no time at all. To top it off, it's made from ingredients you probably have in your pantry right now! To be more efficient, I recommend making a big batch, freezing portions in muffin trays, and transferring to freezer bags. This way, you have it on hand whenever you need it.

In a high-powered blender, combine the tomato sauce, coconut sugar, honey, vinegar, Worcestershire sauce, mustard, garlic, oregano, chili powder, and black pepper. Blend on high until the sauce thickens and steam comes out of the top, about 5 minutes. Store in a covered glass jar in the refrigerator for up to 6 days.

NOTE: If you do not have a high-powered blender, you can make the sauce on the stovetop. Bring all of the ingredients to a boil in a saucepan over medium-high heat. Lower to a simmer and cook, whisking occasionally so nothing burns on the bottom, for 5 minutes. Remove from the heat and let cool to room temperature before storing.

MAKES 2½ CUPS

1 (15-ounce) can tomato sauce

2 tablespoons coconut sugar

2 tablespoons raw honey

1 tablespoon apple cider vinegar

1½ teaspoons reduced-sodium Worcestershire sauce

1½ teaspoons Dijon mustard

1 clove garlic, minced

½ teaspoon dried oregano

½ teaspoon chili powder

½ teaspoon ground black pepper

TACO SEASONING

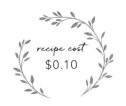

recipe cost
$0.10

Make your own taco seasoning at home! Store-bought brands can have added sugar, preservatives, and fillers. This homemade seasoning is just as delicious as the commercial stuff and more cost effective, too.

MAKES ¼ CUP

4½ teaspoons chili powder
2 teaspoons dried minced onion
1 teaspoon garlic powder
1 teaspoon ground cumin
1 teaspoon fine sea salt
½ teaspoon cayenne pepper
½ teaspoon paprika

1. In a wide-mouth jar, combine the chili powder, dried onion, garlic powder, cumin, salt, cayenne, and paprika. Screw the lid on tightly, then shake to combine.

2. Label and store in your spice cabinet.

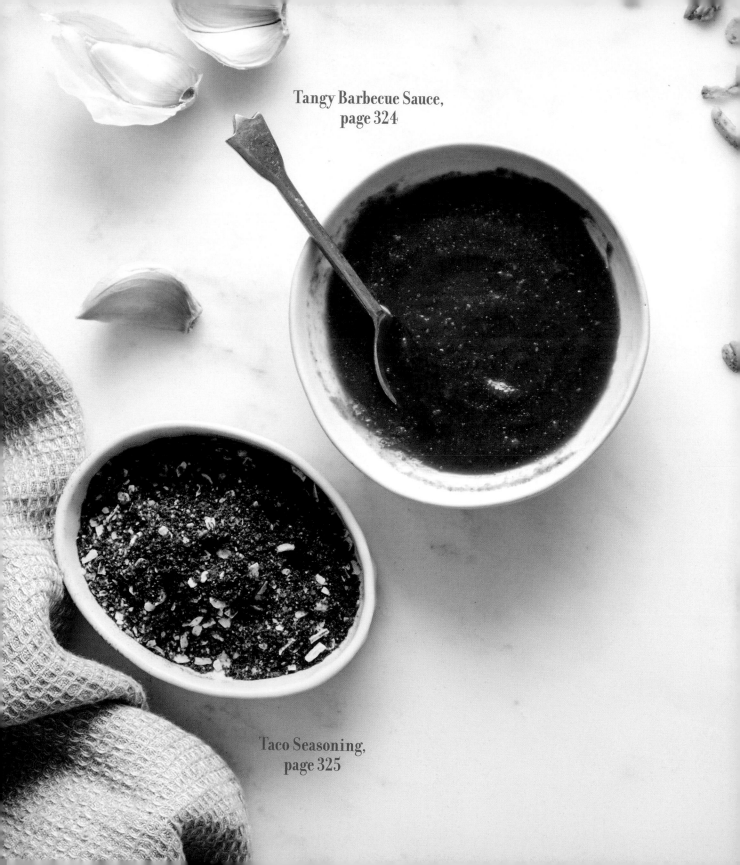

Tangy Barbecue Sauce,
page 324

Taco Seasoning,
page 325

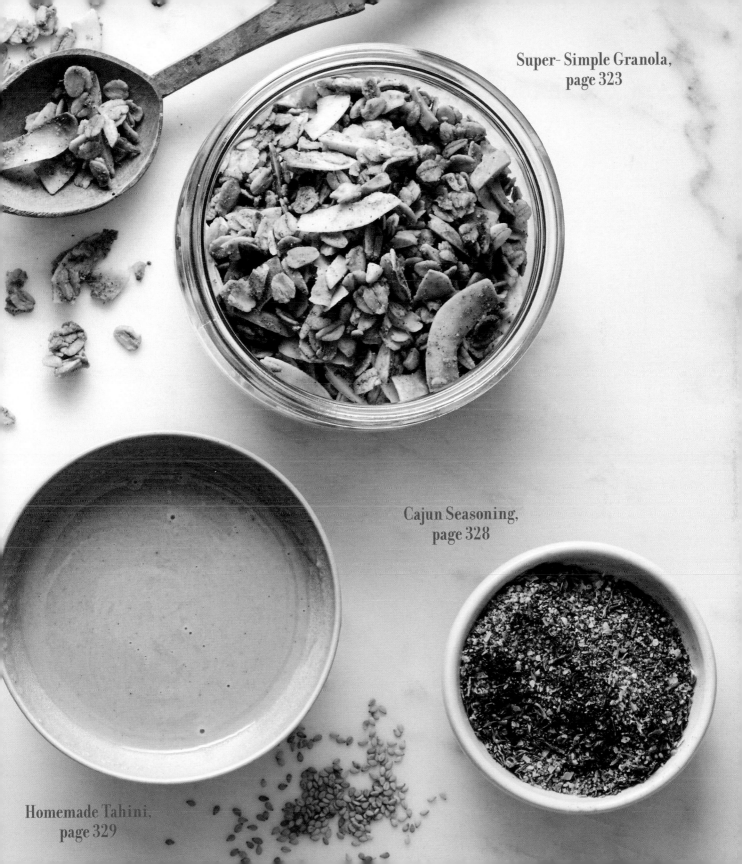

Super-Simple Granola,
page 323

Cajun Seasoning,
page 328

Homemade Tahini,
page 329

CAJUN SEASONING

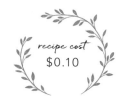

recipe cost
$0.10

Store-bought seasonings can have added sugars and anticaking agents. I enjoy making my mixes at home because I know exactly what goes into them and they come together so quickly! It's also a creative process to taste the new flavors created by combining different spices!

MAKES ¼ CUP

2½ teaspoons smoked paprika

2 teaspoons fine sea salt

2 teaspoons garlic powder

1¼ teaspoons dried oregano

1¼ teaspoons dried thyme

1 teaspoon ground black pepper

1 teaspoon onion powder

1 teaspoon cayenne pepper

½ teaspoon red pepper flakes

1. In a wide-mouth jar, combine the paprika, garlic powder, oregano, thyme, black pepper, onion powder, cayenne, and red pepper flakes. Screw the lid on tightly, then shake to combine.

2. Label and store in your spice cabinet.

HOMEMADE TAHINI

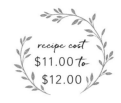

recipe cost
$11.00 to
$12.00

Tahini is a delicious sesame seed butter often used as a nut butter alternative. Use it in any recipe that calls for peanut or almond butter. You can also add a little bit of your favorite sweetener and enjoy it on an English muffin.

MAKES 2 CUPS

2 cups raw sesame seeds

5 tablespoons extra-virgin olive oil, plus more if needed

¼ teaspoon fine sea salt

1. Heat a cast-iron skillet over medium heat.

2. Add the sesame seeds to the skillet and toast for 2 to 3 minutes, stirring constantly to prevent burning, until they have a nice golden color.

3. Transfer the seeds to a small food processor or high-powered blender (see Note page 51). Add the olive oil and salt. Blend on high until smooth and creamy, about 2 minutes. Add more olive oil, if needed, to thin.

4. Store in tightly sealed container in the refrigerator for up to 2 months.

HOMEMADE MAYO

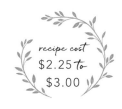

recipe cost
$2.25 to
$3.00

I put off making our own mayo for years! It just sounded too difficult, but really, it's one of the quickest things to whip up in my kitchen. Just combine everything in a jar and blend. You'll need to use an immersion blender though—this won't work by simply whisking. You can also use a blender with variable speeds, but there is more chance for error. Make sure all of your ingredients are at room temperature and that you keep the immersion blender blade low and submerged. Do that and you'll be just fine!

MAKES 1 CUP

1 large egg, at room temperature (see Note)

1 cup avocado oil

¼ teaspoon dried ground mustard

¼ teaspoon red wine vinegar

¼ teaspoon fine sea salt

1. In a wide-mouth jar, combine the egg, avocado oil, ground mustard, vinegar, and salt. Blend on high using an immersion blender. As you blend, very slowly raise the blender up through the mixture, keeping it submerged and letting oil in and around the blades. Once the mixture has started to emulsify, you may have to move the blender up and down through the mixture to blend in any remaining oil.

2. Store in a tightly sealed container in the refrigerator for up to a week.

NOTE: Eggs can be run under warm water to reach room temperature more quickly. Because of the raw eggs, this mayonnaise should be kept no longer than 1 week.

BONE BROTH

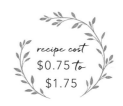

recipe cost
$0.75 *to*
$1.75

Low-sodium, sugar-free bone broths can be difficult to find in the grocery store for less than $6.00 a carton. This can make stirring up soups and stews more expensive than it needs to be. A few years ago, I decided to begin making my own broths at home in an electric pressure cooker. Not only is it a big budget saver, but it's also a great way to utilize vegetables on their way out and leftover bones from rotisserie chicken, beef, lamb, or pork!

MAKES 4 QUARTS

3 pounds meaty bones (chicken, beef, lamb, or pork)

4 quarts water

4 stalks celery, diced

2 large carrots, diced (see Note page 51)

1 medium yellow onion, thinly sliced

¼ cup fresh flat-leaf parsley

1 tablespoon apple cider vinegar

1 teaspoon fine sea salt

1. In an electric pressure cooker, combine the bones, water, celery, carrots, onion, parsley, vinegar, and salt.

2. Place the lid on the cooker and make sure the vent valve is in the SEALING position. Using the display panel, select the MANUAL/PRESSURE COOK function and HIGH PRESSURE. Use the +/− buttons until the display reads 90 minutes.

3. When the cooker beeps, let it naturally release the pressure (this should take about 25 minutes).

4. Once the liquid has cooled to warm or room temperature, carefully strain through a fine-mesh strainer into a bowl. Discard the bones and vegetables. Ladle the broth into quart-size glass jars.

5. Store in the refrigerator for up to 6 days, or freeze in tempered glass jars (with at least 2 inches of space at the top) for up to 6 months.

VEGETABLE BROTH

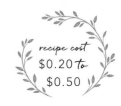

recipe cost
$0.20 to
$0.50

This is one of my favorite Instant Loss recipes of all time! It's certainly one I make the most frequently. Simply collect your kitchen vegetable scraps, clean them well, and freeze them in an airtight freezer bag until the bag is full and you're ready to make this staple. If you don't have time to accumulate scraps, simply use 4 cups of roughly chopped vegetables—mainly carrots, celery, and onions.

MAKES 4 QUARTS

4 cups vegetable scraps (onion ends, carrots tops, celery ends, bell pepper tops, sweet potato ends, etc.)

4 quarts water

5 cloves garlic, crushed

1 bay leaf

1 tablespoon dried parsley flakes

1 tablespoon extra-virgin olive oil

1 teaspoon dried rosemary

½ teaspoon fine sea salt

¼ teaspoon ground black pepper

1. In an electric pressure cooker, combine the vegetable scraps, water, garlic, bay leaf, parsley, olive oil, rosemary, salt, and black pepper.

2. Place the lid on the cooker and make sure the vent valve is in the SEALING position. Using the display panel, select the MANUAL/PRESSURE COOK function and HIGH PRESSURE. Use the +/− buttons until the display reads 40 minutes.

3. When the cooker beeps, let it naturally release the pressure (this should take about 25 minutes).

4. Once the liquid has cooled to warm or room temperature, carefully strain through a fine-mesh strainer into a bowl. Discard the vegetable scraps and bay leaf. Ladle the broth into quart-size glass jars.

5. Store in the refrigerator for up to 6 days, or freeze in tempered glass jars (with at least 2 inches of space at the top) for up to 6 months.

SPAGHETTI SQUASH

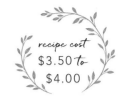

recipe cost
$3.50 to
$4.00

I used to avoid making spaghetti squash at all costs because those things are so gosh darned hard to cut into! Enter the pressure cooker. Not only is it faster to make your squash in the pressure cooker, but there's no hacking required. Simply place the whole thing inside and watch the magic happen!

SERVINGS VARY

1 cup water

1 small to medium spaghetti squash (that fits inside an electric pressure cooker)

1. Pour the water into an electric pressure cooker and place a trivet inside. Set the squash on the trivet.

2. Place the lid on the cooker and make sure the vent valve is in the SEALING position. Using the display panel, select the MANUAL/PRESSURE COOK function and HIGH PRESSURE. Use the +/− buttons until the display reads 30 minutes.

3. When the cooker beeps, switch the vent valve from the SEALING to the VENTING position, administering a quick release. Use caution while the steam escapes.

4. Let the squash cool on the counter for 15 minutes. Cut in half and scrape out and discard the seeds. Using a fork and holding one half of the squash, pull shreds outward from the peel to make squash "spaghetti." Repeat with the remaining half.

NOTE: A 3-pound spaghetti squash will yield about 4 cups of squash "spaghetti."

INDEX

NOTE: Page references in *italics* refer to photos of recipes.

C

cabbage
  Asian Chicken Salad, 152, *153*
  Barbecue Beef and Beans, 172
  Cabbage and Quinoa Bowl,
    282, *283*
  Cabbage Steaks, 244, *245*
  Kale and Cabbage Chicken-
    Bacon Salad, *148,* 149–150
  Turkey Cabbage Cups, 254,
    255
  Veggie Lo Mein, 218, *219*
cage-free poultry, 15
Cajun Popcorn Shrimp, *112,* 113
Cajun Seasoning, *327,* 328
cakes. *see* baked goods
Caprese Frittata, 89–90, *91*
Caramel Sauce
  Bread Pudding with, 304, *305*
  Plantain Pancakes with, 92,
    93
  recipe for, 306
Carrot-Ginger Soup, *130,* 131
Carrots (Citrus-Glazed) with
    Chives, 176, *177*
Casamiento, 173
cashews
  Cashew Milk, 288
  Cashew Parmesan, 266
  Cashew Ricotta Cheese, 137
  Cauliflower Cheese Bisque,
    134, *135*
  Cauliflower Mac and Cheese,
    236
  Chocolate-Mocha Nut
    Clusters, *310,* 311
  No-Queso Queso, 121
  Poppin' Jalapeño Poppers
    with Cilantro-Lime Aioli,
    106, *107*
  Salsa Verde Chicken Nachos
    and Mexican Lasagna,
    258–259

cassava flour
  about, 47–48
  in recipes, 70, 72, 108, 113
Casserole, Tuna-Noodle, 200
cauliflower and cauliflower rice
  Cauliflower Cheese Bisque,
    134, *135*
  Cauliflower Mac and Cheese,
    236
  Smoothie Bowl Parfaits, 76
  Spicy Buffalo Cauliflower
    with Creamy Ranch
    Dressing, 108, *109*
  Summer Pineapple Chicken
    over Cauliflower Rice, *256,*
    257
Cereal, Cinnamon Toast, *96,* 97
certified humane, 13
chicken
  Asian Chicken Salad, 152, *153*
  Balsamic-Dijon Chicken over
    Zucchini Noodles, *196,* 197
  Barbecue Chicken with
    Cilantro-Lime Coleslaw,
    248, 249–250
  Chicken Parm Zucchini
    Boats, *246,* 264, *265*
  Chicken Salad, 22
  Chicken Tinga Tacos, *260,*
    261
  Chicken Waldorf Salad, 151
  Cilantro-Lime Chicken, 267
  definitions, 12–15
  Dry-Rubbed Chili Chicken
    Wings, *116,* 117
  Easy Weeknight Chicken and
    Potatoes, 262, *263*
  Greek Lemon-Chicken Soup,
    132, 133
  Honey-Ginger Chicken, 213
  Jambalaya, *226,* 227
  Kale and Cabbage Chicken-
    Bacon Salad, *148,* 149–150

Lemon-Pepper Chicken with
    Asparagus, 198, *199*
  Salsa Verde Chicken Nachos
    and Mexican Lasagna,
    258–259
  Savory Garlic-Herb Chicken
    Waffles with Maple-Chili
    Syrup, *204,* 205–206
  Southwest Chicken Fajita
    Soup, 138, *139*
  Summer Pineapple Chicken
    over Cauliflower Rice, *256,*
    257
chickpeas
  chickpea flour in recipes, 143,
    318
  Cinnamon Toast Cereal, *96,* 97
  Crunchy Chickpea Caesar
    Salad, 162, *163*
  Curried Chickpea Salad
    Cups, *146,* 154, *155*
  Kung Pao Chickpeas, *214,* 215
  Summer Vegetable
    Ratatouille, 128, *129*
  Sweet Heat Crunchy
    Chickpeas, 118, *119*
children, whole foods for, 16–17.
    see also healthy eating
chives
  Citrus-Glazed Carrots with
    Chives, 176, *177*
  Garlic-Chive Mashed
    Potatoes, 184, *185*
chocolate
  Chocolate Brownie Donuts,
    58, *59*
  Chocolate Frosting, 322
  Chocolate-Mocha Nut
    Clusters, *310,* 311
  Chocolate Pecan Cookies, 72,
    73
  Frozen Chocolate–Peanut
    Butter Pie, *302,* 303